FRACTURED MINDS

FRACTURED MINDS

A Case-Study Approach to Clinical Neuropsychology

Second Edition

Jenni A. Ogden

OXFORD
UNIVERSITY PRESS

2005

OXFORD
UNIVERSITY PRESS

Oxford University Press, Inc., publishes works that further
Oxford University's objective of excellence
in research, scholarship, and education.

Oxford   New York
Auckland   Cape Town   Dar es Salaam   Hong Kong   Karachi
Kuala Lumpur   Madrid   Melbourne   Mexico City   Nairobi
New Delhi   Shanghai   Taipei   Toronto

With offices in
Argentina   Austria   Brazil   Chile   Czech Republic   France   Greece
Guatemala   Hungary   Italy   Japan   Poland   Portugal   Singapore
South Korea   Switzerland   Thailand   Turkey   Ukraine   Vietnam

Published by Oxford University Press, Inc.
198 Madison Avenue, New York, New York 10016

www.oup.com

Oxford is a registered trademark of Oxford University Press

Library of Congress Cataloging-in-Publication Data

Ogden, Jenni A.
  Fractured minds : a case-study approach to clinical neuropsychology / Jenni A. Ogden.—
2nd ed.
    p. ; cm.
  Includes bibliographical references and index.
  ISBN-13: 978-0-19-517135-8; 978-0-19-517136-5 (pbk)

    1. Clinical neuropsychology—Case studies. I. Title.
  [DNLM: 1. Nervous System Diseases—Case Reports. 2. Neuropsychology—Case
Reports. WL 140 O34f 2005]
  RC359.O36 2005
  616.89—dc22

                                                            2004053118

9   8   7   6   5   4

Printed in the United States of America
on acid-free paper

In memory of my mother,
who taught me that the mind and
spirit can rise above even the
most disabling illnesses,
and for my first two granddaughters,
Sophie and Belize,
born during the revision
of this book and with
their whole lives ahead of them.

PREFACE

The second edition of *Fractured Minds* follows the same format as the previous edition, with two introductory chapters followed by 17 chapters that each focus on a different neurological disorder. In each of these chapters a theoretical section precedes an illustrative case study. All the chapters from the first edition have been revised to include pertinent new research findings, new treatments, and further discussion of many issues important to the discipline and profession of clinical neuropsychology. The original cases have, with one exception, been retained, and for some cases additional recent case material has been added. Thus the reader can discover what has happened to Rangi, following many years free of epilepsy, and Mark, the (now middle-aged) man with visual object agnosia and prosopagnosia. A new case has replaced the original case in the subarachnoid hemorrhage chapter, allowing the inclusion of an illustrative neuropsychological assessment report that includes the latest Wechsler scales.

Three entirely new chapters on multiple sclerosis, Parkinson's disease, and Huntington's disease have been added. These not only make the range of neurological disorders covered much broader but also provide a vehicle for describing and exploring motor disorders, neurosurgical treatment to alleviate motor symptoms, genetically inherited disorders, genetic counseling, gene therapy, and some of the many difficult ethical issues that go hand-in-hand with new technology and knowledge.

Throughout, my aim has been to reveal the people who stand behind each disorder: patients, families, clinicians, support groups, and researchers. I hope that their courageous and sad stories will enhance the reader's understanding of neurological disease processes and modern treatments, as well as add depth and color to my descriptions of how clinical neuropsychologists go about their business of unraveling the mysteries of brain–behavior relationships.

Preface to the First Edition

I wrote this book for two reasons. My first reason was to relate the stories of some of the neurological patients who, over the years, have graciously admitted me into their lives, albeit in most cases for a brief time. The primary reason for my acquaintance with these people was either to assess their cognitive and psychological functioning and assist them with rehabilitation or to involve them in research projects with the goal of increasing our understanding of higher-level brain functioning.

My personal gain from contact with neurological patients is immeasurable. I have not only been privileged with intriguing glimpses into the human mind, but these people have also humbled me with their courage, humor, generosity of spirit, and determination to triumph over their illnesses, and for some, their uncomplaining acceptance of irretrievable losses and the certainty of an untimely death. As a PhD student new to neurosurgery and neurology ward rounds, I sometimes had to turn away from the bed so that the patient (and doctors) would not notice the tears in my eyes. Over the years I have conquered this "unprofessional" behavior and replaced it with a more subtle lump in my throat in response to the tragic stories, often masked by the brisk medical protocol that is commonplace in these wards. By sharing my experiences of how these "ordinary" folk cope with the extraordinary stress of a brain disorder, I hope to pass on something of their lives to the readers of this book.

My second reason for writing this book was to satisfy a need for an introductory text in clinical neuropsychology that would capture the attention of students and other health professionals interested in gaining a broad understanding of clinical neuropsychology, but without being required to learn "how to do it." The experiences of people with damaged brains and disordered minds seem to be intrinsically interesting to most people, perhaps because we can all relate in some small way to forgetting important information, not being able to say a word although we know we know it, or becoming clumsy and inefficient when we are overtired or intoxicated. Neurological disorders of one sort or another are common, and few people reach midlife without being touched by a family member or close friend with a head injury, dementia, stroke, or other neurological problem.

My own university teaching has convinced me that relating stories about real people as a pathway into the mysteries of neurological disorders and how they affect the mind generally works better than describing complex research studies and force-feeding facts about neuroanatomy and neuropathology. For example, an excursion into the world of patient H.M. not only results in an "emotional" understanding of what it might be like to have no memory but also introduces the reader or listener to the medial temporal lobes, epilepsy, and the many ways memory can be categorized.

Important theories and research studies pertinent to H.M.'s amnesia and other memory impairments can be included to give a general overview of the area and to encourage the interested reader to pursue them in more detail. Some of the neuropsychological tests commonly used to assess memory and other cognitive impairments can be described in general terms, and ethical, cultural, and other issues that are part and parcel of the clinical neuropsychologist's practice can be presented and discussed when they arise in the "natural" course of the case presentation.

This book thus represents a series of readings in introductory clinical neuropsychology. I hope that by the end of the book, the reader will have a broad view of clinical neuropsychology that will be sufficient in itself for many readers and that will encourage and prepare others for more advanced study. Each chapter includes a moderate number of references so that students can use the book as a springboard for further serious study. Chapters can be read (or used as a basis for a lecture, laboratory, or tutorial) in any order. However, for those new to this field, reading Chapters 1 and 2 first will provide a basis for understanding the following 14 chapters, each of which is centered around a particular neuropsychological disorder as experienced by one or two patients. Chapter 1 provides an overview of many different aspects of neuropsychology, including basic neuroanatomy, important assumptions and concepts understood by neuropsychologists, and a demystification of the "jargon" used in this field. Chapter 2 takes the reader through the steps of a neuropsychological assessment and briefly describes the more common tests referred to in the case studies.

Each case study is preceded by a section covering the main theoretical and neuropathological aspects of the disorder that often includes a sample of the relevant research in the area. Some chapters focus on the clinical assessment, treatment, and rehabilitation of common disorders, such as head injury, epilepsy, and dementia; others describe in straightforward language the research that is conducted to understand less common but fascinating disorders, such as the inability to recognize faces and objects by sight.

Although this book was written primarily for college and university students, it may also be of interest to health professionals who work with neurological patients. For example, practicing as well as student clinical psychologists; physical, speech, and occupational therapists; nurses; and junior doctors who work with neurological patients need to understand the kinds of cognitive impairments and other difficulties experienced by these people without needing to know in detail how to assess and rehabilitate the problems themselves. Increasingly, a multidisciplinary approach is taken in the assessment, treatment, and rehabilitation of neurological patients. For such an approach to work effectively, it is important that each professional understands, at least in a general way, the concepts and assessment measures used by other professionals. In addition, many of the ethical and professional issues discussed in the book are common to all health professionals. Sometimes patients (and their families) ask for books they can read to help them better understand their disorders. I hope one or more of the chapters in this book will assist in fulfilling that need for some people.

This is not a test manual or a text to prepare the reader to practice as a clinical neuropsychologist, but its breadth and detail may be sufficient to convey the richness and fascination of working with this population. Individual cases are of real people whose names and other personal details have been changed to protect their identity. In no specific case has the patient or client's gender been changed, as this is often an important factor in that patient's assessment and rehabilitation. When writing in general terms about patients, clients, and health professionals, however, to avoid the clumsy and impersonal use of *she/he* and *her/his*, I have used one or the other pronoun in a fairly random manner. Of course, generally speaking, in all these instances I could have used the alternative pronoun just as easily.

I must accept responsibility for the ways in which I have expressed the different aspects of neuropsychology in this book, and I am sure many readers will disagree with me on a number of issues. Indeed, given the ever-increasing body of neuropsychological knowledge that pours out of scientific journals every month, many of the ideas expressed in this book may well be outdated by the time it appears on the shelf. That aside, I could not have written this book without the massed wisdom and help of numerous people over the years.

ACKNOWLEDGMENTS

I am indebted to all the patients and their families who willingly gave up their time and cooperated with my tests and interviews, often when they themselves were going through one of the most significant crises of their lives. Although I am especially grateful to the 18 people and their families whose particular stories I have told here, I also thank the hundreds of patients who have, over the years, taught me much of what I know. I especially thank my own academic teachers and mentors, Michael Corballis and Suzanne Corkin, and Dorothy Gronwall, whose death in 2001 was a sad occasion, but whose legacy lives on. My mentors have supported me as well as taught me, and have even put up with my argumentative nature with good grace. Every clinical neuropsychologist needs a neurosurgeon or neurologist alongside, and Edward Mee has fulfilled that role for me. Not only has he taught me much about neuroanatomy, neuropathology, neurology, and even neurosurgery, but he has also maintained my belief that all health professionals, even busy surgeons, can take the time to care about the whole person, and not just the disorder that person endures.

I thank the staffs of the University of Auckland Department of Psychology, the Department of Neurology and Neurosurgery of Auckland Hospital, and the Clinical Research Center at Massachusetts Institute of Technology, all of whom have assisted my clinical, academic, and research endeavors in numerous ways over the years. The New Zealand Neurological Foundation, Inc., and the Health Research Council of New Zealand have supported many of my research projects, some of which have found their way into this book. Many of my colleagues and students have in various ways influenced and guided my neuropsychological thinking and clinical practice, encouraged me to write this book, and read drafts of chapters. In particular, I acknowledge Joe Bogen, Edith Kaplan, Muriel Lezak, Garry McFarlane-Nathan, Anne Aimola Davies (nee Maguire), Erana Cooper, Jennifer Hume, Laurie Miller, Gill Rhodes, Fred Seymour, Jon Simcock, Lynette Tippett, Guy Von Sturmer, and Kevin Walsh. I thank Meryl Hawkins, who drew the brains in Chapters 1 and 5, and my editor at Oxford University Press, Jeffrey House, who took a punt on a new author who wanted to write a novel disguised as a textbook, and who then asked for a second edition. I thank Fiona Stevens for all her guidance in the production of the second edition.

Finally, I thank my husband, John, and my children, Caroline, Jonathan, Josie, and Joachim, who have been listening to my stories about H.M., Michael, and others over the dinner table for more years than they care to remember. They may not feel obliged to take the second edition of the book to bed, but perhaps they will read it to my grandchildren to put them to sleep!

CONTENTS

FRACTURED MINDS

1

■

Introduction to Clinical Neuropsychology

A Definition of Clinical Neuropsychology and Its Aims

This book is concerned with the lives of real people whose behavior, emotions, or thinking abilities have become disordered, disrupted, or unusual as a result of some type of brain disorder or damage. The study of human behaviors, emotions, and thoughts and how they relate to the brain, particularly the damaged brain, is the subject matter of clinical neuropsychology.

Clinical neuropsychology has both applied and academic aims. Applied aims include learning more about neurological disorders and diseases so that we can more accurately and usefully diagnose, treat, and rehabilitate people who suffer such disorders and, along with other disciplines, ultimately find ways to prevent their occurrence. The primary academic aim is to learn more about how the undamaged or "normal" human brain and mind work by carrying out experiments, usually in the form of cognitive tests, on brain-damaged people.

This introductory chapter describes the similarities and differences between clinical neuropsychology and other related disciplines. It then touches on functional neuroanatomy, important neuropsychological terms and concepts, the interaction of clinical practice and research, the roles of a clinical neuropsychologist, and cross-cultural issues in neuropsychology. Each of these topics demands a chapter or book to itself, and a few paragraphs on each will act only as a reminder of knowledge you already have or provide just enough material to help you understand most of the information in the case studies. To provide a general sense of the basic tools the neuropsychologist uses to understand what is going on in the minds of brain-damaged patients or clients, Chapter 2 describes the different aspects of the neuropsychological assessment. Chapters 3 to 19 each present one or two case studies chosen to illustrate particular neuropsychological disorders, such as aphasia, visual agnosia, and dementia. A number of other issues important to the clinical neuropsychologist are raised throughout the case studies. At the end of this introductory chapter is a list of topics keyed to the chapters that provide further information about them.

Relationship of Clinical Neuropsychology to Other Disciplines

A number of disciplines are closely related to clinical neuropsychology and overlap with it (Fig. 1-1). The main ones can best be conceptualized as a continuum with the brain at one end (neurology) and the mind at the other (cognitive psychology). *Neurology* is the study of the medical aspects of central nervous system disorders and treatments. Compared with neuropsychologists, neurologists tend to be more concerned with clinical symptoms and signs as indications of underlying neuropathology in the brain, spinal cord, and peripheral nervous system and less concerned with the details of the higher behaviors and cognitions mediated by the brain and how the detailed study of their breakdown can inform us about normal higher cognitive processes.

At the other, more academic, end of the spectrum lies *cognitive psychology*, a popular subdiscipline of academic psychology. Its aim is to understand the workings of the human mind by analyzing the higher cognitive functions and their components. Participants in cognitive psychology experiments are unimpaired people (usually undergraduate university students) rather than brain-damaged patients, and cognitive psychologists have developed many important experimental paradigms that allow measurement of minute differences in cognitive performance under controlled conditions. For example, the time required to perform different tasks or a single task under different conditions might be measured in milliseconds, and from these results inferences can be made about the cognitive processes underlying the behaviors.

Cognitive neuropsychology is a relatively recent label for a type of research that many neuropsychologists have been conducting for years. It is, as the name suggests, a hybrid of cognitive psychology and clinical neuropsychology. It concentrates on the detailed analysis of higher cognitive functions, often using similar paradigms to those used in cognitive psychology, but it studies brain-damaged patients rather than "normals" (McCarthy and Warrington 1990). In their hypotheses and analyses of deficits and their implications for the normal functioning of the brain, cognitive neuropsy-

Figure 1-1 The discipline of clinical neuropsychology in relation to neurology and psychology.

chologists, although certainly not ignoring the brain entirely, tend to be less interested than clinical neuropsychologists in where the damage is and how it might be related to the impairment. Similarly, they are not interested in brain pathology, disease, and treatment on their own per se, but only as a means to the end of understanding the workings of the normal mind.

Thus, *clinical neuropsychology* positions itself between neurology and cognitive neuropsychology. It has a neurological interest in brain pathology and the resulting symptoms and a psychological interest in the analysis of higher cognitive functions, both to understand the workings of the normal mind and to develop better rehabilitation methods for patients. In practice, all the disciplines in Figure 1-1 overlap considerably, and many practitioners and researchers straddle two or more of these. Some neurologists specialize in clinical neuropsychology, and they are often known as *behavioral neurologists*. Clinical neuropsychologists who have an affiliation with a university psychology department as well as a hospital often carry out research that would best fit into the cognitive neuropsychology category. This is well illustrated by some of the case studies in this book that are more closely aligned with cognitive neuropsychology than clinical neuropsychology (see Chapters 3, 6, 8, and 19).

Other important areas that contribute to clinical neuropsychology include animal psychology and neuroscience, neuropharmacology, and human neurophysiology. This latter discipline measures the electrical brain waves of patients using electroencephalographs (EEG) and evoked potentials. In recent years rapidly developing neuroimaging technology has changed the face of neuroscience, and clinical neuropsychology has been one of the greatest beneficiaries. Computed tomography (CT) (see Chapters 6, 7, and 19 for examples) and magnetic resonance imaging (MRI) (see Chapter 8 and 14 for examples) permit us to visualize the anatomic structures and damage in the living brain, while cerebral blood flow techniques, positron emission tomography (PET), and functional MRI allow us to visualize the changing metabolism of the working brain. The relevance of these latter techniques lies in their potential to confirm and extend our hypotheses about brain–behavior relations. That is, when a non-brain-damaged person is speaking, does Broca's area (hypothesized to mediate speech) "light up" on a PET scan? Alternatively, when a patient has a large lesion in Broca's area (as confirmed on a CT brain scan) but still manages to speak, what area of the brain "lights up" when a PET scan is carried out on this patient?

Finally, but importantly, a practicing clinical neuropsychologist should first be an accomplished clinical psychologist, as will become evident in many of the case studies that follow. Even clinical neuropsychologists who restrict themselves to assessment and do not take an active part in rehabilitation and therapy require some clinical skills to enable them to build the rapport necessary to achieve a valid and useful assessment and to discuss in a sensitive manner the often distressing information about a patient's performance. In addition, patients often express strong emotions about their illness and their wider situation during their assessment, especially during the initial interview, and the clinical neuropsychologist should be able to respond professionally and sensitively. People with stable, long-term lesions who have volunteered as research subjects are also entitled to sensitive treatment that does not exploit or disempower them.

Functional Neuroanatomy

The human brain is the most complex system in the animal kingdom, and it is well beyond the scope of this book to cover neuroanatomy in any detail. This section provides a brief, simplistic overview of the cortical areas and other neuroanatomical structures that are most closely related to the disorders of higher cortical functioning covered in this book. This section should serve as a reminder for readers who have studied neuroanatomy and provide some background for those who have not. For readers who wish to learn more about this important area, the neuropsychology texts by Lezak (1995) and Walsh (1994) have excellent, easy-to-read sections on neuro-atomy for neuropsychologists; more detailed descriptions of neuroanatomy can be found in Mesulam (1985).

Gross Structure of the Brain

The brain has three major divisions: the cerebral hemispheres, the cerebellum, and the brain stem. Neuropsychology is most concerned with the cerebral hemispheres. Figure 1-2 shows lateral (from the side) and medial (split down the middle from front to back) views of the human brain. The *brain stem*, an upward extension of the spinal cord, consists of four parts: the medulla oblongata, pons, midbrain, and diencephalon. It is the life-support part of the brain as it controls respiration, cardiovascular function, and gastrointestinal function. It also contains the nuclei for the cranial nerves connected with the special senses, but it is not directly concerned with higher cognitive function. The *cerebellar hemispheres* are paired structures at the base of the cerebral hemispheres and are concerned mainly with motor coordination, muscle tone, and balance.

The *cerebral hemispheres* are paired structures above the midbrain and pons. They are covered by a highly convoluted layer of nerve cells called the *cerebral cortex*, or *grey matter*. The "hills" of the cortex are called *gyri* (singular, gyrus) and the "valleys" are called *sulci* (singular, sulcus). The axons or fiber tracts that connect the nerve cells to the rest of the brain form a layer directly below the cortex called the *white matter*. Deep within the hemispheres are further paired structures of grey matter called the *basal ganglia*. Chapter 15, which describes Parkinson's disease, provides more detail about the basal ganglia and their connections. The two hemispheres are separated by the *longitudinal fissure*, a deep groove that runs from the anterior frontal lobes to the posterior occipital lobes. The other main fissures are the *central (or rolandic) fissure* or sulcus, which separates the frontal from the parietal lobe, and the *lateral (or sylvian) fissure* or sulcus, which separates the temporal lobe from the frontal and parietal lobes. A tough band of interhemispheric fibers called the *corpus callosum* forms the major

Figure 1-2 The upper figure is a lateral view of the left hemisphere; the lower figure a medial view of the right hemisphere of the human brain.

7

functional connection between the two hemispheres. Within each hemisphere, fiber tracts connect different parts of the hemisphere.

A system called the ascending *reticular formation* (RF) controls the overall arousal level of the cortex. The RF is a diffuse system of multisynaptic neuron chains traveling up through the brain stem. All the major sensory pathways send impulses via collateral axons to the RF, which relays them to a group of nuclei in the *thalamus*, paired grey matter structures deep in the brain on either side of the midline at the upper end of the brain stem. The thalamus serves as a relay center for motor pathways, many sensory pathways, and the RF. On reaching the thalamus, the impulses are relayed to the cerebral cortex, where they influence the level of mental alertness or sleep.

Within the brain lies the *limbic system*, which includes the hippocampus and amygdala, which lie medially to the temporal lobes; the cingulate gyrus, which lies along the medial surface of the frontal and parietal lobes; and some deep, midline structures in the brain, including the mamillary bodies. The limbic system is involved in emotion, motivation, and memory.

The brain has three coverings, called the *meninges*. The outermost thick, tough, covering is called the *dura mater* ("tough mother"), which adheres to the inner surface of the skull. The delicate, filamentous middle membrane, called the *arachnoid mater* ("spider mother"), is attached by cobweb-like strands of tissue to the fine *pia mater* ("little mother"), which adheres closely to the cortex. The *subarachnoid space* lies between the arachnoid mater and the pia mater and is filled with *cerebrospinal fluid* (*CSF*). Blood vessels also lie within the subarachnoid space and dip down in the sulci to supply deeper parts of the brain.

An inflammation of the meninges is called *meningitis*; one symptom of meningitis is a stiff neck, caused by the muscles of the neck contracting strongly (called guarding) to prevent bending of the neck and the subsequent painful stretching of the inflamed meninges.

The *ventricles* are lakes of CSF located deep within the hemispheres. The lateral ventricles, large paired structures in the center of each hemisphere, connect in the middle to form the third ventricle and, below that, the fourth ventricle. The CSF is continually formed by the choroid plexus within the ventricles and circulates through the ventricles and around the outside of the brain and spinal cord within the subarachnoid space. Excess CSF drains into the venous system from the subarachnoid space. If one of the small apertures between the ventricles becomes blocked, the CSF cannot flow out and the ventricles increase in size, causing increased intracranial pressure. This condition, known as *hydrocephalus*, can be corrected by a neurosurgeon placing a valve, or shunt, into the blocked ventricle to allow the CSF to flow through a tube into a body cavity.

The *cerebrovascular system* is too complex to describe in detail here, but in simple terms it involves two pairs of cerebral arteries: the *internal carotid arteries*, which supply the anterior parts of the brain, and the *vertebral arteries*, which supply the posterior parts of the brain. The two internal carotid arteries enter the skull and ascend on either side of the optic chiasm, where each artery branches to form the *anterior cerebral arteries* (ACA) and *middle cerebral arteries* (MCA), one set in each hemisphere. The ACAs sweep forward to supply the medial and lower (inferior) surfaces of the frontal lobes, the medial surfaces of the parietal lobes, and the corpus callosum. The MCAs travel laterally within the lateral fissure and branch to supply much of the lateral surfaces of the frontal, temporal, and parietal lobes as well as parts of the inferior surfaces of the frontal lobes and medial surfaces of the temporal lobe. The MCA also branches to form the *striate arteries*, which supply the deeply situated *internal capsule*, the main passageway for the fiber tracts between the motor cortex and the spine (the *corticospinal tract* or *pyramidal tract*). The tiny diameter of the striate arteries makes them vulnerable to blockage, resulting in damage to the corticospinal tract and subsequent paralysis of the opposite side of the body. The MCA supplies 75% or more of the blood supply to the cerebral hemispheres.

The paired vertebral arteries enter the skull at the point where the spinal cord becomes continuous with the brain stem and join to form the single *basilar artery* on the undersurface of the brainstem; the basilar artery then divides to form paired *posterior cerebral arteries*, which supply the occipital lobes and parts of the medial and inferior surfaces of the temporal lobes, including the hippocampus. The internal carotid and vertebral arterial systems are linked at the base of the brain by a single *anterior communicating artery* and two *posterior communicating arteries*, forming a ring of vessels lying in the subarachnoid space, called the *Circle of Willis*. If one of the main arteries becomes blocked, the blood can pass around the circle to reach the deprived area. The Circle of Willis is a frequent site of weakenings on the artery wall, called *aneurysms*. If an aneurysm bursts, it expels blood around the brain in the subarachnoid space, causing a *subarachnoid hemorrhage* (see Chapter 12). A blockage in a vessel away from the Circle of Willis can result in the blood and oxygen supply being cut off to the part of the brain that vessel supplies, resulting in an area of brain death, called a *stroke* (see Chapter 5).

The venous system involves *superficial veins*, which drain the lateral and lower (inferior) surfaces of the hemispheres, and *deep veins*, which drain the internal area of the brain. The cerebral veins empty into channels within the dura mater called *venous sinuses*, which in turn empty into the large internal jugular vein.

Cerebral Cortex

Cortical zones   The cortex of each hemisphere can be divided in various ways, two of which are particularly useful for neuropsychologists. By dividing the cerebral hemispheres into primary, secondary, and tertiary cortical zones, as illustrated in Figure 1-3, the anatomical-functional relationships of the cortex can be conceptualized (Luria 1973; Mesulam 1985). The parietal, temporal, and occipital lobes lying behind the central sulcus constitute the *posterior cortex* and are involved mainly in a person's awareness of what is happening in the world. Each of these lobes can be divided into three zones.

The *primary zones* are primary projection areas in which incoming sensory in-

Figure 1-3 A diagram of a lateral view of the left hemisphere of the human brain divided into primary, secondary, and tertiary cortical zones. CS, central (rolandic) sulcus; LF, lateral (sylvian) fissure; M, motor strip; PM, premotor cortex; PF, prefrontal cortex; PS, primary sensory cortex; SS, secondary sensory cortex; PA, primary auditory cortex; SA, secondary auditory cortex; PV, primary visual cortex; SV, secondary visual cortex; TC, tertiary (multimodal) cortex.

formation is projected to sense-modality-specific neurons. Each side of the body is mapped topographically onto the primary sensory strip of the opposite (contralateral) hemisphere. Thus, a touch on the index finger of the right hand is projected to specific neurons in the primary sensory cortex of the left *parietal lobe* (the postcentral gyrus lying directly behind the central sulcus). The position of the finger would be projected to other specific neurons in the primary zone. The topographic pattern of neurons within the primary sensory strip of the parietal lobe can be conceptualized as a person hanging upside down with his foot hanging over the longitudinal fissure into the medial side of the hemisphere, with the trunk and hand represented on the lateral surface of the hemisphere and the face represented at the lower edge of the lateral surface at the edge of the lateral or sylvian fissure. The primary zone of the temporal lobes is concerned with sounds, and different frequencies are represented in different parts of the primary zone. Similarly, the primary zone of the occipital lobes represents specific parts of the visual field. Damage to specific areas of the primary cortex results in highly specific deficits of sensation in the topographically related body part or sense organ.

The *secondary zones* (also called the *association cortex*) lie adjacent to the primary zones. The neurons in these zones, unlike those in the primary zones, do not have a direct topographic relationship with sensory information relayed from a particular body part or sense organ. Instead, they receive the modality-specific information from their primary cortex and integrate it into meaningful wholes. Thus, the secondary cortex is concerned with perception and meaning within a single-sense modality. Damage to parts of the secondary cortex can therefore result in an inability to perceive or comprehend what one is touching or hearing or seeing, depending on whether the damage is in the parietal, temporal, or occipital secondary zones.

The *tertiary zones* lie at the inner borders of each lobe so that the parietal, temporal, and occipital tertiary zones overlap. At this level, modality specificity disappears, and integration of information across sense modalities occurs. Damage to the tertiary zones can lead to complex higher cognitive disorders that involve transmodal integration (e.g., writing to dictation). The tertiary zones also have links with the limbic system, which is involved in emotion and memory; therefore, disorders resulting from damage to the tertiary cortex may also involve abnormal emotional components.

The *frontal lobes* lie anterior to the central sulcus and are concerned mainly with acting on knowledge relayed to the posterior part of the cerebral cortex from the outside world. The frontal lobes can also be divided into three zones. The *primary zone*, or *motor strip*, is on the precentral gyrus, immediately anterior to the central sulcus, and parallels the sensory strip in that each side of the body is mapped topographically (like a person hanging upside down) onto the primary motor strip of the opposite (contralateral) hemisphere. The *secondary zone* (association cortex), also called the *premotor cortex*, mediates the organization of motor patterns, such as riding a bicycle.

The *tertiary zone*, also called the *prefrontal cortex*, is a large area situated at the anterior pole of the brain; it includes both the lateral cortex and the *basomedial* (or orbitomedial) cortex, which lies between the two hemispheres and extends to the underside of the frontal lobes above the eyes. The *tertiary cortex* is involved in executive functions, including planning, organization, and abstract thinking. Because they also have rich connections with the limbic system, the prefrontal lobes are intimately involved with mood, motivation, and emotion, and damage to them can result in many and varied impairments involving the interactions of motivational and emotional states and executive functions.

Cortical lobes   The division of the cortex of each hemisphere into four lobes is the most often used concept in clinical neuropsychology. Although the lobes are often viewed as separate areas and are frequently linked to specific functions, they are in fact divisions of convenience rather than true anatomic divisions. Nevertheless, these divisions serve a useful purpose in discussions of brain–behavior relations. The four cortical lobes of the left hemisphere are labeled in Figure 1-2, and the right hemisphere is divided up in the same way. The large frontal lobes form the anterior part of the brain, and the parietal, temporal, and occipital lobes make up the portion posterior to the central sulcus.

All three posterior lobes (in each hemisphere) are involved in the awareness, perception, and integration of information from the outside world, although their connections with the limbic system ensure that the way the world is experienced is influenced by the individual's mood, motivation, and past experiences. Generally, the *parietal lobe* is involved in functions involving tactile sensations, position sense, and spatial relations. The *left* parietal lobe has a bias toward sequential and logical spatial abilities, such as perceiving the details within a spatial pattern, whereas the *right* parietal lobe is more involved with the holistic appreciation of spatial information. The left parietal lobe also appears to mediate the ability to calculate, which involves both logical and spatial concepts. The right parietal lobe is especially good at conceptualizing complex spatial relations, and people with right parietal lesions often have extreme difficulty copying complex patterns or working out how to put jigsaw puzzles together.

The *temporal lobes* are concerned primarily with auditory and olfactory abilities, but they are involved in integrating visual perceptions with other sensory information. They also mediate some memory functions, especially those involved in new learning. Their intimate connections with the hippocampus, a part of the limbic system, allow the integration of emotion and motivation with the sensory information relayed from the outside world to the posterior lobes of the hemispheres. The *left* temporal lobe is concerned more with verbal and sequential functions; it includes the language comprehension area and is involved in new verbal learning and memory. The *right* temporal lobe tends to be more concerned with nonverbal functions, such as the interpretation of emotional voice tone and emotional facial expression and the appreciation of music and nonlanguage sounds. It also appears to play a part in nonverbal learning and memory, although this role is not as clear as the left temporal lobe's role in verbal memory.

The *occipital lobes* are the visual lobes, and they mediate sight, visual perception, and visual knowledge. A patient with a large lesion of the right occipital lobe may have a complete left-visual-field defect (loss of vision) in the visual fields of both eyes (called a homonymous hemianopia), and a patient with bilateral lesions of the primary visual cortex at the very pole of the occipital lobes will be unable to see although his eyes function normally. This condition is termed *cortical blindness*. Visual-field defects can also occur if the visual pathways are damaged at other points. A lesion in the right temporal lobe that damages the optic radiation as it travels from the optic chiasma to the occipital cortex will result in a visual-field defect in the upper left quadrant of both eyes. A lesion of the right parietal lobe that damages the optic tract will result in a visual-field defect in the lower left quadrant of both eyes. Visual-field defects are straightforward sensory defects resulting from damage to the primary projection cortex and the optic fibers traveling to them.

Lesions of the occipital secondary or association cortex can result in a number of strange disorders, particularly when the lesions are bilateral. For example, the patient described in Chapter 8 has bilateral medial occipital lobe lesions; although he can see and describe the form of objects, he is unable to recognize what it is he is seeing. This condition is called *visual agnosia*. Again, there is some functional division between the occipital lobes of the left and right hemispheres, with the *left* occipital lobe being more concerned with visual language functions such as reading, and the *right* occipital lobe being more concerned with visually judging the orientation of lines or objects in space.

The *frontal lobes*, which are anterior to the central sulcus, are concerned with motor functions and executive functions such as forming abstract concepts and planning and executing actions based on the information received from the posterior cortex. Motor functions are mediated by the primary and premotor frontal cortex, and the left frontal lobe includes the speech area *Broca's area*. The executive functions are mediated by the prefrontal lobes and are integrated with emotional and motivational states via part of the limbic system (the *cingulate cortex*), which forms the medial parts of the frontal lobes.

The functional verbal–nonverbal division between the left and right prefrontal lobes is less marked than in the posterior lobes, but it nevertheless can be demonstrated with some neuropsychological tasks. For example, patients with left frontal lesions are frequently less able to produce words beginning with a specific letter under time pressure than those with right frontal lesions; conversely, patients with right frontal lesions are sometimes less able to create different designs than patients with left frontal damage.

Other deficits resulting from frontal-lobe damage include recent memory deficits (*frontal amnesia*), wherein the patient is unable to use memory strategies (e.g., logically structuring the material he wishes to memorize) and as a result has difficulty learning and recalling new information. The other main area of disturbance found after frontal-lobe lesions is related to the close anatomic and functional connections between the limbic structures and the frontal lobes and is often described as a *personality change* (see Chapter 9). This can be the onset of an apathetic, aspontaneous, or even mute state or an increase in aggression or the display of inappropriate behaviors.

Functional Systems

Simple motor and sensory functions, and even some more complex perceptual functions, are mediated by a particular group of neurons; therefore, damage to these neurons results in an unambiguous deficit. For example, damage to the area of motor cortex that mediates hand movements results in a paralysis of the hand on the opposite side of the body. Many of our higher cognitive functions, such as reading or memory, are, however, the result of quite complex *functional systems*, composed of a number of different brain areas working together to produce a behavior. The concept of a functional system was proposed by Luria (1973), who further proposed that in terms of double dissociation, damage to area *A* will result in the impairment of a factor or subcomponent *a*, and all functional systems that include this factor will suffer. Likewise, when area *B* is damaged, all functional systems that include subcomponent *b* will suffer.

As an example, damage to the right parietal lobe may impair the ability to conceptualize spatial relationships. In turn, this impairment may disrupt many functional systems and result in a wide range of behavioral deficits. The patient may no longer be able to do jigsaw puzzles, may become easily lost in an unfamiliar environment, may have difficulty learning and remembering new tasks that have a spatial component, and may no longer be able to perform calculations on paper or mentally that involve carrying figures from one column to another (a spatial task).

The concept of functional systems suggests one possible way of overcoming an impairment. If the patient can find a new way to reach the same endpoint while avoiding the necessity to include the impaired subcomponent, then recovery of function is possible. For example, he may be able to overcome his calculation difficulty by using a calculator that does not require a spatial ability but that simply requires pressing the right numbers and mathematical symbols in the correct order. In some cases of spontaneous recovery of function, the impaired functional system may restructure itself, perhaps by bypassing the damaged neurons. Nearby undamaged neurons can sprout new dendrites that "fill the gap" left by the dead or damaged neurons and connect with the dendritic trees of undamaged neurons in other cortical areas. The new cortical area could either "learn" the cognitive subcomponent that was previously mediated by the now-damaged neurons or could supply a different cognitive subcomponent that allows the functional system to remain viable, albeit using a slightly different process. This restructuring would, of course, take place outside the awareness of the patient, although he may unknowingly assist the process by continuing to practice the impaired behavior.

Disconnection Syndrome

A number of disorders are thought to result from an anatomic disconnection between two cortical areas (Geschwind 1965). One example is provided by a type of apraxia (ideomotor apraxia; see Chapter 6), wherein the patient is unable to perform skilled movements to verbal command but can perform them spontaneously. Several mechanisms have been put forward to explain this condition, but one disconnection explanation is that it is caused by damage to the fiber connection (the *arcuate fasciculus*) between the language comprehension area in the posterior left temporal lobe and the motor association cortex in the left frontal lobe.

The disconnection can be within one cerebral hemisphere as in the above example, or it can be between hemispheres, as in the case where the corpus callosum connecting the hemispheres is damaged. For example, damage to the anterior section of the corpus callosum can result in a disconnection between the verbal comprehension area in the left hemisphere and the motor strip in the right hemisphere. As a consequence, the patient may not be able to comb his hair on verbal command with his left hand (innervated by the right motor strip) but can do so with his right hand, as the left motor strip is still connected to the left verbal comprehension area.

Experiments with split-brain subjects who have had the corpus callosum cut as a treatment for epilepsy have produced many examples of a "pure" disconnection syndrome (see Chapter 18). For example, an object flashed in the right visual field (and therefore projected to the left hemisphere) can be described or named by the split brain subject because the speech faculty is also in the left hemisphere. An object flashed in the left visual field (and therefore projected to the right hemisphere) cannot be described in speech or writing, but the isolated right hemisphere, via the left hand, can respond nonverbally to the object it sees by pointing to a matching stimulus or to the name on a list (Sperry et al. 1969). The finding that the right hemisphere can point to a name on a list demonstrates that it does have the ability to comprehend simple language, although it cannot express itself in words.

Neuropsychological Terminology

In the company of most medical and scientific disciplines, neurology and neuropsychology are well endowed with their own jargon. Although jargon should be avoided wherever possible, to understand the vast neurological and neuropsychological literature it is necessary to have a grasp of the most common of these terms. For example, *deficit, dysfunction, symptom, impairment*, and *disorder* are used synonymously and can refer to any motor, sensory, perceptual, behavioral, psychological, emotional, or cognitive abnormality. A *syndrome* refers to a group of symptoms that characteristically occur together after brain damage (see Chapter 6). In many cases, jargon terms can provide shorthand descriptions for complex disorders. Fortunately, a few simple rules can simplify their interpretation for the beginner; indeed, it can even be fun trying to work out what deficits a patient should have by breaking down the diagnostic label into its component parts.

Any label containing *phasia* refers to a speech disorder; *graphia* refers to writing, and *lexia* to reading. *Praxia* means to work or perform purposeful actions, and *gnosia* means to know. If the base word is prefixed by an *a*, strictly speaking it means that that function is completely absent (e.g., *agnosia* means not to know); prefixed by *dys*, it means partial impairment (e.g., *dyslexia* means to have a marked reading difficulty). However, these conventions are often not adhered to, and a patient labeled as having expressive aphasia may not be totally mute but more accurately may be dysphasic.

Sometimes the main label is preceded by a common English word that signifies the specific type of disorder. Therefore, *visual agnosia* means not to know what one is seeing, and *tactile agnosia* means not to know what one is touching. A patient with *dressing apraxia* has difficulty with the actions related to dressing and may try to put his left leg into the right sleeve and his right leg into the left leg of the garment, thus getting into an impossible tangle. In addition, many terms can be partially, if not fully, understood if the base of the word is known. For example, *prosopagnosia* denotes an inability to recognize or know faces, and *anosognosia* is to deny knowledge, as in the case of a patient who denies she has paralyzed limbs. Some patients who suffer from cortical blindness deny that they are blind; this disorder is termed *visual anosognosia*. Many of these terms appear in the following case studies and are defined when they first arise.

Other terms commonly used to describe brain–behavior relations include *unilateral* and *bilateral*, which refer to damage in one hemisphere or both hemispheres, respectively, and *contralesional* and *contralateral*, which refer to impairments (or body parts) and lesions that are opposite each other. For example, a paralyzed right arm is caused by a lesion in the contralateral (left) motor strip; alternatively, a lesion in the arm section of the left motor strip causes paralysis of the contralesional (right) arm. In another example, a patient may ignore or neglect stimuli in the contralesional hemispace (the side of space opposite the brain lesion).

Assumptions that Underlie Clinical Neuropsychology

The study of brain-damaged patients to understand the workings of the normal brain and mind relies on two important assumptions. The first is that the brain of the patient was normal before the brain damage, an assumption that is often challenged when patients with long-term neurological conditions are used as experimental subjects in an attempt to understand normal brain functioning. For example, patients with long-standing epilepsy who later in life undergo neurosurgery in an attempt to cure their epilepsy often participate in experiments to discover what impairments result from removing the temporal lobe (see Chapters 3 and 4). The argument that their brains may have been organized differently from normal as the result of their epilepsy can to a large extent be dismissed as we assess more patients without epilepsy who demonstrate the same sort of impairments after traumatic temporal lobe injury.

Experiments with patients who have undergone a surgical splitting of the *cerebral commissures* (the large band of fibers connecting the two cerebral hemispheres), again in an attempt to control severe, long-term epileptic seizures, face similar criticisms (see Chapter 18). Fortunately, the results of experiments on normal people, in which stimuli are briefly flashed to one hemisphere or the other, generally support the findings of the split-brain studies, suggesting that their brains do not differ greatly from normal.

The second assumption underlying both cognitive and clinical neuropsychology experiments is that we can generalize about brain–behavior relations from one "normal" human to another. The main criticism of this assumption is the evidence that not all patients with a lesion to a specific area of the brain suffer the same impairments. For example, most but not all adult patients who sustain damage to the inferior, posterior left frontal gyrus (Broca's area) suffer impairment of language. Nevertheless, as the result of numerous studies of the impairments of brain-damaged people, it is generally accepted that it is valid to make broad generalizations about brain–behavior relationships from one human to another. The most obvious of these generalizations is that the left cerebral hemisphere is dominant for speech in most people.

Making generalizations in the case of children is more difficult, as the brain develops functions at different rates as the child grows older. Thus, the practice of child clinical neuropsychology and experiments with brain-damaged children, although having much in common with adult neuropsychology, require different tests with age-appropriate normative data and different clinical methods and skills. A number of good books have been written about this subject area for readers with a particular interest in the neuropsychological problems of children (Anderson et al. 2001; Sattler 1992; Spreen, Risser, and Edgell 1995).

Focal Lesions and Diffuse Brain Damage

A *focal lesion*, as its name suggests, is damage restricted to a circumscribed area of the brain. *Lesion* is a general term used to describe any type of focal brain damage. *Infarct* or *infarction* refers to any area of dead brain. The most common cause of a focal lesion is a stroke, caused by a blockage or spasm of a cerebral artery and a loss of blood and oxygen to the part of the brain that artery supplies (see Chapter 5). Focal lesions can also be caused by a circumscribed area of bleeding that forms a blood clot within the brain substance (an intracerebral *hematoma*; see Chapter 5).

In an open head injury the skull is fractured, and an object may penetrate the skull and underlying brain (e.g., bone fragments, bullets, or metal from an automobile accident), damaging the brain tissue through which it passes. The neurosurgeon usually cleans the wound, removing the object and any damaged tissue and debris, and leaving a clean focal lesion that does not affect the rest of the brain. Studies of the impairments demonstrated by patients with lesions from penetrating objects or focal strokes have contributed a great deal to our understanding of the functional organization of the brain (e.g., Luria 1970; Newcombe 1969). Neurosurgical operations to remove or resect tumors or to remove parts of the brain that cause epilepsy (as in the case of temporal lobectomies) also result in focal lesions (see Chapters 3 and 4).

Some viruses attack specific areas of the brain, causing focal damage, often bilaterally. For example, the herpes simplex encephalitis virus usually targets the medial temporal lobes and sometimes attacks the inferior temporal and frontal areas as well, resulting in severe memory deficits and, in some cases, executive deficits (Utley, Ogden, Gibb, McGrath, and Anderson 1997). Brain tumors and brain abscesses are also focal lesions in the sense that they cause neural death by destroying neurons directly or via pressure effects. However, malignant tumors, while appearing to have a circumscribed boundary on a CT brain scan, may be widespread with no clear division between diseased and healthy brain. It is therefore important to be cautious when proposing associations between a tumor lesion in a specific area of the brain and the impairments that the patient demonstrates (see Chapters 6 and 7).

Diffuse brain damage refers to damage that affects many areas of the brain, as in

Alzheimer's disease and other dementias (see Chapter 17). The damage can often be visualized on a CT or MRI scan or at postmortem as *atrophy*, which is shriveled or shrunken cortex and white matter, signifying neuronal death, and usually affecting large areas of the cortex. Brain atrophy decreases the brain mass and allows the fluid-filled ventricles in the middle of the brain and the subarachnoid space around the brain to expand. Other disease processes such as meningitis and encephalitis can also result in widespread brain damage that is sometimes transient and sometimes permanent.

Progressive diseases other than AD, such as Huntington's disease (HD), Parkinson's disease (PD), and multiple sclerosis (MS), cause increasing impairment of motor and cognitive functions as time goes on. HD (see Chapter 16) is a progressive degenerative genetic disorder, and 50% of the children of a parent with HD will develop the disease (Mendelian autosomal dominant inheritance) and inevitably will become demented. The caudate nucleus, putamen, and globus pallidus become severely atrophied, but as the disease advances, brain atrophy is widespread and thus diffuse.

PD (see Chapter 15) is a disease of unknown cause that usually becomes apparent in the sixth decade and involves neurotransmitter deficits (dopamine) as a result of loss of dopamine-producing neurons in the substantia nigra of the basal ganglia. Although the majority of PD patients suffer from severe motor disorders and a number of mild to moderate cognitive impairments, only a small percentage become demented. As the dopamine deficits stemming from the atrophied basal ganglia result in widespread deficits in other parts of the brain, especially the prefrontal cortex, on functional and neuropsychological assessment, especially in advanced cases, PD patients may display a picture that is typical of diffuse damage.

MS (see Chapter 14) is an autoimmune, inflammatory disease that often first becomes apparent in adults in their 30s. As it results in the episodic occurrence of many plaques of demyelination of white matter pathways in the CNS that can later recover or remain as plaques, it causes a range of fluctuating focal motor and cognitive deficits. In many cases, as the disease progresses, the numerous focal lesions that are present at any one time can result in a functional picture that is more typical of diffuse damage. This damage is rarely sufficient to result in dementia, but it often causes memory impairments, poor sustained attention, and slowed information processing.

Diffuse damage can also occur after closed head injury, when the head hits a moving object and the brain accelerates inside the skull. This can cause stretching and tearing of neural axons, as well as numerous small areas of bleeding and infarction where the brain scrapes against the skull (see Chapters 10 and 11). A type of stroke called a *subarachnoid hemorrhage*, caused by the rupture of a cerebral artery and the expelling of blood into the subarachnoid space around the brain, can also result in diffuse cortical damage (see Chapter 12), as can severe and chronic cases of neurotoxicity caused by long-term exposure to organic solvents (see Chapter 13).

Many brain pathologies cause swelling in the vicinity of the damage; this swelling is termed *edema*. Edema, particularly common in association with malignant tumors, has the effect of increasing the area of dysfunctional brain. As the edema resolves (often when the patient is treated with steroids), the area of dysfunctional brain decreases, and often impairments subside dramatically (see Chapters 6 and 7). Massive brain swelling, most common after severe head injury, can compress the brain stem, resulting in the patient's death.

Cerebral Dominance, Lateralization of Function, and Specialization

The idea that in humans the left hemisphere has a strong relationship with language functions was first suggested by Broca (1861), who discovered that speech was impaired following damage to the posterior portion of the third convolution of the left frontal lobe (often called *Broca's area*). This discovery was followed closely by Wernicke's (1874) observation that a lesion in the left superior temporal gyrus (often called *Wernicke's area*) resulted in difficulties with comprehending language. Since that time, numerous studies on brain-lesioned patients have proved beyond doubt that in at least 92% of right-handers and 69% of left-handers (Milner 1975), the left hemisphere is specialized not only for the verbal functions of speech, language comprehension, reading, writing, and verbal memory but also for a number of other functions as well: functions that involve sequential, logical thinking, such as the ability to conceptualize mathematical relationships, and other functions, such as the ability to tell left from right or to carry out skilled acts on verbal command (Strub and Geschwind 1983).

For many years, the left hemisphere was viewed as the dominant hemisphere, and the right hemisphere as the minor or nondominant hemisphere, implying that the right hemisphere did not have its own, equally important areas of specialization. More recently, it has been established that the right hemisphere is "better" at some tasks than the left; in particular, tasks involving stimuli that cannot be readily verbalized. Included are nonverbal memory functions (Milner 1968b), interpretation of nonverbal emotional expression (Gainotti 1984), and visuospatial functions generally (De Renzi 1982). Some researchers also believe that the right hemisphere is dominant for some forms of attention in light of evidence that it has the ability to attend to both sides of space, whereas the left hemisphere is confined to attending to the right side of space (Heilman 1982).

Information from studies on commissurotomized (split-brain subjects) carried out by Sperry et al. (1969) and their many followers have generally confirmed the verbal/ sequential specialization of the left hemisphere and the nonverbal/visuospatial specialization of the right hemisphere, although it is now clear that these distinctions are far from absolute (see Chapter 18). The left hemisphere is capable of quite complex spatial tasks, although many such tasks may be performed better by the right hemisphere; the right hemisphere has some ability to comprehend simple language and is involved in extralinguistic aspects of language, such as voice tone (Searleman 1977). In general, however, the specialization of the left hemisphere for language functions is more pronounced than the specialization of the right hemisphere for visuospatial functions, which have a greater degree of bilateral (both hemispheres) representation.

The term *lateralization of function* is simply another way to express hemispheric specialization in the sense that language is lateralized to the left hemisphere. The term *specialization* is also used to describe the mediation of particular functions by specific cortical areas within a hemisphere. For example, the occipital cortex is specialized for visual perception.

The old concept of absolute left cerebral dominance is hard to put to rest. It has even been extended in the popular press to include an absolute specialization of the right hemisphere for "creative thinking," the ability to draw, and "female" traits of sensitivity and gentleness. The now-popular right hemisphere is also often publicized as the seat of the subconscious, controlled and subdued by the left hemisphere with its overpowering "male" traits of competitiveness, logical reasoning powers, and poor ability to show emotion. Although this makes a good story and sells parapsychology books and even cars ("Buy a car for your right creative and passionate hemisphere") and may be fostered by the political correctness of emphasizing "female" attributes and criticizing "male" attributes, there is no solid evidence for these extreme claims. As an example of the absurdity of such views, the idea that creativity per se is the specialized realm of the right hemisphere appears quite incongruous when one considers the great literary writings of humankind. Why these should be considered less creative than great art or architecture is decidedly unclear. There is even evidence to suggest that musical appreciation, intuitively a nonverbal function, is mediated predominantly by the right hemisphere in nonmusicians but by the left hemisphere in musicians. It has been suggested that for musicians, music is conceptualized as a sequential, logical "language," thus explaining its mediation by the left hemisphere (Sergent, Zuck, Terriah, and MacDonald 1992).

The current scientific view, backed by considerable evidence, is that whereas each hemisphere has certain specialist abilities (often also represented to a lesser degree in the other hemisphere), in the unimpaired brain the two hemispheres work as a team, and neither should be considered dominant. When the term "cerebral dominance" is used, it should be justified by the addition of the specialist functions to which it refers; for example, the (left) hemisphere is dominant for language.

Functional Plasticity

The concept of *plasticity of function* is, in one sense, the reverse of specialization. It refers to the ability of some areas of cortex to take on functions not normally attributed to them. The clearest examples of this occur in the case of hemispherectomy, where an entire hemisphere is removed or stripped of its cortex because it is so badly damaged or diseased that it no longer functions normally. These damaged hemispheres often cause uncontrollable seizures and disturbed behaviors and inhibit the normal functioning of the healthy hemisphere (see Chapter 19).

When brain damage or hemispherectomy occurs in childhood, the other intact hemisphere is often able to take over many of the functions of the damaged hemisphere. Damasio, Lima, and Damasio (1975) studied a child whose right hemisphere was damaged at the age of 5 years, resulting 7 years later in uncontrollable seizures and disturbed behavior. After a right hemispherectomy, her seizures stopped, her behavior improved, and assessments demonstrated that her left hemisphere could perform many of the visuospatial tasks usually mediated primarily by the right hemisphere, in addition to language functions. Similarly, when left hemispherectomies are performed after damage in childhood, the right hemisphere can take over sophisticated language functions (Ogden 1996), although it appears that some visuospatial abilities are compromised (Ogden 1988a, 1989; see also Chapter 19). Doubt continues over whether plasticity, at least for language, is possible only following childhood damage (perhaps up to the age of 12 to 15 years) or whether it can occur at any age if enough time has elapsed to allow new areas of brain to take over the functions. This issue has not been resolved because of the lack of patients who survive for long recovery periods after massive damage or disease to one hemisphere in adulthood (St. James-Roberts 1981).

Plasticity also refers to the concept that there can be a window of opportunity in development during which a particular function becomes established. Put in these terms, the hemispherectomy studies suggest that language becomes established up to the age of 12 years or so, primarily in the left hemisphere, but in the right hemisphere if the left is damaged. If the child is isolated completely from language during those first 12 years, they will never be able to establish normal language thereafter—in either hemisphere. Other functions may also develop preferentially only within a particular age range. One study that assessed visual imagery in blind people provided some evidence for plasticity for this function (although not for hemispheric specialization), as people who were blind from birth or went blind before about 12 years of age reported little or no visual imagery (including visual dreams) in adulthood, whereas people who went blind after the age of 12 years still commonly utilized visual imagery (and reported visual dreams) in adulthood after many years of total blindness (Ogden and Barker 2001).

Double Dissociation of Function

An individual patient with brain damage in a particular area may show impairment on one test and not on another. Although this discrepancy may indicate that the impaired ability is mediated by the lesioned area of cortex, and the unimpaired ability is not (a single dissociation), an alternative explanation is that the test used to assess the impaired function was simply more difficult than the test used to assess the unimpaired function. That is, if the tests were of equal difficulty, both would be impaired by damage in this area and possibly by damage in other areas as well. This ambiguity can be overcome by a method called the *double dissociation of function* (Teuber 1955). Simply put, it states that to confirm the independence of functions, symptom *a* must appear in association with lesions in area *A* but not with those in area *B*, and symptom *b* must appear with lesions in area *B* but not with those in area *A*.

This principle is particularly useful in discriminating functions that appear very similar. For example, if a patient with damage in a particular area of his brain is impaired with respect to a specific cognitive ability (e.g., he cannot memorize verbal information) but is not impaired in other components of the same general ability (e.g., he can memorize nonverbal, visuospatial patterns), and a second patient demonstrates the reverse pattern (e.g., he can memorize verbal material but not nonverbal material), this proves that the two types of memory are dissociable and do not simply vary with respect to difficulty level. In addition, the areas of the brain damaged in each case must be associated in some way with the impaired function. Indeed, verbal memory difficulties frequently occur after damage to the medial part of the left temporal lobe (called the *hippocampus*), and there is some evidence that nonverbal memory is affected by right hippocampal damage in some patients (see Chapters 3 and 4).

It should be noted, however, that failure to find double dissociations does not necessarily mean that specific associations do not exist between the impaired function and the area of damaged brain: Performance on a particular task can be influenced by a number of factors, such as the multiple discrete functions involved in a test or the level of test difficulty (Walsh 1985, p 26). In addition, if two neural structures that each mediate separate, discrete functions are anatomically close together, the chances of finding two patients with lesions (and therefore the associated impairments) confined to only one of these neural structures becomes very small. An example is the difficulty of deciding whether a *syndrome* (a cluster of symptoms that appear together following brain damage to a particular area of the brain) is the result of one underlying cognitive deficit causing many symptoms or results from many separate deficits, each mediated by different neural structures that lie very close together (see Gerstmann's syndrome, Chapter 6).

Neuropsychological Research and Clinical Practice

One of the most stimulating aspects of clinical neuropsychology is the continual interplay between research and clinical practice. In part, this interplay is a function of the relatively recent emergence of clinical neuropsychology as a discipline separate from neurology and psychology, but it is also related to the intrinsic nature of clinical neuropsychology. For example, neuropsychology researchers who are not interested in the clinical assessment and rehabilitation of patients with neurological conditions nevertheless require excellent clinical skills and knowledge if they use neurological patients as their research subjects. A patient who is excessively anxious will not produce valid results on neuropsychological experiments, and first must be helped to relax. The researcher who is unaware of the more subtle psychological effects of depression, fatigue, and head injury on higher cognitive functions may unknowingly produce research that is seriously flawed. It is important for researchers to keep abreast of the clinical literature to ensure that they are aware of new clinical findings about neurological disorders that may have implications for their own research.

Research skills are just as important for the practicing clinical neuropsychologist as clinical skills are for the researcher. First, it is important to obtain up-to-date normative data on many of the tests clinicians use, and these data are often gathered by clinicians working as researchers. Second, clinicians need a good grasp of appropriate research methods to design and evaluate specific tests to examine complex higher cognitive functions in different patients because the importance of individual differences increases with the complexity of the cognitive function being assessed. Third, the neuropsychological experimental literature can provide clinicians with new tests and paradigms that they can adapt for their own clinical purposes.

Roles of a Clinical Neuropsychologist

An individual clinical neuropsychologist not only can fulfill diverse roles as a clinician in an acute or outpatient neurosurgical–neurological service, in a rehabilitation service, or in private practice but also can become involved in research. This research can involve either intensive study of interesting single cases (see Chapters 3, 6, 8, and 19) or large group studies of neurological patients (e.g., Ogden 1985a; Ogden, Mee, and Henning 1993a; Ogden, Utley, and Mee 1997; Utley et al. 1997). In the setting of an acute or outpatient service, the clinical neuropsychological investigation may make an important contribution to the diagnosis of a disorder. For example, it might be important to establish whether a patient is depressed or in the early stages of dementia. Patients who are possible candidates for a temporal lobectomy as a cure for temporal lobe epilepsy must be carefully assessed by a neuropsychologist to ensure that the temporal lobe that will be left intact after neurosurgery is undamaged, and therefore capable of mediating memory (see Chapter 4). Patients in trials of new drug regimens can benefit from cognitive testing before and after the drug regimen is established (See Chapter 15). Assessments over time that monitor the changing cognitive status of patients with progressive diseases (see Chapters 14, 15 and 17) or following treatments such as neurosurgery (see Chapters 4 and 12) and radiotherapy can provide information to guide the patient's rehabilitation and, in addition, can provide data on long-term prognosis for future patients with similar conditions. The methodology required for carrying out longitudinal studies assessing interventions (e.g., drug treatments, neurosurgery, psychotherapy) for the symptoms of neurological disorders is fraught with difficulties and challenges, as many factors such as spontaneous recovery independent of the intervention, and practice effects that occur if the same neuropsychological test is given to the patient on multiple occasions, must be taken into account. In addition, even when assessing patients with the same neurological disorder, the patient group is likely to be heterogeneous on numerous variables such as age, educational level, and ethnicity (Towgood, Ogden, and Mee 2004).

The neuropsychologist is often a key staff member in rehabilitation programs, and in a head injury or stroke rehabilitation service, the neuropsychologist will usually work within a multidisciplinary or interdisciplinary team. In the multidisciplinary team, a number of different disciplines (e.g., occupational and physical therapists, speech pathologists and clinical psychologists and neuropsychologists) independently assess the needs of the patient and accordingly plan a rehabilitation program within their discipline. Although regular team meetings are usually held to discuss the patient's progress and ensure all team members are aware of what other team members are trying to accomplish, it sometimes happens that many different goals are being worked toward simultaneously, which can cause confusion and overload for the patient.

In the interdisciplinary team, the patient is often assessed in a more holistic way, often by a key therapist on the team, who will then request more specialized assessments as necessary. The key therapist, in collaboration with other team members, then establishes and prioritizes goals for rehabilitation toward which each therapist then works, but within their own discipline. This ensures that the patient's progress toward the stated goals is reinforced by all the therapists and avoids the situation in which one therapy discipline might unknowingly interfere with the program or goals of another therapist. In either team situation, in addition to assessing the client and planning and supervising the cognitive and psychological aspects of the client's program, the neuropsychologist may also act as rehabilitation coordinator or key therapist with responsibility for overseeing the total rehabilitation program of particular clients.

In many countries the demand for neuropsychological expertise in medicolegal cases is growing. A neuropsychological report on an accident victim with a possible head injury may be required to support claims for compensation. In legal suits involving neurologically impaired clients, before a court hearing, the neuropsychologist may be asked to prepare a written submission based on the neuropsychological assessment of the client and to act as an expert witness at the hearing. For example, a head-injured client may bring a charge against a person whose actions caused the head injury or against a person he believes has taken advantage of his reduced cognitive abilities to exploit or abuse him. In the reverse situation, a client with neurological damage may be accused of a deed his lawyer argues he should not be held responsible for because of his cognitive disabilities. Whatever the reason for the court case, the neuropsychologist who acts as an expert witness must be ready to put forward a reasoned and tight argument based on her professional observations and opinion that is supported by the established body of knowledge in the relevant area.

Understanding Neuropsychology through Case Studies

The detailed examination of a selection of interesting case studies can provide not only a relatively user-friendly, jargon-free description of a range of neurological disorders, both common and rare, but can also serve to highlight the clinical and human aspects of the patients who suffer these disorders. Telling the stories of individual victims of brain damage allows their patterns of cognitive functioning and rehabilitation to be described within an ecological context. Throughout the case studies, issues that commonly arise in the practice and research of neuropsychology are introduced. Such issues include patient-centered concerns (e.g., cultural and psychosocial aspects, family involvement, patient rights), and clinician-centered concerns (e.g., personal involvement and burnout, interaction with other health professionals, conflicts between research and clinical objectives, ethical issues).

The purpose of broadening the case studies in this way is to stimulate thinking and discussion about these issues. Another aim is to highlight the importance of conceptualizing problems and assessing and rehabilitating patients, their families, and their caregivers as an integrated "system" with all the humanistic and ethical aspects that entails, rather than as a disorder in isolation. By the end of the book, in addition to coming to know individuals and their families who have suffered and coped with brain damage, the reader should have gathered an overview of the theory and practice of neuropsychology. The reader should also have some idea about the types of rehabilitation programs and levels of recovery that are possible with different types of brain damage.

To understand the case descriptions, a sophisticated knowledge of neuroanatomy and specific neuropsychological tests is not necessary. Brief descriptions of the main tests mentioned can be found in Chapter 2. When it is helpful to do so within the context of a particular case study, the purpose of the neuropsychological tests used and their results are described in general terms.

I suggest that Chapters 1 and 2 be read before the individual case studies, but each case study chapter stands on its own and can be read in isolation from the others and in any order. Different topics, concepts, and issues are distributed through the case studies, depending on where they best fit within the context of the case. A list of some of the main topics and the chapters that include substantial discussion of them follows.

Neuropsychological Impairments

Agnosias (autotopagnosia, visual object agnosia, prosopagnosia): Chapters 6 and 8.

Amnesia and memory impairments: Most chapters refer to memory impairments as they are so common and important in a wide range of neurological disorders; however, Chapters 3, 4, 9, 10, and 17 are the most informative.

Aphasia and language disorders: Chapter 5. Chapters 18 and 19 provide discussions of language abilities in split-brain and hemispherectomized people.

Apraxia: Chapter 6.

Dementia: Chapters 16 and 17.

Diffuse brain-damage impairments: Chapters 10, 11, 12, 13, 14, 16, and 17.

Disconnection syndromes: Chapters 5, 6, and 18.

Focal brain damage impairments: Chapters 3, 4, 5, 6, 7, 8, 9, and 12.

Frontal-lobe (executive) syndrome: Chapters 9, 10, 15, 16, and 17.

Gerstmann's syndrome: Chapter 6.

Postconcussion syndrome: Chapter 11.

Hemineglect (unilateral inattention): Chapters 7 and 12.

Hemispherectomy: Chapter 19.
Left-hemispheric disorders: Chapters 5 and 6.
Organic solvent neurotoxicity impairments: Chapter 13.
Right-hemispheric disorders: Chapter 7.
Split-brain syndrome (commissurotomy): Chapter 18.

Neuropathology

Basal ganglion disorders: Parkinson's disease, Chapter 15; Huntington's disease, Chapter 16.
Benign tumors (meningioma): Chapter 7.
Cerebrovascular accidents (CVAs): Intracerebral hematoma, Chapter 5; stroke, Chapter 5; subarachnoid hemorrhage, Chapter 12.
Coma: Chapters 8 and 10.
Dementias: Korsakoff's syndrome, Chapter 3; Huntington's disease, Chapter 16; Alzheimer's disease, Chapter 17
Demyelination: Multiple sclerosis, Chapter 14.
Epilepsy: Chapters 3, 4, 18, and 19.
Genetic disorders: Huntington's disease, Chapter 16.
Infarctions (dead brain tissue): Chapters 8, 9 and 12.
Korsakoff's syndrome: Chapter 3.
Malignant tumors (metastatic carcinomas, glioma, astrocytoma): Chapters 6 and 7.
Motor Disorders: Chapters 14, 15, and 16.
Neurosurgical lesions: Chapters 3, 4, 15, 18, and 19.
Neurotoxicity: Chapter 13.
Traumatic (closed) brain injury: Chapters 8, 9, 10, and 11.

Other Topics

Behavior modification and cognitive-behavior therapy: Chapters 2, 4, and 10.
Cross-cultural issues: Chapters 2, 4, 5, and 11.
Death and dying: Chapters 6, 7, 16, and 17.
Ethical issues: Chapters 2, 6, 8, and 16.
Family-centered rehabilitation and family therapy: Chapters 10, 11, 12, 13, and 17.
Gene therapy: Chapter 15.
Genetic counseling: Chapter 16.
Multidisciplinary and interdisciplinary rehabilitation teams: Chapters 10, 14, and 16.
Radiotherapy: Chapter 7.

Rehabilitation, including self-help: Chapters 4, 5, 7, 9, 10, 11, 12, 13, 14, 15, 16, and 17.

Research-oriented assessment: Chapters 3, 6, 8, 18, and 19.

Single case study design: Chapter 5.

Social stigma and brain damage: Chapters 4, 14, 15, and 16.

Wada (sodium amytal) test: Chapter 4.

2

The Neuropsychological Assessment

Different Approaches to Neuropsychological Assessment

Quantitative Method

In its extreme form, the quantitative method of assessment involves the standardized use of a set group, or battery, of tests. These tests are scored quantitatively, and the resulting data are compared with normative data from a group of non-brain-damaged people, preferably matched to the patient in regard to important variables such as age, sex, socioeconomic group, culture, and years of formal education. To establish whether a patient's scores are typical of the scores of other people with similar disorders, comparisons with the scores of groups of patients with similar disorders or lesions in a similar area of the brain can sometimes be made. The advantage of the quantitative method is that the assessment can be conducted by a trained technician (psychometrist) who does not necessarily need to understand the concepts underlying the tests or their interpretation; a computer can score the tests and even interpret them according to the most likely pathology based on the best fit with normative and research data. The Halstead-Reitan Battery (Halstead 1947; Reitan and Davison 1974) is designed to be used in this way.

The pitfalls of this approach are that it does not allow for individual differences in brain–behavior relations and considerably restricts the possible interpretations. Also, a deficit may be missed because there is no test that covers it, or time may be wasted assessing many functions that are clearly intact. In addition, an enormous wealth of qualitative information is lost, information that may be essential to the correct interpretation of the data. For example, if the patient is very tired by the end of the test session and clearly having difficulty concentrating, the purely quantitative approach will ignore this and the lowered test score will be interpreted as an impairment.

Qualitative Method

This method of assessment, which was introduced by the great Russian neuropsychologist Aleksander Luria (1966, 1973) and described by Christensen (1979), emphasizes the uniqueness of every case. Assessment follows a hypothesis-testing approach in which the subject may be given particular tests, depending on the information available to the neuropsychologist (e.g., information that the patient has had a minor closed-head injury or has a parietal tumor). Then the patient is given increasingly more specific tests, depending on the results of previous tests, until the pattern of spared and impaired functions becomes clear. Throughout the assessment, use is made of qualitative information, such as the different steps and errors the patient makes when performing a task, as well as the final (quantitative) result. Other information taken into account includes the contextual factors that may influence a patient's performance, such as emotional state, learning history, other medical and physical problems, and so on.

The main drawback of the qualitative approach is that it relies on the training and experience of the neuropsychologist. To some extent, it is true to say that the results achieved by such a method can never be repeated exactly, especially by another neuropsychologist. As some critics of the qualitative approach comment, "The only person who can carry out an assessment by the Luria method is Luria!"

Flexible Assessment Method

This approach, also known as the qualitative-flexible approach, is the one favored by Edith Kaplan, Muriel Lezak, Kevin Walsh, and many other prominent clinical neuropsychologists and authors (Kaplan 1988; Lezak 1995; Walsh 1994). In essence, this approach uses a flexible battery or range of tests that often includes many of the subtests of a standard quantitative test battery, such as one of the Wechsler Intelligence Scales (WIS). These tests have been revised over the years; the most recent version for adults being the Wechsler Adult Intelligence Scale-III (WAIS-III) (Wechsler 1997a). Earlier editions include the Wechsler Adult Intelligence Scale (WAIS) (Wechsler 1955) and the Wechsler Adult Intelligence Scale–Revised (WAIS-R) (Wechsler 1981). The WIS has also been developed for children and revised over the years. This is titled the Wechsler Intelligence Scale for Children (WISC), with the most recent edition being the WISC-IV (Wechsler 2003).

The WAIS-R is used in some of the case studies in this book, and although there are some quite significant differences between the WAIS-R and the WAIS-III, which will be briefly described later in this chapter under *Neuropsychological Tests*, it is not important to understand these differences in any detail in the context of this book. The other series of Wechsler batteries assess verbal and visual memory functions, and the first edition was titled the Wechsler Memory Scale (WMS; Wechsler 1945). As for the WAIS, a number of revised editions have followed, with the most recent being the WMS-III (Wechsler 1997b).

The principles underlying the different editions of the Wechsler batteries remain the same; the changes include changing subtest items or adding or deleting whole subtests to improve the validity and sensitivity of the tests to the abilities they are aiming to measure, improving the scoring and introducing new ways of interpreting patterns of scores, and updating normative data.

With each new edition of the WAIS, WISC and WMS, their relevance to neuropsychological assessment rather than to the assessment of intelligence as a concept, often in neurologically normal people (e.g., students, army recruits, etc.), becomes greater. Each improved edition involves a large group of psychometrists, neuropsychologists, and statisticians working together in developing new test items, carrying out research on the new items, improving scoring and interpretation strategies, and gathering normative data. These widely used test batteries measure performance quantitatively by using standardized scores for each of its component subtests, allowing them to be readily compared with normative data.

Each new edition of one of the Wechsler batteries often takes a few years to become established as the most commonly used edition. This is a result of a number of factors: the cost of acquiring the new battery; the fact that the clinical neuropsychologist may have built up a great deal of knowledge based on their administration, scoring, and interpretation of the older edition; the lack of research published in peer-reviewed scientific journals on the new edition; and in many cases the belief that some of the revised or new subtests are not as useful as the older versions of the tests. The flexibility of the clinical neuropsychologist to pick and choose between Wechsler batteries and the subtests within them is another hallmark of the flexible assessment method. It is the selection of appropriate tests for the particular client and the specific referral questions that the assessment is designed to answer, along with the interpretation of the pattern of test results, that is important, rather than administration of the latest test battery simply because it has been published.

The flexible assessment also takes into account the methods used and errors made by the patient in performing the task as well as other contextual information from the patient's history and current situation. Tests might also be given in a nonstandardized manner; for example, a patient may be encouraged to continue beyond the time limit so that his optimal ability can be assessed when he is not under time pressure. Depending on the results of these initial tests, the patient is often given additional tests to prove or disprove hypotheses and to delineate more fully the parameters of any impairments.

Edith Kaplan and her colleagues developed a method of using qualitative information in a consistent way when employing the WAIS-R. They call this method the WAIS-R NI (the WAIS-R as a Neuropsychological Instrument; Kaplan, Fein, Morris, and Delis 1991), which elegantly formalizes what qualitative-flexible neuropsychologists have been doing informally for many years; that is, they specify and provide interpretations for the different process errors individuals make when doing the tests. New ways of administering some of the tests allow different cognitive impairments to be distinguished.

The case studies in this book all follow the qualitative-flexible assessment approach. In the good company of many other neuropsychologists, I almost always begin the testing part of assessment by giving all or some of the subtests in one of the WAIS batteries (usually, but not always using the latest edition), in addition to tests of verbal and nonverbal memory. Some, but rarely all, of the memory tests may come from an edition of the WMS.

Neuropsychological Assessment Process

Referral

Referrals for a neuropsychological assessment can come from any health professional, but most come from general practitioners, neurologists, neurosurgeons, psychiatrists, and therapists involved in rehabilitation (e.g., clinical psychologists and speech, occupational, and physical therapists). The legal profession also uses neuropsychological assessments. The referral question should specify the aim of the assessment: to aid with diagnosis, as in the case of suspected dementia (Chapter 17), to provide an up-to-date picture of the patient's impairments and deficits so that the therapist or rehabilitation team can better plan a rehabilitation program (Chapters 10–16), or to monitor a patient's recovery (Chapter 11) or progression of disease (Chapters 14–17). Other aims of assessment are to provide a baseline measure of cognitive functioning before neurosurgery or drug treatment and a follow-up assessment, as in the case of temporal lobectomy for epilepsy (Chapter 4); to provide an assessment of disability that can be used for insurance or compensation purposes; or to assist in preparing a legal case, as, for example, in a case where a person with frontal-lobe damage is raped or is charged with neglecting her children.

Clinical Interview

Usually the assessment would begin with an interview to enable the neuropsychologist to form a picture of the patient's difficulties and intact abilities from the point of view of the patient (and, if possible, other family members). A medical and psychological history is also taken, with the neuropsychologist especially alert for possible causes for the patient's problems that may not have been noted by the referring agency. Psychological and contextual factors, such as depression and suicide risk, high levels of stress, financial hardships, marital and family problems, and family and community support, are assessed to aid the neuropsychologist in interpreting the test data and in making recommendations regarding rehabilitation.

Assessment Procedures and Context

Following the interview, which should also serve to relax the client, inform him of his rights, and clearly explain the aim and format of the assessment he is about to undergo, the patient is given the various tests that the neuropsychologist has selected. The assessment is often carried out in one session of 3 hours or longer, including regular breaks, or if the patient tires easily or loses concentration, the tests can be carried out in two or more sessions. Often the aim of the assessment is to determine what the patient can and cannot do when he is performing to his best ability. To do so requires that the testing take place in a quiet room with good lighting and few distractions, such as interesting sights outside a window or extraneous noises. However, if the aim of the assessment is to evaluate the patient's readiness to return to work or school, testing his concentration, memory, and ability to perform work-related tasks in a noisy work or school environment will be of more value.

There is little point in testing a patient who feels unwell, overly anxious, tired, or moderately to severely depressed, as the results will not reflect the patient's true cognitive abilities. People who are actively psychotic are also untestable. If a comprehension deficit is suspected, a patient can be tested with special aphasia batteries to assess his language abilities, but he should not be given a general test battery if it becomes clear that he is unable to understand the test instructions. There are, however, special techniques and tests that can be used to assess patients with only a minimal ability to comprehend or respond; these techniques are outside the scope of this book.

Neuropsychological Assessment Report

On completion of the testing, the neuropsychologist writes a report for the referral agency, and many neuropsychologists provide the client or patient with this report as well, preferably in a follow-up session so that the results and the neuropsychologist's interpretation and recommendations can be carefully and sensitively explained. Therefore, the report should be written in straightforward language that makes the neuropsychologist's interpretations clear (see Chapter 12 for an example of a report).

Some neuropsychologists include the patient's raw or standardized test scores along with normative data in their report. Others prefer to keep these in a separate confidential file to be made available, with the patient's permission, to other professionals who have the training to interpret the scores. Neuropsychological test scores usually have little meaning to people not thoroughly trained in clinical neuropsychology and should always be accompanied by a clearly written interpretation to lessen the possibility of misinterpretation by lay people and health professionals without adequate neuropsychological knowledge. When deciding to whom scores or even the written report should be released, it should be kept in mind that the occasional professional with doubtful ethics and little or no neuropsychological training might, for example, label a person as "retarded" if the patient's IQ scores fall somewhat below "average."

Neuropsychological Tests

General Remarks

Literally hundreds of neuropsychological tests exist and are currently used; new tests are constantly being developed and old ones revised. Therefore, it is well beyond the scope of this book to even scrape the surface in this area. Readers who intend to learn how to conduct a neuropsychological assessment must undergo appropriate training and become familiar with a wide selection of these tests. Detailed descriptions and normative data for many tests can be found in books written for that purpose. Two of the best such test manuals are those by Muriel Lezak (1995) and Otfried Spreen and Esther Strauss (1998).

The following section describes, in rather broad terms, some of the most commonly used tests and general categories of tests usually included in a basic neuropsychological assessment. In the case studies that follow, for the purposes of simplification, I have generally restricted myself to the tests described below, with the exception of specialist tests designed more for experimental than basic clinical assessment purposes (e.g., Chapters 6, 8, and 19).

Tests of General Intellectual Ability

The most commonly used general ability test is the Wechsler Adult Intelligence Scale (WAIS) and its revised editions (grouped together as the Wechsler Intelligence Scales, or WIS). Although the various editions of the WIS share 11 subtests, each assessing a different cognitive ability, the most recent version, the WAIS-III, includes a further three subtests. The raw score for each subtest is converted to a scaled score, standardized for the age group of the individual, with a mean of 10 and a standard deviation (SD) of three. Conversion tables allow the sum of the subtest scores to be converted to IQ scores and, in the latest version, to additional index scores.

Six of the WIS tests assess different verbal functions, such as general knowledge, vocabulary, comprehension, and verbal abstract thinking, and are grouped together to form the *Verbal IQ*. Five of the tests assess a range of performance abilities, including complex visuospatial function, perceptual organization, and psychomotor speed, and bonus points are gained for fast performance on most of these tests. They are grouped together to form the *Performance IQ*. In the WAIS-III there are three further supplementary tests. These are given if further information is required or if the additional summary index scores are to be calculated. Some of the WIS subtests also tap attention, concentration, short-term memory, memory for past facts, and conceptual ability. A *Full-scale IQ* can be derived from the combined Verbal and Performance IQ. The Full-scale IQ, Verbal IQ, and Performance IQ each have a mean of 100 and a SD of 15. As these IQ scores are the result of averaging subtest scores over many different abilities, they are often misleading; the lowest and highest subtest score, even in normal adults, can differ by 5–9 points (Matarazzo and Prifitera 1989). Full-scale,

Verbal, and Performance IQ scores, compared with premorbid ability, can nonetheless provide an estimate of the extent of overall decline in some patients, such as those with dementia or severe head injury.

Sometimes when a patient is assessed more than once over a long time period, two different editions of the WIS will be used. In such cases it is important to note that each edition of the WIS yields IQ scores that are lower (by up to 7 points) than the previous WIS. Thus if the patient gains a Verbal IQ of 100 on the WAIS-III, but gained a Verbal IQ of 107 on the WAIS-R 10 years earlier, this probably means that his Verbal IQ remained stable over that time period. The reason that people tested on the current version of the WIS have to get higher raw scores than on a previous version to get the same IQ is that the abilities of the normative group from which the standardized scores are derived, have improved. Thus, a 20 year old in 2004, on average, knows more (in relation to the current WIS tests) than a 20 year old in 1980, but as the average IQ remains at 100, everyone must do better to keep pace with the changing knowledge base in the population. Of course, if there were subtests on "surviving without electricity" or "sewing one's own clothes," the older generation would probably dramatically increase their test scores (and any IQ scores derived from these) on current versions of the WIS, which are standardized against the abilities of the population in 2004.

The WAIS-III goes beyond the previous versions in that addition to the IQ scores, four index scores can be derived from the subtest scores. These are labeled Verbal Comprehension, Perceptual Organization, Working Memory, and Processing Speed. These indices can make interpretation of the pattern of scores for neuropsychological purposes more objective.

Each WIS subtest does not, in fact, test a single "cognitive" function but, rather, assesses a complex of functions. Thus, there can be a number of different reasons for obtaining a poor score on any one subtest. The qualitative-flexible approach encourages observation of how an individual approaches the test and the errors he makes, thereby providing valuable clues about why he ultimately obtains a poor score. This hypothesis can then be tested by giving him another test that taps abilities that seem not to be impaired but that also involve the ability that was hypothesized to be impaired on the previous test. If the hypothesis is supported, then he will also have difficulties with this test.

Language Abilities

Because of the many complex ways it can break down, language is often seen as a specialist's area for both assessment and treatment. Many clinical neuropsychologists do not have specialist expertise in assessing language impairments and will refer patients with these problems to speech pathologists, or therapists who deal exclusively with these disorders. Language impairments include speech fluency, naming, repetition, comprehension, reading, spelling, and writing deficits, and many test batteries have been designed to assess the various aspects of linguistic ability.

If comprehension difficulties are suspected, it is important to assess basic auditory comprehension before carrying out any further neuropsychological tests. The Short Token Test (De Renzi and Faglioni 1978) fulfills this function. Using colored tokens, the patient is asked to carry out commands of increasing length and complexity. For example, she will be asked to "touch the large white circle and the small green square." A number of aphasia batteries have been developed to enable a detailed evaluation of a wide range of language abilities. The Boston Diagnostic Aphasia Examination (BDAE) (Goodglass and Kaplan 1983) and the Neurosensory Center Comprehensive Examination For Aphasia (NCCEA) (Spreen and Benton 1977) are two widely used aphasia batteries. Other batteries, such as the Communicative Abilities in Daily Living (CADL) (Holland 1980, 1984), are designed to assess the patient's problems in trying to communicate in normal living situations. An assessment of the patient's ability to communicate nonverbally is also included.

Highly specialized tests and batteries of tests are also available for evaluating, in careful detail, the intricacies of one or more aspects of language, such as reading and spelling. These tests can be useful for research and are often developed as a result of years of research with different types of reading and spelling problems. The Psycho-linguistic Assessments of Language Processing in Aphasia (PALPA) (Kay, Lesser, and Coltheart 1992) is such a battery.

Visuospatial Perceptual Abilities

Some of the WIS subtests (e.g., Block Design and Object Assembly) assess complex visuospatial functions that are often impaired following brain damage. Another commonly used test of visuospatial perception is the copy of the Complex Figure (Meyers and Meyers 1995; Osterreith 1944; Rey 1941; Taylor 1969). The top line of Figure 2-1 shows Rey's version of this figure, and copies of it can be seen in the middle line. On the left is the copy by a non-brain-damaged man (whose score of 32 fell at the 50th percentile); on the right, the copy of a man with right parietal lobe damage (whose score of 20 fell below the 10th percentile). The drawing is scored out of 36, and the individual's score is compared with normative data.

Executive and Control Abilities

The frontal lobes of the brain are often referred to as the *executive lobes* because their main function is to formulate goals, to organize and plan, to carry out goal-directed plans, and to solve problems. Patients with damage to the frontal lobes often have difficulty with abstract concepts and think in a concrete or literal manner. Executive functions can also be impaired by damage in other parts of the brain, although severe executive problems are almost always associated with dysfunctional frontal lobes. Some subtests of the WIS batteries tap executive functions to a degree (e.g., Similarities, the proverbs of the Comprehension subtest, and the process by which Block Design, Object Assembly, and Picture Arrangement are carried out).

Other tests sensitive to executive functions involve sorting objects into categories according to rules that the individual must discover by attending to his errors. At different points in the test, the rules are changed by the examiner, often without warning, and the individual must discover from his new errors the new rules and change his sorting behavior accordingly. The most commonly used of these tests are the Wisconsin Card Sorting Test (WCST) (Heaton 1981) and the simpler Modified Wisconsin Card Sorting Test (MWCST) (Nelson 1976). These tests use a set of playing cards that can be sorted by the number, color, or form of the symbols on each card. Such tests tap the ability to form abstract concepts, to problem-solve, to plan a strategy, to learn from one's errors and change one's behavior accordingly, and to change mental set. People with frontal-lobe damage often have extreme difficulty with this test, and the type of errors they make can provide information about their particular deficits. For example, some cannot grasp the abstract idea that they must sort to a particular category, some cannot learn from their new errors when the rule and category change, and some perseverate (return to the previous category), even though they know the rule has changed. People in this last group have difficulty changing their mental set. The Halstead Category Test (HCT) (Halstead 1947), in which the individual must decide which object or stimulus in a set differs from all the others, is another task that taps the ability to figure out abstract principles.

Another, much simpler test that involves changing mental set is the Trail Making Test (Reitan 1958). In Part I of this test, the patient must connect consecutively numbered circles scattered over a page. In Part II the same number of consecutively numbered and lettered circles must be connected by alternating between the two sequences. The examiner corrects the patient each time an error is made, and the score is simply the time taken to complete each part. This test is very sensitive to any brain damage because it depends on the speed of response and mental tracking; if, however, in part II the patient clearly has difficulty changing mental set, frontal-lobe dysfunction should be suspected and further examined.

A third group of tests sensitive to executive and particularly frontal-lobe dysfunctions include Controlled Oral Word Fluency tests (Benton and Hamsher 1976; Borkowski, Benton, and Spreen 1967) and Design Fluency tests (Jones-Gotman and Milner 1977). Typically, the patient is asked to produce, in 1 minute, as many words or designs that fall within a specified category (e.g., words starting with a particular letter, often F, A, and S, or designs that are not scribbles but not recognizable objects or symbols). Set rules must be followed; for example, with word fluency, no proper names must be used; with designs, no more than one straight line must be used. The final score is the number of correct and different responses, and it can be compared with normative data from a similar age, sex, and socioeconomic group. Equally important are the qualitative or process data, including rule-breaking errors and perseverative errors (giving the same word or word stem or same design many times). Although poor scores on fluency tests alone cannot point to frontal-lobe damage, patients with left frontal lesions often perform more poorly than patients with damage in other areas on word fluency tests (Perret 1974), and there is some evidence to suggest that some patients with right frontal damage perform more poorly on design fluency tests (Jones-Gotman and Milner 1977).

More recently, batteries of tests that assess different aspects of executive functioning have been published. One interesting test battery called the Behavioural Assessment of the Dysexecutive Syndrome (BADS; Wilson, Alderman, Burgess, Emslie, and Evans 1996) includes subtests that require the sort of initiative, problem-solving, planning, and organization that are essential for day-to-day functioning. This battery attempts, with some success, to get away from the highly structured, rule-bound context that is typical of most psychometric assessments. Given that patients with executive problems may function quite adequately if they are told what to do, are given an external structure to guide them, or are completing well-learned tasks, many common psychometric tests will not tap into the essentials of impaired executive functioning, even in patients who demonstrate clear executive deficits in their daily lives.

Another recently published battery, the Delis-Kaplan Executive Function System (D-KEFS; Delis, Kaplan, and Kramer 2001), brings together a number of well-established tests of executive function in addition to new tests, and it also provides data on the correlation of this battery with other commonly used IQ and memory tests. Such batteries take considerable time to administer in full (e.g., the D-KEFS is estimated to take 90 minutes), so they should only be used when executive difficulties are particularly debilitating. Such batteries might be used before developing a rehabilitation program for an individual client, on the basis that the profile of impaired and spared executive functions would provide guidance on which deficits require rehabilitation and which functions are intact, and could be utilized to enhance the client's abilities.

Memory Tests

Memory involves many different abilities, such as attention, concentration, sensory memory, short-term memory, working memory, encoding, long-term store, recall, and recognition. People with memory impairments most often have difficulties with one or more of the functions involved in learning and retrieving or recalling new information, usually termed *anterograde* or *recent* memory impairment, as it affects the memory for material learned since the brain damage occurred. A few patients, such as those with dementia, have *retrograde amnesia*, referring to the inability to recall memories learned and stored before the onset of the brain disorder. There are numerous tests for each of these memory types and subcomponents, and it is often important to attempt to delineate the specific difficulties experienced by a patient with memory impairment. More details about the different forms of memory impairment can be found in Chapter 3.

The WAIS batteries include the Digit Span subtest, which assesses short-term memory; that is, the number of units we can hold in our memory over a period of about 7 seconds (seven units plus or minus two items). This subtest is often seen as a measure of attention and concentration rather than of memory. If short-term memory is impaired, it will obviously affect the ability to learn new information. The WAIS batteries do not contain any tests of new learning, and as this is the most common memory problem following brain disease, screening tests for recent verbal and non-verbal memory are almost always given in the initial stages of assessment. The most commonly used memory battery is the WMS (Wechsler 1945) and its substantially revised and expanded versions, the Wechsler Memory Scale–Revised (WMS-R; Wechsler 1987) and the Wechsler Memory Scale–III (WMS-III0; Wechsler 1997b). The original WMS was woefully inadequate with regard to tests of nonverbal, vis-uospatial memory, but the new editions go some way toward correcting this problem. One of the most important aspects of the WMS-III is that it was developed in harness with the WAIS-III, and standardization of the two batteries included a proportion of the standardization samples being assessed on both batteries. The 350-page Technical Manual on the WAIS-III and WMS-III that accompanies the substantial administration and scoring manuals for each battery provides a wealth of data on each battery and the ways in which both batteries can be used together.

The enormous amount of time and expertise that has gone into each new edition of these test batteries has surely improved the validity and reliability of these instru-ments, but even so, individual clinicians sometimes find that an older edition of a subtest is more useful for their purposes, or for the assessment of a particular neu-ropsychological disorder, and will mix and match across batteries. This highlights the fact that neuropsychological assessment cannot be carried out to a formula, by a skilled technician or psychometrist, but requires the knowledge and experience that is essential to the training of a clinical neuropsychologist.

The main verbal memory subtests of the WMS batteries are Logical Memory, Paired Associates, and learning a list of unrelated words. Logical Memory involves asking the patient to repeat two one-paragraph stories immediately after being read them and then to recall them again after a delay in which other distracting items are presented. In Paired Associates, the patient is read a list of paired words, which are not usually commonly associated (e.g., school–grocery). The patient is read the list four times, and after each reading, he is given the first word of each pair and asked to give the second. Later, after a delay, the first word of each pair is given again to see whether the patient can still recall the recently learned word associations. If he can, this implies that these word pairs were stored in long-term memory store and can be retrieved. In the list-learning test, he learns a list of 12 words over four trials and, as for the other tests, is tested after a delay. The patient is also given a second list after he has learned the first to see whether this affects the subsequent recall of the first list. Other commonly used list learning tests include the Oral Selective Reminding Test (SRT) (Buschke and Fuld 1974) and the Rey Auditory-Verbal Learning Test (RAVLT) (Rey 1964). Nonverbal memory tests include reproducing simple designs immediately after viewing them and following a delay; viewing pictures of faces and picking them out from a series of faces, and viewing a drawing of a scene and then answering questions about it.

There are many other memory tests that can be used to assess the different types and components of memory. One list-learning test uses a shopping list with groups of different types of items on it, such as clothes, herbs, and household utensils (the California Verbal Learning Test (CVLT) (Delis et al. 1987), instead of the list of unrelated words used in the WAIS-III. This format is considered more applicable to the real-life difficulties patients experience, is thus less tedious to do and provides additional information about the ability of the patient to aid his memory by grouping together items from the same category.

A frequently used nonverbal memory test is the recall of the Rey Complex Figure (Fig. 2-1). This is often used as a test of incidental learning, as when the patient initially copies the figure, he is not told he will later be asked to recall it. The bottom row on the figure shows the recall attempts of a "normal" man (whose score of 26 fell at the 70th percentile) and a brain-damaged patient (whose score of 10.5 fell below the 10th percentile).

Recall of material is often improved if the patient is cued in some way, suggesting that the patient did store the material but has difficulty in retrieving it spontaneously. Recognition memory tests take advantage of this and require the patient to recognize items that were recently seen that are dispersed among similar items not seen before. Persons who fail this task are suspected of having an impairment of storage of information and are therefore less likely to respond to rehabilitation strategies aimed at "jogging their memory." One test of this type is the Recognition Memory Test (Warrington 1984). In the verbal trial, the patient reads a list of 50 high-frequency words and is then shown a list of 50 pairs of words, one of each pair coming from the list just read, the other a distractor. The patient's task is simply to decide (or guess) which of the two words she has just seen. The nonverbal version is the forerunner to the face recognition test now in the WMS-III and uses photographs of unfamiliar men's faces instead of words; after the patient has viewed 50 faces, she must choose which face in each of 50 pairs is the one she has just seen. This test sounds difficult, but for people with normal memory abilities it is, in fact, surprisingly easy. The idea of using faces as the nonverbal memory items is an excellent one, as it is extremely difficult to "learn" faces in a verbal fashion. That is, although one can provide a general description of a face, the particular form and spatial arrangement of the features is too complex and subtle to allow us to distinguish between two superficially similar faces verbally.

Retrograde memory loss is more difficult to assess than recent memory because to do so effectively, it is important to know what experiences the patient has had in the past and to what information she has been exposed. Some tests have been developed that require the patient to select from a number of choices the occupations of famous people whose fame is restricted to a single decade. Many items from across many decades are used. Other tests that assess autobiographical or personal memory loss use an interview format to try to establish the richness and reliability of the patient's memory for incidents that happened in each phase of her development (e.g., The Autobiographical Memory Interview; AMI; Kopelman, Wilson, and Baddeley 1990). If possible, these events should be confirmed by family members.

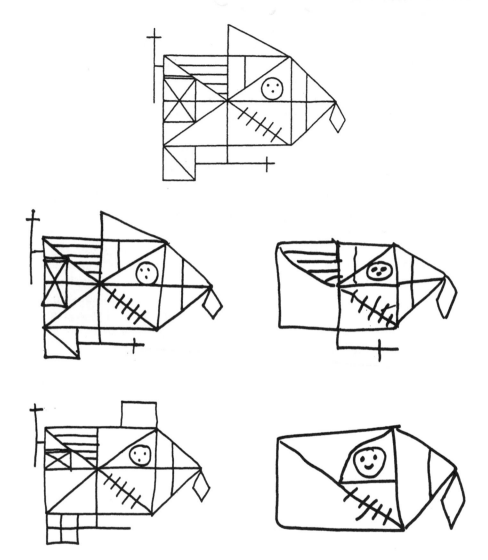

Figure 2-1 The Rey Complex Figure. At the top is the model the individual is asked to copy. On the left of the middle row is the copy of a normal middle-aged man, and below that is his recall of the figure 40 minutes later. On the right of the middle row is the copy of a middle-aged man who had suffered a right parietal stroke, and below that is his recall of the figure 40 minutes later.

Estimation of Premorbid Abilities

It is essential to estimate a patient's *premorbid abilities* (i.e., abilities before the brain damage occurred) before a valid interpretation of current functioning can be made. For example, a man who, after a head injury, gains WIS subtest scores and IQ scores in the "average" range is clearly significantly impaired if before his head injury he was a university professor with an estimated IQ in the "very superior" range. Premorbid IQ is ideally estimated by taking account of the person's highest educational qualification, occupation, hobbies, and any other information that signals "intelligence." A prison inmate with little formal education, drug dealing as an occupation, and petty burglary as a hobby could be estimated as possessing above average to superior intelligence if he had successfully masterminded an escape from a high-security prison and remained free for some months.

It is often difficult to estimate with confidence the premorbid IQ from life experiences. Certain types of test results can provide a reasonable estimate, in that they rely on overlearned factual material that is very resistant to brain damage. For example, two of the verbal subtests of the WIS batteries (Information and Vocabulary) can often serve this purpose; again, these subtests rely to some extent on formal education, and for patients with left-hemispheric damage and language deficits, even these tests can produce very impaired scores. Sometimes the highest subtest score or, more validly, the average of the three highest subtest scores on the WAIS battery is taken as an indication of premorbid IQ. The National Adult Reading Test (NART) (Nelson and O'Connell 1978) and the National Adult Reading Test-Revised (NART-R) (Nelson and Willison 1991) are tests that have been designed specifically for assessment of premorbid IQ. They rely on the fact that the ability to pronounce irregularly spelled English words is highly correlated with the WIS IQs and does not deteriorate, except in advanced dementia, even when the patient can no longer remember or explain the meaning of words.

Equations that use a range of demographic measures and that predict the WIS IQ of non-brain-damaged people have also been used to estimate premorbid intelligence of brain-damaged people. The Barona Equations are examples of this method (Barona, Reynolds, and Chastain 1984; Barona and Chastain 1986). Whereas these equations may provide a reasonable estimate for the demographically average individual, they do not respect individual differences, such as the person who lives in poor socioeconomic circumstances and attends school irregularly but who later in life demonstrates a high IQ by planning and carrying out complex crimes.

Intelligence, an ill-defined and global concept, is the result of genetic, environmental, and educational factors as well as a construct of the way we choose to define and measure it. Clearly, some people have more talents in some areas than in others; and to discover these variations is an important part of the premorbid estimation. An artist or draftsman who obtains a slightly below average score when copying a complex design (e.g., the Complex Figure) should engender more concern than an English teacher who obtains the same score but who, according to his wife, has always been a hopeless artist.

Follow-Up Assessment

Some patients require only one assessment, but others need a follow-up assessment to determine recovery, further deterioration, or a change in abilities after neurosurgery, radiation, or drug treatment or after withdrawal or a period free of neurotoxic organic solvents. Tests demonstrated to have a minimal practice effect can be repeated, or parallel versions of tests can be given at the second assessment. Sometimes completely new tests are given to test hypotheses suggested by the first assessment. At all stages of follow-up, psychosocial factors and changes should be taken into account, and when appropriate, updated rehabilitation and therapy recommendations should be made.

Limitations of Neuropsychological Assessment

A competent neuropsychological assessment requires a competent neuropsychologist, suitable tests for the purposes of that particular assessment and client, and a cooperative client. Clearly, an assessment carried out by an inadequately trained or inexperienced assessor can be very damaging to the client. Test scores obtained as the result of incorrect testing procedures, incorrect scoring, and incorrect interpretation may not be obviously incorrect to other health professionals. Reports placed in the client's medical file, and thereafter viewed as "expert opinion" by the client, family, and other health professionals, may be written on the basis of incorrect interpretation of test patterns and without knowledgeable integration of quantitative and qualitative data.

Often there are limited normative data available for even the better known tests, especially for minority ethnic groups, the elderly, and many clinical populations (e.g., spina bifida, developmentally retarded people, and others). If tests must be used for individuals who fall outside the population group on which the tests were normalized, they must be interpreted with caution, and qualitative data become even more important. Assessments are unlikely to be valid if carried out on clients who are uncooperative or unmotivated either because of poor rapport between client and assessor or because their neurological disorder or psychological state prevents them from cooperating or focusing on the tests. Other factors, such as a noisy and disruptive testing environment, a client who is "malingering" to gain financial compensation or to avoid returning to work or school, or a neuropsychologist who is perceived by the client to be officious and uncaring or culturally inappropriate, will also diminish the validity of the assessment findings.

A neuropsychological assessment must be carried out and interpreted within the context of other assessments and information gathering (e.g., neurological, psychological, family, work, socioeconomic, cultural) if our aim is to gain an in-depth and broad understanding of the client and the problems he is experiencing. If rehabilitation is a goal, assessment of the client's strengths and intact abilities is as important as assessment of his weaknesses.

Neuropsychologists who view themselves as one member of a multidisciplinary or interdisciplinary system are more likely to prove useful to neurologically impaired clients than are those who work in isolation. The multidisciplinary system does not necessitate working within a cohesive team, but it does require an awareness and respect for the assessments and opinions of other professionals as well as those of the client and family.

Like all professionals, ethical neuropsychologists will ensure that they keep current with the research literature and regularly consult with peers about professional issues, difficult cases, new assessment methods, and so on.

Cross-Cultural Issues in Neuropsychology

The man often dubbed the Father of Modern Neuropsychology, Alexsandr Luria (1902–1977), was Russian; since his time, clinical neuropsychology has become widely practiced and researched throughout the United States, Canada, Europe, and Australasia, as well as within the white and Westernized populations of Asia, South America, and South Africa. Clinical neuropsychological research with nonwhite cultural groups is increasing (Ardila, Rosseli, and Ostrosky 1992; Ardila, Rosseli, and Rosas 1989; Ogden, Cooper, and Dudley 2003; Ogden and McFarlane-Nathan 1997), but Western concepts and systems, and white neuropsychologists, still dominate.

Superficially, it might seem that the findings of clinical neuropsychology should be generalizable to all ethnic and cultural groups, which is probably the case when we consider the overall picture. It seems likely, for example, that medial temporal lobe damage will potentially give rise to problems with learning and remembering new material, and parietal lobe damage to visuospatial impairments, regardless of ethnicity. It is at the level of detail that we must question our assumptions about cross-cultural brain–behavior similarities. For example, many Australian aborigines demonstrate an uncanny ability (from the point of view of white cultures) to navigate (without a compass) their way across vast deserts and to track animals by recognizing footprints. Most white Australians have no idea how the aboriginal people achieve this, let alone be able to do it themselves. The Footprint Recognition Test (Porteus 1931) is thus culturally biased in favor of aborigines. Likewise, the Horse Recognition Test (Dubois 1939), is culturally biased toward Pueblo Indians. As neuropsychologists, we must ask whether the Australian aborigines and Pueblo Indians have evolved highly sophisticated and specialized topographical orientation and visuospatial abilities or whether they learn these skills as children. Either way, this finding has implications for brain–behavior relationships.

In the case of specialist evolution, we might expect to find in aborigines a cortical area or neural system specialized for this ability that is absent in races not possessing this skill. Perhaps this skill is associated with a greater development of parietal lobe systems or is mediated in part by the same system that enables a city dweller to find his way around a new city. If each individual must learn the skill anew, questions arise about the way the functional systems of the developing brain are organized and whether, given the same learning environment, the brains of aborigines have a greater potential for developing these skills than the brains of people of other races.

In practical terms, the different abilities of different ethnic groups, whether innate or learned, should influence how we interpret impairments after brain damage. To interpret test results correctly, we require normative data for that particular group of people. Most normative test data are grouped according to age, sometimes gender, and sometimes level of formal education and socioeconomic group. Ideally, we should also have normative data on the performance of different ethnic, cultural, and even subcultural groups; this area of neuropsychology that has been largely overlooked.

Normative test data alone will not solve the problem of cross-cultural assessment, as the manner in which tests are given, the cultural similarity of the neuropsychologist to the patient or client, the content and format of the tests themselves, and the way both the qualitative and quantitative assessment data are interpreted also contribute to a valid, reliable, and helpful assessment. Some pioneers have begun to map this vast territory (e.g., Ardila et al. 1989, 1992), but there is a long and difficult road ahead for these committed researchers, and they deserve our full support and cooperation.

The form an assessment should take to optimize its usefulness for a particular individual is an important but difficult issue in a country that includes many ethnic groups in various stages of assimilation by the dominant culture. Commonly, all we have available for a client of an ethnic minority are European or white-American assessment tests to be given by a white neuropsychologist. The validity of giving a person from another cultural group a European or American-based assessment will increase as a function of the client's level of acculturation into the dominant culture. For example, a part-Maori man who has been raised in a large New Zealand city by a pakeha (white) mother, who has succeeded in the pakeha education system, and who identifies primarily with pakeha will probably be reasonably well served by the same test battery and conditions as his pakeha peers.

The New Zealand neuropsychologists must come to terms with the fact that many of the Maori or part-Maori clients who require neuropsychological assessments following, for example, head injuries, are unlikely to have succeeded in a pakeha school system based on European values, skills, learning conditions, and assessment measures. In addition, many Maori, forced into close social contact with pakeha, may not feel truly comfortable in a pakeha world and have long since given up hope that their pakeha friends and acquaintances could understand that their worldview is fundamentally different from that of the pakeha. The danger here lies in the pakeha neuropsychologist's interpretation of the Maori client's test performance as well as the qualitative information that is gathered from an interview (Ogden 2001a). These cautionary remarks are not, of course, restricted to the situation in New Zealand but are equally appropriate for many Westernized countries in which the indigenous people and minority ethnic groups have been (and often still are) oppressed and dominated by the dominant white culture.

The separate question of the morality of giving a client of another culture no choice regarding the ethnicity of his assessment (however acculturated he is) is one that rightly concerns many neuropsychologists. Usually, faced with a client from a different culture, our choices are limited to not performing an assessment at all or to performing one as sensitively as we can while consulting with people of the client's culture who may be able to advise us about how best to put the client at ease during the assessment as well as to suggest culturally appropriate interpretations of some of the data.

I have included this brief discussion of cross-cultural issues because I believe the broadening of clinical neuropsychology to include all ethnic groups and cultures that it can serve is the most pressing need in neuropsychology today. The fact that this text is primarily about white neuropsychology is another reflection of the current state of clinical neuropsychology and my own limited experience. Although the issue of culturally sensitive assessment is addressed in a limited way in Chapters 4, 5, and 11, my hope is that in time many neuropsychologists from different cultures will be writing their own books based on their own research and clinical practice.

3

■

Marooned in the Moment

H.M., a Case of Global Amnesia

H.M. is perhaps the most famous of all neurological cases. As a result of a neurosurgical procedure carried out in an attempt to reduce his epileptic seizures, H.M. became globally amnesic. From the time of his operation when he was 27 years old until the present (H.M. is in now in his late 70s), he has been unable to learn consciously or remember any new information (*anterograde amnesia*). In addition, he has suffered a dense memory loss for a period of 11 years preceding his surgery (*retrograde amnesia*). In essence, H.M.'s knowledge base remains as it was when he was a teenager, although his intelligence in other areas is largely unimpaired. It is as though time stopped for H.M. around the age of 16 years, and today he lives in a timeless vacuum, interacting intelligently minute by minute with whatever stimuli impinge directly upon him.[1]

The operation performed on H.M. was a gamble that went dreadfully wrong. Parts of the anterior medial temporal lobes were removed, and although this procedure was indeed successful in substantially reducing H.M.'s seizures, the tragic consequences of the operation motivated his neurosurgeon to campaign widely against its future use (Scoville 1968). In 1953 it was unknown that the temporal lobes had anything to do with memory, and the irony is that through many years of intensive research on H.M.'s memory impairments, we have learned much about memory and how different memory processes relate to the temporal lobes. Innumerable research articles have been written, and are still being written, about all the possible aspects of H.M.'s memory deficits and about his functioning in other areas.[2]

1. I am grateful to Brenda Milner and Suzanne Corkin for their permission to study H.M. This chapter is based on a chapter entitled "Memories of H.M." by J.A. Ogden and S. Corkin, in *Memory Mechanisms. A Tribute to G.V. Goddard*, W. Abraham, M. Corballis, and K. White, eds., pp 195–215, 1991, Hillsdale, NJ: Lawrence Erlbaum. Conversations between J.A.O. and H.M. are reprinted from this chapter with kind permission from Lawrence Erlbaum Associates Inc., Publishers, 365 Broadway, Hillsdale, NJ, 07642, USA.

2. For a historical view of the early research on memory, read the special 1968 issue of the journal *Neuropsychologia, vol 6*, no. 3, in which five of the nine articles were devoted to H.M. Some general review articles providing a broader perspective on H.M. include Corkin 1984; Milner, Corkin, and Teuber 1968; and Ogden and Corkin 1991.

Like many other single case studies, research papers on H.M., while systematically exploring the parameters of his memory, usually do not describe in detail the rich qualitative data gathered by the researchers during their extended interactions with H.M. In clinical neuropsychology generally, qualitative observations and anecdotal evidence not only serve to lighten the tedium that often accompanies long sessions of testing in an experimental situation but, more important, may also enrich our under-standing of the neuropsychological functions we are attempting to measure experi-mentally. The same experiment can be repeated time after time without H.M. showing any signs of boredom because each time the experiment is new to him. Repeating the same experiment numerous times would certainly become tedious for H.M.'s experi-menters except for the delightful personality of their subject and the conversations and interactions that occur during the testing session.

At the Clinical Research Center at Massachusetts Institute of Technology (MIT), where H.M. has undergone most of his assessments over the last 30 or more years, he is a great favorite with researchers and clinical staff alike, not because of his now famous initials and the intensively studied amnesia associated with them, but because of his endearing nature, sense of humor, and willingness to be helpful. Perhaps if his personality were less agreeable, fewer researchers would be willing to spend numerous hours with him, and we would know considerably less about his memory and memory functions in general. In this chapter, I try to paint a picture of H.M. as a person; a view that is usually masked in the research literature by the technical descriptions of the experiment that is the focus of the article. In addition, I also hope to illustrate one of the most important aspects of studying a single case: how qualitative as well as quantitative data can contribute to our theoretical knowledge about cognitive, emo-tional, and other neuropsychological processes.

Theoretical Background

Impairments in new learning and memory can occur for verbal material after damage to the medial temporal lobe of the hemisphere dominant for language (usually the left hemisphere) and, to a lesser degree, for nonverbal material after damage to the medial temporal lobe of the other hemisphere. Although either type of memory impairment can cause severe disability, the person can usually continue to live independently, is well aware of the passage of time, and can often use intact memory abilities to com-pensate for those lost. For example, someone with a verbal memory impairment may not be able to recall a new name but will remember the face. Thus, the problems these people experience are in no way as debilitating as the problems faced by one with global amnesia, such as H.M. Global amnesia is global in the sense that it pervades every aspect of the victim's life. It includes an inability to learn new information, whether verbal, nonverbal, visual, or auditory, and it also usually includes a period of memory loss for events and facts that occurred before the brain damage occurred (retrograde amnesia).

Global amnesia usually results from bilateral damage to particular structures on the internal aspects of the cerebral hemispheres. Included are the medial temporal structures and structures surrounding the ventricles, including the thalamus and the mamillary bodies of the hypothalamus. H.M.'s global amnesia was caused by the bilateral removal of the anterior medial temporal structures. Patients who survive herpes simplex encephalitis may also demonstrate global amnesia because this disease can destroy the medial temporal lobe structures bilaterally. Korsakoff's disease, which is caused by a deficiency in thiamine (usually as a result of alcoholism), also results in global amnesia, but in this case it is the mamillothalamic region that is destroyed bilaterally. The amnesia of Korsakoff's disease appears to be qualitatively different from the amnesia suffered by H.M. and survivors of herpes simplex encephalitis. H.M. has a "pure forgetting" problem, and providing cues to assist recall is of no benefit. In Korsakoff's disease cues can aid recall, which suggests that new material can be stored and, under some circumstances, retrieved. Korsakoff's patients have great difficulty using higher-order concepts to organize material to be remembered (e.g., grouping different object names in a memory task by category), and this is likely to be associated with the frontal-lobe atrophy that many alcoholic Korsakoff's patients also display. When they are provided with ways to group memory items for storing them in a logical fashion, a reminder later of those groupings will improve their recall. Unlike H.M., Korsakoff's patients frequently *perseverate* (i.e., repeat actions or words) and *confabulate* (i.e., produce unconsidered, inconsistent, and sometimes exotic explanations, perhaps to fill memory gaps). These behaviors are also seen in people with bilateral damage to the frontal lobes, and in Korsakoff's patients they may be associated with frontal-lobe atrophy rather than with the mamillothalamic lesions. For a clear explanation of the connections between the various anatomical structures that have been implicated in the different amnesic disorders, read Bauer, Grande, and Valenstein (2003).

Case Presentation

Background

Born in 1926, H.M. had a normal, uneventful childhood until he was nine, when he was knocked down by a bicycle and became unconscious for about 5 minutes. He began having absence seizures when he was 10 years old (possibly as a result of his earlier minor head injury). He remembers riding in a car on his 16th birthday when he had his first generalized seizure. He left high school because he was teased by his peers about his seizures, but he returned later to a different high school and graduated at the age of 21, having taken the "practical" course. He enjoyed roller-skating and hunting and even today, in his late 70s, often reminisces about these activities and talks with obvious pleasure about the different guns in his father's gun collection. After he completed high school, he was able to work for a while on an assembly line and as a motor-winder before his seizures became too frequent. He was apparently uninterested in girls and never married or had a girlfriend. H.M.'s apparent disinterest in sexual relationships may be associated with sexual dysfunction caused by antiepileptic therapy, or perhaps it was in part a result of his embarrassment because of his epilepsy. His lack of interest in sexual relationships or conversation about sexual topics has not changed since his operation, and it is possible that the medial temporal resection exacerbated a preexisting hyposexuality.

From the age of 16 until his operation 11 years later, he was having about 10 absence seizures a day and one generalized seizure a week; these seizures could not be controlled by large doses of antiepileptic medications (phenytoin). Electroencephalography (EEG) did not show any localized epileptogenic area but did indicate abnormal diffuse slow activity. During a minor seizure, bilateral generalized EEG abnormalities were recorded, with a predominance in the centrotemporal areas of both hemispheres. At the age of 27, a bilateral medial temporal lobectomy was performed, removing what the surgeon believed was eight centimeters of each of the medial temporal lobes and the amygdalae on both sides; the temporal neocortex was left almost intact. H.M. was awake and talking during the procedure (Corkin 1984; Scoville 1968). As a result of the operation, his generalized seizures were reduced to less than one a year and about five absence seizures a month. He has remained on antiepileptic medication to this day.

Since his operation, H.M. has had a profound anterograde amnesia and a retrograde amnesia for the 11 years preceding his surgery, but his other cognitive functions remain largely unaffected. A magnetic resonance imaging (MRI) brain scan carried out when H.M. was 66 (Corkin, Amaral, Gonzalez, Johnson, and Hyman 1997), shows that the neurosurgeon overestimated the area and amount of medial temporal-lobe tissue that was removed. The resection in fact bilaterally ablated the medial tips of the temporal lobes and extended medially back 5.4 centimeters (cm) on the left and 5.1 cm on the right. Most of the amygdaloid complex, entorhinal cortex, and anterior 2–2.5 cm of dentate gyrus, hippocampus, and subicular complex were removed, leaving approximately the posterior 2 cm of these medial structures intact but shrunken (Fig. 3-1). Outside these temporal regions, the only abnormality is a marked cerebellar atrophy, which has been evident from computed tomography CT scans since H.M. was 58. This atrophy is likely to be a result of long-term phenytoin treatment, as he demonstrated symptoms of toxicity to this drug as early as age 36. His antiepileptic medications were changed to Tegretol when he was 58 years old, and other antiepileptic medications have been added since that time.

After his operation, H.M. lived with his parents. After the death of his father in 1967, he attended a rehabilitation workshop daily for 10 years. He lived with his mother until 1977, and she died in a nursing home in 1981 at the age of 94. H.M. has lived in a nursing home since 1980. When asked where he lives, he often replies that he lives in a house with his mother. He is clearly unsure about whether his parents are still alive. If asked, "Where are your parents?" he replies by giving the name of the town in which they lived. If asked more directly, "Are your parents living?" he replies that he is not sure.

Two or three times each year H.M. spends 1 or 2 weeks living in at the Clinical

Figure 3-1 A magnetic resonance imaging scan (a T2-weighted series of axial images) of H.M.'s brain carried out when he was aged 66 years. Horizontal sections were taken through the brain from the base of the brain, through the cerebellar hemispheres (section A), and upward through the temporal lobes. The nose and eyes would be at the top of the scans. The eyes can be seen in sections E and F. The white signal indicating increased fluid space shows that the neurosurgical resection extensively damaged the anterior medial temporal polar cortex bilaterally (sections C–F). The subcortial white matter associated with the most anterior portions of the superior, middle, and inferior temporal gyri may also have been damaged. Extensive atrophy of the cerebellum is also apparent. (From Corkin, Amaral, Gonzalez, Johnson, and Hyman, 1997. *The Journal of Neuroscience* 17, p. 3970, by permission of *The Journal of Neuroscience*. Copyright 1997 by the Society for Neuroscience.)

Research Center at MIT to have a medical checkup and to participate in memory and other psychological experiments. He seems to enjoy his visits and greets everyone with a smile and readily engages in conversation. When asked whether he would be willing to participate in an experiment, he always agrees immediately and is completely cooperative and pleasant throughout the test session. Over the many years that he has been coming to MIT, he has learned to associate the hospital environment with the institution; when asked where he is, he can accurately reply "Massachusetts Institute of Technology." He always appears pleased to have got this right. He knows he has a memory problem, although it is unlikely that he is aware of its extent or that he has been the subject of a great deal of research.

I spent a considerable amount of time with H.M. around his 60th birthday and did not meet him again until he was 66. In the intervening 6 years, he had gained a little weight and was finding it increasingly difficult to walk, probably as a result of cerebellar atrophy. Otherwise, he seemed exactly the same as before. His facial expressions, the ways he expressed words, the stories he told, and his mannerisms were uncannily identical to those of 6 years previously. My life had moved on, but H.M.'s had not.

Neuropsychological Outcome

General intellectual abilities   On the day before his operation, H.M. was assessed on the Wechsler-Bellevue Scale, and on this test his Verbal IQ was 101 and his Performance IQ was 106. He was not given any memory tests at that time, presumably because there was no reason to believe that his memory would be affected by the operation. Since his operation he has been assessed on the Wechsler Intelligence Scales and the Wechsler Memory Scale six times. He falls in the average range for Verbal IQ and in the average to superior ranges for Performance IQ. His Memory Quotient consistently falls 35 points or more below his Full-scale IQ, and his delayed recall scores on the Logical Memory and Paired Associate (verbal) and Visual Reproduction (nonverbal) tests are always severely depressed.

In 1983, when H.M. was 57, his IQ scores were 10 to 11 points lower than 10 years previously. This lowering of his scores most likely reflects the fact that the older versions of the Wechsler scales on average produce IQ scores that are about 7 IQ points higher than later revisions. Over the years, H.M. has been assessed on all the revisions of the Wechsler Intelligence Scales, and it is to be expected that his IQ score will drop with each new revision, even if his intellectual abilities have not changed.

Memory functions   Memory is complex, and studies of H.M.'s dense amnesia along with studies of other patients with amnesias have resulted in numerous theories about memory functioning. One method used to conceptualize and simplify memory is to categorize the various aspects of memory into dichotomies. Using this approach, it becomes apparent that H.M.'s memory disorder generally fits all of the following dichotomies, the first process being largely spared and the second being severely impaired:

   a. Immediate memory versus long-term memory (new learning)
   b. Remote memory versus anterograde memory
   c. Implicit memory versus explicit memory.

In addition, HM has demonstrated impairments since his operation on both processes of the following dichotomies:

d. Verbal memory versus nonverbal memory

e. Semantic memory versus episodic memory.

The following descriptions of each of these aspects of H.M.'s memory illustrate the richness qualitative information can add to the interpretation of quantitative findings in a single case study.

Immediate versus long-term memory: H.M.'s immediate memory span for digits and block patterns has been borderline normal since 1955 (Corkin 1982), although in recent years his digit span has dropped from six digits to five. Decay of immediate or short-term memory as measured by recognition (Wickelgren 1968) or recall (Corkin 1982) is normal. As soon as H.M.'s span is exceeded by one item, if he is distracted, or if he is unable to rehearse the material verbally, he forgets it (Drachman and Arbit 1966; Milner 1968a; Prisko 1963).

One day H.M. was given five digits to repeat and remember, and then the experimenter was called away. An hour or more later, she returned to H.M.'s room; on seeing her, H.M. accurately repeated the five digits. He had not been distracted and had been rehearsing the numbers the entire time, thus containing them in immediate or working memory. Because time is measured by the memories that are laid down as it passes, H.M. was presumably unaware of the time that had elapsed since the experimenter had left the room.

His long-term memory (new learning) for verbal and for nonverbal material in all modalities is severely impaired. He demonstrates an inability to learn stories, verbal and nonverbal paired associates, block patterns, songs and drawings, new vocabulary words (Gabrieli, Cohen, and Corkin 1988), visual and tactual stylus mazes (Corkin 1965; Milner 1965), digit strings (Drachman and Arbit 1966), object names (Smith and Milner 1981), object locations (Smith 1988), and nonsense syllables and shapes (Penfield and Milner 1958). He also performs poorly on a forced-choice recognition task using faces, houses, words, and tonal sequences.

There is evidence, however, that H.M. has some ability to store and use new information. This evidence comes from experiments using repetition priming; that is, the influence of prior processing of material on later purposeful performance with that material. For example, without being told that he was to be given a memory test, H.M. was shown words such as *DEFINE*; to ensure that he had processed the words, he was asked to decide whether each word had the letter *A* in it. He was later given the stem *DEF* and asked to complete it with the first word that came to mind. He usually responded with the previously experienced word but he was unable to pick out the words he had just seen from a list of words (Keane, Gabrieli, and Corkin 1987). Normal people also demonstrate this priming effect. Similarly, if asked to draw a figure by connecting five dots in a matrix of nine dots and then later asked to draw the first pattern that came to mind using a matrix of nine dots, he responded by drawing the previously drawn figure as often as control subjects (Gabrieli 1986). If shown the patterns among other patterns, however, he could not recognize the ones he drew earlier. He also gets faster at recognizing incomplete line drawings of objects with repeated exposure, although he cannot recognize which drawings he has previously seen (Milner, Corkin, and Teuber 1968).

Remote versus anterograde memory: Milner et al. (1968) reported that H.M.'s retrograde amnesia extended back 2 years before his operation. This estimate came from the neurosurgeon's notes and postoperative interviews with H.M. Since that time, a number of objective tests of remote memory given to H.M. support an 11-year period of retrograde amnesia. These tests use the recall or recognition of famous tunes, public events, and famous scenes taken from the 1920s to the 1960s (Corkin 1984). H.M.'s personal memories are nearly all from the age of 16 years or earlier, also suggesting a loss of memories or inability to retrieve them for an 11-year period before his surgery (Sagar, Cohen, Corkin, and Growdon 1985). It may be that H.M.'s seizures and high doses of antiepileptic medications resulted in an inability to store new memories before his operation, and there may be an increasing loss of remote memories because of impoverished rehearsal of them. H.M. can, however, retrieve some memories from the 11-year period before his surgery, usually via a recognition or cueing procedure rather than via spontaneous recall. For example, if given the first two letters of the name of the surgeon who carried out his operation, whom he knew in the years immediately preceding the operation, he quickly produces the surgeon's complete name. He also occasionally remembers information he must have stored after the operation. For example, he knows that as a result of the surgery he has memory problems and that the operation has not been done on anyone else since.

The remote memories that are intact seem detailed and clear, presumably because to H.M. they are relatively recent memories and have not been subject to interference from new memories. When asked about various actors and singers famous during his childhood, he can often describe them, the films they were in, and who their costars were. He knows the names of the friends he had in second grade, remembers his first major seizure, and relates pleasurable memories of hunting with his father and roller-skating. When asked at the age of 60 about roller-skating, he said he gave it up about 13 years ago. He also relates stories about his parents' families, presumably told to him by his parents when he was young. He talks about his mother's trip to Ireland as a girl to be confirmed into the Catholic church and of an aunt who emigrated to Australia. This latter story was often cued when I told him I came from New Zealand.

Constant retelling of old memories, whether they are factual or not, does not change them significantly for H.M. because, unlike most of us, he is unable to update his memories and recall the slightly changed version. As a result, the many researchers who have assessed H.M. over 30 years can all repeat stories told by H.M. with very similar words and intonations. When H.M. is distracted while telling one of his stories, he can be cued into retelling it a few minutes later and will repeat it using not only the same verbal expressions, but also the same facial expressions and gestures. Occasionally he appears to lose the thread of the story and inserts a different line but then quickly returns to the old story. For example, when asked about his operation, he will usually launch into a story about wanting to be a brain surgeon. The following transcript of a conversation I had with H.M. illustrates these points.

In this particular conversation, the first time he told the story he changed it slightly (indicated by italics). Near the end of the story, he forgot he had just been telling it but cued himself into telling it again, this time using the phrases he normally uses. This conversation also gives some insight into the way H.M. thinks about his own operation and its results.

JAO: Do you know why you are here at MIT?

HM: I wonder at times, but I know one thing. What is learned about me will help other people.

JAO: Yes, it has helped other people.

HM: And that is the important thing. Because at one time that's what I wanted to be, a brain surgeon.

JAO: Really? A brain surgeon?

HM: And I said "no" to myself, before I had any kind of epilepsy.

JAO: Did you? Why is that?

HM: Because I wore glasses. I said, suppose you are making an incision in someone— (pause)—*and you could get blood on your glasses,* or an attendant could be mopping your brow and go too low and move your glasses over. You could make the wrong movement then.

JAO: And then what would happen?

HM: And that person could be dead, or paralyzed.

JAO: So it's a good job you decided not to be a brain surgeon.

HM: Yeah. I thought mostly dead, but could be paralyzed in a way. You could make the incision just right, and then a little deviation, might be a leg or an arm, or maybe an eye too; on one side in fact.

JAO: Do you remember when you had your operation?

HM: No, I don't.

JAO: What do you think happened there?

HM: Well I think I was ah—well, I'm having an argument with myself right away. I'm the third or fourth person who had it, and I think that they, well, possibly didn't make the right movement at the right time, themselves then. But they learned something.

JAO: They did indeed.

HM: That would help other people around the world too.

JAO: They never did it again.

HM: They never did it again because by knowing it—(pause)—and a funny part, I always thought of being a brain surgeon myself.

JAO: Did you?

HM: Yeah. And I said "no" to myself.

JAO: Why was that?

HM: Because I said an attendant might mop your brow and might move your glasses over a little bit, and you would make the wrong movement.

JAO: What would happen if you made the wrong movement?

HM: And that would affect all the other operations you had then.

JAO: Would it? How?

HM: Because if that person was paralyzed on one side, or you made the wrong movement, in a way, and they possibly couldn't hear on one side, or one eye, you would wonder to yourself and that would make you nervous.

JAO: Yes, it would.

HM: Because every time you did you would try and be extra careful and you might be detrimental to that person; to perform that operation right on that time because you'd have that thought and that might slow you up, then, because you were making a movement and you should have continued right on.

JAO: Do you remember who the surgeon was who did your operation?

HM: No, I don't.

JAO: I'll give you a hint. Sc—.

HM: Scoville.

JAO: That's right. You got that fast.

HM: Well, because I couldn't remember fully, but the little hint.

When H.M. was given a test designed to assess his ability to recall or recognize personal events, there was an absence of personal memories after the age of 16 years (Corkin 1984; Sagar et al. 1985). On a test designed to assess the content and temporal context of public events over five decades, H.M. demonstrated normal performance for events from the 1940s but impaired performance for the 1950s to 1980s (Corkin 1984; Corkin, Cohen, and Sagar 1983; Gabrieli et al. 1988). His occasional recall of famous people and events that were publicized after his operation in 1953 is spasmodic at best, and he tends to confuse these memories with other events, or he confuses them in time. In the following conversation, he confuses Elvis Presley's death with the assassinations of President John Kennedy and Robert Kennedy. An Elvis Presley recording was first played on radio in 1954, one year after H.M.'s operation.

JAO: Do you know who Elvis Presley is?

HM: He was a recording star, and he used to sing a lot.

JAO: What sort of things did he sing?

HM: Jive.

JAO: Do you like to jive, or did you like to jive?

HM: No.

JAO: Why not?

HM: I liked to listen, that was all.

JAO: Do you think he is still alive, Elvis Presley?

HM: No, I don't think so.

JAO: Have you any idea what might have happened to him?

HM: Well I believe he got the first bullet I think that was for Kennedy, I think it was.

JAO: You remember Kennedy?

HM: Yes, Robert.

JAO: What was he?

HM: Well, he was the president. I think about three times. He was appointed to president too.

JAO: He got a bullet. What was that all about?

HM: Well, they were trying to assassinate him.

JAO: And did they? Did they kill him or not?

HM: No they didn't.

JAO: So is he still alive?

HM: Yes, he is still alive, but he got out of politics in a way.

JAO: I don't blame him.

HM: No, guess not.
JAO: How long ago was he the president do you think?
HM: He became the President after Roosevelt. 'Course there was Teddy Roosevelt. That
     was a long time before that.
JAO: What is Franklin Roosevelt's wife's name?
HM: I can't think of it.
JAO: It starts with *E* I think—Eleanor. You were going to say that?
HM: No, I wasn't. I was going to say Ethel. (Ethel was Robert Kennedy's wife.)

H.M. spends much of his day watching television and reading the newspapers; therefore, he hears, sees, and reads reports of major news items many times over. It appears that many repetitions of significant events makes it more likely that H.M. will recall them in part, at least over a period of days. Two weeks and massive media coverage after the American space shuttle *Challenger* exploded shortly after it was launched, H.M. replied to my question, "What is a space shuttle?" with the following description: "Well, I think it is a spaceship they shot up and after it is shot up, then it turns itself on. And also there is another part to it that can be sent back. After they've shot off, and shot off the second one, they can return. They use part of it again." Further questions about specific details of the *Challenger* tragedy cued no clear memories, and when he was asked the occupation of the first American civilian, a woman teacher, to go into space, he replied, "I think of working for the Army." This illustrates the dense nature of H.M.'s anterograde amnesia. Although H.M. had some knowledge of the space shuttle program generally, his memory of the *Challenger* explosion specifically was at best fragmented and incomplete despite constant media coverage, which emphasized the tragic death of the civilian teacher.

Although H.M. occasionally demonstrates fragments of recall about events and people that came into the public arena following his operation (e.g., Elvis, the Kennedy brothers, and the space shuttles), the most memorable aspect of his memory impairment remains his dense anterograde amnesia for nearly all episodic information since his operation. He does not recognize anyone he has met or seen since 1953 and cannot even recognize current photographs of himself. He cannot say what he was doing 5 minutes ago; with whom he lives; what day, month, year, or season it is; or his age.

Implicit memory versus explicit memory. This dichotomy perhaps fits H.M.'s memory disorder better than any other. It is purely descriptive and may not apply to all learning and memory phenomena. Explicit memory describes traditional tests of recognition and recall, and implicit memory describes a range of memory abilities that do not require the explicit conscious recollection of previous experiences (Schacter 1987). In 1962 Milner reported that H.M. decreased his error rate and time scores on a mirror-drawing task over 3 days of training. He never recognized the apparatus or that he had done the task before. This achievement could be classified as both motor learning and learning a new procedure. Certainly it could be described as implicit learning without explicit knowledge. Since then, his ability to learn new procedural skills (knowing how to do something) without explicit knowledge that he has performed the task before has been demonstrated many times (Corkin 1968; Mickel et al. 1986; Nissen, Cohen, and Corkin 1981). He improves on mirror reading and reading words presented briefly on a tachistoscope (Nissen et al. 1981), which are both perceptual skills. H.M. has also demonstrated an improvement on the Tower of Hanoi puzzle, a task that involves cognitive skills (Cohen and Corkin 1981).

H.M.'s normal ability to learn how to perform new tasks is evident in his daily routine. For example, at the age of 60 he broke his ankle and was obliged to use a fold-up wheelchair to get around. He learned how to open it and was also able to explain to me how to do so; he also learned the most effective way to position himself to get into it from another chair. Later, when he advanced to a walking frame, he acquired the procedure for dealing with that equipment as well. Although he used the walker with considerable skill, he could not remember why he needed it.

d. Verbal versus nonverbal memory: Since his operation, H.M. has been unable to recall or recognize verbal or nonverbal material presented in the visual, auditory, or tactile modality (Corkin 1965; Drachman and Arbit 1966; Jones 1974; Milner 1965; Scoville and Milner 1957). Since the consequences of his bilateral medial temporal lobectomy became known, many studies involving brain-damaged patients have confirmed that essential processes involved in verbal memory are mediated predominantly by the medial temporal structures of the hemisphere dominant for language (usually the left) (Meyer and Yates 1955; Milner 1966). Some rather less convincing evidence suggests that some aspects of nonverbal memory are mediated by the temporal-lobe structures of the other, nonverbal, hemisphere, usually the right (Milner 1968b). It seems clear that H.M. has both verbal and nonverbal memory impairments because he has lost a significant portion of the medial temporal-lobe structures of both hemispheres.

e. Semantic vs episodic memory: Tulving (1972, 1983) proposed a dissociation between context-free generic knowledge of the world (semantic memory) and autobiographical records of personal experience associated with a particular time and place (*episodic memory*). Within the framework of the implicit/explicit memory dichotomy, semantic and episodic memory can be seen as components of explicit memory and therefore should both be impaired in global amnesias (Cohen 1984; Cermak, Talbot, Chandler, and Wolbarst 1985; Squire 1986; Zola-Morgan, Cohen, and Squire 1983).

An important episode from H.M.'s life illustrates his almost immediate forgetting of personal events. He was staying at MIT at the time of his 60th birthday, and the staff and researchers at the Clinical Research Center organized a birthday party for him. It was a very jolly occasion, and H.M. clearly enjoyed himself. The next day I went to see him, sitting in his room surrounded by birthday cards. "Do you remember anything special happening to you yesterday?" I asked. "No, I can't say that I do," replied H.M. I pointed to all the birthday cards on his table and said, "Look at all these. I wonder what they are here for." H.M. replied, "They are birthday cards, aren't they?" "Oh", I rejoined, "I wonder whose they can be?" "Well," replied H.M. with a twinkle, "they could be mine. Perhaps it was my birthday!" The very next day when I asked H.M. his age, he replied that he was about 34. When I told him he had celebrated his 60th birthday two days before, he commented, "See, I don't remember."

Most formal studies have addressed the episodic components of explicit memory while neglecting the ability of people with amnesia to learn new facts. Studies assessing semantic knowledge have tested explicit knowledge about public events and figures (Cohen and Squire 1980; Marsel-Wilson and Teuber 1975), and such studies have demonstrated that semantic learning is impaired in amnesia.

Gabrieli et al. (1988) argued that these findings may be a result of the recognition or recall procedures used to assess new semantic knowledge. People with amnesia, including H.M., demonstrate preserved learning only when it is assessed without the subject's explicit knowledge, and Gabrieli et al. (1988) devised a way to assess new semantic learning in H.M. using implicit measures of performance. They carried out a series of experiments using uncommon words and words new to the English language since H.M.'s operation in 1953. In one experiment, H.M. and control subjects were taught definitions of eight uncommon English words, and learning was assessed by improved performance over trials with the same words. Subjects were never asked whether they had seen the words before. H.M. was unable to learn the meaning of any word he did not already know.

A second experiment examined the possibility that H.M. would learn new words better if they were presented in a real-life "ecological" rather than laboratory context. He was tested on the recall and recognition of words that had entered a standard English dictionary between 1954 and 1981. All the words were commonly known to high-school students and were interspersed with similar, pronounceable nonwords. H.M. was asked to decide whether each letter string was a word or nonword (a lexical decision task) and to give the meanings of the real words. He demonstrated normal recall of definitions of words entering the English language before 1950, borderline recall for 1950s words, and severely impaired recall for post-1950s words. These results were paralleled on the recognition and word decision tasks. H.M. was also asked to pronounce words and nonwords presented visually in a perceptually difficult condition. A control subject read new words 17 faster than nonwords, but H.M.'s reading of post-1950s words was no faster than his reading of nonwords.

Another experiment examined whether H.M. could recognize names of famous people when they were interspersed among names of nonfamous people. He scored normally on famous names before the 1950s, was mildly impaired on names that became famous during the 1950s, and severely impaired on names that had become famous in the 1960s to 1980s. This series of experiments provides good evidence that H.M. has suffered a markedly impaired ability to encode and store semantic information since his operation. Even so, H.M.'s ability to recall or recognize a famous name or face occasionally demonstrates that he has stored some semantic information since 1953. Because he has the posterior half of the hippocampus remaining bilaterally, this spared tissue may be sufficient to mediate some new memories. Alternatively or in addition, memory circuits that bypass the hippocampus and amygdala may be able to mediate new memories, albeit in a very impoverished way.

Psychological Consequences

H.M.'s personality can best be described as placid, happy, and uncomplaining. As Suzanne Corkin (1984) wrote, "One of H.M.'s most striking characteristics is that he rarely complains about anything. In 1968, his mother stated that "the trouble with H. is that he doesn't complain—ever. There could be something seriously wrong with him, but you would have to guess." (p. 251). To his caregivers, in some ways, looking after H.M. is rather similar to looking after a baby. They have to rely on their observations of his behaviors to assess whether he is feeling unwell, hungry, thirsty, or tired. To work out what H.M. is feeling is not as difficult as with a baby because H.M. will respond to direct questions. If asked, "Where do you have a pain?" however, he usually will not answer with a specific location but must be asked, "Is it in your head? your tooth?" and so on until the right body part is mentioned.

The inability to comment spontaneously on his state seems to extend to H.M.'s tendency not to initiate new topics of conversation. Rather, he responds readily to a conversational stimulus from another person, and from then on the conversation is maintained and changed to different topics by the person talking with him or by H.M. cueing himself into the recitation of a story from his first 16 years of life. Impoverished conversational spontaneity is usually associated with bilateral frontal-lobe damage, but frontal damage is unlikely the cause in the case of H.M., as both neuropathological evidence (CT and MRI scans) and behavioral evidence (his normal ability to perform tests of frontal-lobe function) suggest that his frontal lobes are intact. Rather, H.M.'s amnesia probably makes it impossible for him to prepare mentally and to retain the information and logical structure necessary to allow him to introduce a new topic of conversation.

It is surprising that H.M. does not react with some degree of confusion, frustration, or anger from continually facing the situation of not knowing where he is, what year it is, what new type of technology or development he is looking at, or who the people are who speak to him. It is tempting to think that because he is unaware of what has just happened and unable to think about what is about to happen that he has nothing on which to base feelings of anger or frustration. That is, it seems reasonable to suppose that an ability to remember is a prerequisite for strong emotional reactions. Other cases with amnesia nearly as dense as that suffered by H.M. do not support this hypothesis, however. Clive Wearing, a noted musician and choir master from England, was left globally amnesic as a consequence of herpes simplex encephalitis. Clive was constantly angry, frustrated, and upset by his experience of living minute by minute in a world he could not remember, and he frequently exclaimed, "I have been dead. I have just woken up this minute" (Wilson and Wearing 1995).

In the case of H.M., it may be that the removal of his amygdalae from both hemispheres resulted in a severe dampening of his emotions, as it is well established in the animal literature that the amygdala is associated with control of the expression of aggression. His many years of antiepileptic medication may also have lowered his threshold for emotional arousal. Alternatively, perhaps he is just a contented and happy person by nature, and his personality has little to do with his epilepsy per se or his brain surgery and drug regimen. His father was apparently very similar to H.M.: good humored and placid.

On rare occasions, H.M. has become briefly annoyed when provoked. He would sometimes become angry when his mother "nagged" him when he lived with her and apparently kicked her in the shin and hit her with his glasses on occasion (Corkin 1984). He sometimes looks and sounds sad when he is retold that his father is dead. I was interested to see whether H.M.'s ability to express and recognize emotional facial and voice expression was normal and attempted to test this experimentally. I recorded my own voice and the voices of a man and child saying "I am going to the movies" in happy, sad, surprised, angry, tearful, and disinterested voices and played each one to H.M. and asked him to judge the emotion in the voice. On all but the angry voice H.M.'s accuracy (75%–100% correct) was as good as same-age control subjects and another globally amnesic subject. He reported the angry voice as sounding surprised, doubly surprised, happy, tearfully happy, or tearful, but never angry, annoyed, or mad. I then asked H.M. to repeat the sentence after me, imitating my voice tones, and later asked him to say the sentence expressing each voice tone I named. He did both tasks reasonably well, including those sentences with angry tones.

I also assessed his ability to interpret facial expressions. I made my face look sad, happy, and so on, and he first named each of my expressions, then copied them, and finally made each facial expression on my command. He found these tasks difficult, primarily because he could not stop smiling. For example, when asked to look angry, he would try by turning his mouth down at the corners, and then he would break into a smile. This experiment was repeated five times over 3 weeks, and H.M.'s performance was quite consistent across all trials. His particular difficulty with interpreting angry expressions and acting out anger is interesting and may be related to the removal of his amygdalae. Alternatively, anger may simply be an emotion so foreign to H.M. that he has difficulty recognizing it in others or pretending to express it.

It has often been said that memory equates with consciousness or even "soul." In spite of the fact that H.M. lives minute by minute with no conscious knowledge of his past beyond his childhood years or what his future will bring, everyone who meets H.M. is impressed by his endearing nature, his appropriate interactions, his sense of humor, and his intelligent problem-solving skills. They are invariably left with no doubt that he is conscious of himself as a whole person and has the full complement of "soul."

Personal and Social Consequences

H.M.'s most obvious personal loss stems directly from his amnesia; that is, with the loss of his memory, he has lost his independence. He appears rather negligent about his self-care and requires supervision to ensure that he washes, shaves, dresses, changes his clothes, and eats. This, of course, may not be negligence but simply a consequence of his amnesia. Without a sense of time of day, it must be difficult to know when to wash and so on, and of course H.M. cannot remember when he last washed. Perhaps, if left to his own devices for a long time, he would shave when his beard became obvious to him, change his clothes when they became obviously dirty, and ask for food when he became hungry. To test this would, of course, be unethical.

More significantly, since the onset of his amnesia, he has not been able to go anywhere unaccompanied and often requires assistance when making important decisions that affect his own life, although he has been judged by a psychiatrist to be qualified to give informed consent for testing. As the world continues to change, H.M.'s knowledge of how to live in it becomes increasingly outdated. Even if he were still physically fit at age 78 years, the world of 2004 is very different from the world of 1942, the year that marks the beginning of H.M.'s retrograde amnesia. It is thus hardly surprising that he needs assistance to make some decisions.

H.M. spends his days doing crossword puzzles (which can have the answers erased so he can do them again), watching television, and reading the newspaper. He is compliant with his caregivers and anyone else who asks him to do anything. He gets up and goes to bed when he is told, eats when he is told, and happily puts away his crossword to be taken to the laboratory for an experimental session. He will go anywhere with anyone, and if he is asked to sit in a particular chair he will sit there all day without moving or complaining, if not told otherwise. Clearly, if he were in the community or not cared for sensitively within the nursing home and at MIT, he could be easily exploited. His identity is therefore very closely guarded, and the scientists who are given approval to carry out experiments with him are kept to a minimum and are closely monitored.

H.M. greets everyone with warmth, and people who are meeting him for the first time as well as those who have spent years with him share an uncanny feeling that he recognizes them and is greeting them like an old friend. Yet when asked the question, "Do you think you have seen me before?" H.M. always replies, "No, I can't say that I have," or sometimes "Well, I don't remember, but as soon as you asked me that I had an argument with myself. I think I might have met you before." H.M. is famous throughout the psychological and neurological world: Most first-year psychology undergraduates have heard about him and answered examination questions about him, numerous people have felt honored to be introduced to him, and a smaller group of people who have cared for him or worked with him, including me, have come to think of H.M. as a dear friend. The poignancy in this is that H.M. is unaware of any of us as soon as our conversation with him ends.

Discussion

The many studies carried out with H.M. continue to confirm the importance of the medial temporal lobes (particularly the hippocampus and adjacent cortical structures) for the encoding and storage of new explicit information, whether it is episodic or semantic. Studies of H.M.'s memory abilities have also shown that with the exception of lexical decision tasks, most tasks requiring implicit learning do not require the amygdalae and anterior hippocampus, whether the learning assesses motor, perceptual, or cognitive skills.

H.M.'s impoverished retrieval of explicit information presumably encoded and stored in the 11 years immediately preceding his operation cannot be so clearly related to the removal of the medial temporal-lobe structures. There is some evidence that semantic information presented immediately before his operation is better recalled than episodic events that occurred during the same time span. For example, H.M.'s personal (episodic) memories are drawn almost entirely from the period when he was less than 17 years old (Sagar et al. 1985), but he demonstrates only moderately impaired recall for definitions of English words (semantic information) that entered the dictionary in the 1950s yet severely impaired recall for 1960s and later words (Gabrieli et al. 1988). Possibly semantic information encoded and stored in the years immediately preceding his operation remains more salient than episodic information stored during the same period because semantic facts (e.g., 1950s words) continue to be presented in H.M.'s day-to-day environment, whereas rehearsal of his personal memories relies primarily on his own initiative and the reminders of others who are aware of the specific episodes. His good recall of episodes before the age of 17 may be in part a consequence of his frequent rehearsal of these childhood memories with his parents and other relatives when they were alive. The most parsimonious explanation for H.M.'s 11 years of somewhat patchy retrograde amnesia may be that his encoding and storage of new information were impoverished but not totally absent as a result of the ongoing seizure activity he suffered during that period. In support of this view, his first generalized seizure occurred on his sixteenth birthday. The weak memory traces laid down in the 11-year period before H.M.'s operation fade if H.M. is not frequently reminded of them and are therefore less likely to be recalled or recognized. Thus, world facts from the 1940s and 1950s that are still commonly used will be better recalled than personal episodes from that period.

For more than 50 years, H.M. has put enormous effort and time into memory research, and the fact that he has no conscious memory of this work does not in any way detract from the debt we owe him. Researchers are still gathering new information about memory processes from him, although as illustrated by the following story, good research practice can sometimes be overlooked in the excitement of the moment.

At 9:30 a.m. on the 14th February, 1986, I went to collect H.M. from his room. He was eating a large chocolate heart that had been given to him by the staff to celebrate St. Valentine's Day. He finished the heart, crumpled up the shiny red paper it had been wrapped in, and put it in his shirt pocket. He then came with me to the testing room, and for the next 2 hours we concentrated on mentally rotating letters and other tasks. At about 11:30 a.m., H.M. put his hand into his shirt pocket to get out his handkerchief and pulled out the shiny red paper at the same time. He held it at arms length and looked at it quizzically, so I asked him why he had the paper in his pocket. "Well," replied H.M., "It could have been wrapped around a big chocolate heart. It must be St. Valentine's Day!" I tried to contain my excitement over this evidence of recall of a personal episode that had occurred 2 hours earlier, and I told

H.M. to replace the red paper in his pocket. I then took him to the lunchroom and went to tell my story to John Gabrieli, an experienced tester of H.M. John said that H.M., being a true American, had been eating large chocolate hearts wrapped in red shiny paper every St. Valentine's Day since he was a year old. This was just a well-learned old association and certainly not evidence of new learning. I insisted that this was not so and took John to the lunchroom, where I asked H.M. to look in his shirt pocket. He pulled out the red, shiny paper, held it at arms length, and looked at it quizzically. I asked him why he had the paper in his pocket, and he replied "Well, it might have been wrapped around a big chocolate rabbit. It must be Easter!"

4
■

Out of Control
The Consequences and Treatment of Epilepsy

One day, while shopping for a present for relatives overseas, I saw displayed in a jeweler's shop a group of intricately carved greenstone pendants. My disappointment on finding that the price of a pendant was too high for my pocket quickly turned to pleasure when I discovered the carver's name. Only a few years earlier I had watched this man struggling to cope with epilepsy, for him a most disabling neurological disorder. Rangi's beautiful pendants were a remarkable personal achievement, attributable not only to his skill as a carver, but also to his courage and determination. As will become apparent when Rangi's story is told, his pendants could also be regarded as an indirect result of current neurological and neurosurgical research, technology, and practice in the treatment of epilepsy.

Epilepsy is an umbrella term for a range of central nervous system disorders that include seizures as a symptom. The exact nature of the neural mechanisms triggering seizures is not known, and researchers interested in the causes of seizures are continually exploring new hypotheses and refining old ones. In simple terms, *brain functioning* can be conceived of as the outcome of electrochemical impulses that travel along neural pathways and that are directed and coordinated by a complex process in which some neurons are excited by an impulse and others are inhibited by it. In some persons, the balance between excitatory and inhibitory neurons is disrupted; as a result, more and more neurons become excited but are not counteracted by inhibitory activity. At some point the seizure threshold is reached, and the storm of electrical activity in the brain results in a seizure. This usually (but not always) causes some transient alteration in consciousness, accompanied by motor, sensory, cognitive, or emotional changes.

Because seizures can be idiopathic (i.e., with no obvious cause) or can occur as a result of many types of brain damage, as a group they have a high incidence. A conservative figure is that 5 people in 1000 will suffer from epilepsy (e.g., a seizure condition rather than an isolated seizure), and about 5 will have a seizure of some sort in their lifetime (Neugebauer and Susser 1979).

Seizures can be debilitating or embarrassing and, in some cases, may indicate or cause brain damage or dysfunction that can result in cognitive and personality disorders or impairments. Thus, almost everyone who suffers from epilepsy seeks a cure. For some a cure occurs spontaneously, but for most the best they can hope for is good control via medication that does not otherwise significantly interfere with their lives. Unfortunately, the antiepileptic medication that is the treatment of choice for most people with epilepsy can itself result in lowered or slowed cognitive function. A small number of sufferers have frequent seizures that cannot be controlled by medication but that can be controlled or even completely cured by surgery that removes the focus of the seizures in the brain.

Theoretical Background

Definitions and Neuropathology

Idiopathic seizures may occur because of an inherited mechanism that leads to a lowered seizure threshold, or in some cases, the causal brain lesion may simply be inaccessible to current technology (e.g., too small to be seen on computed tomography [CT] or magnetic resonance imaging [MRI] scans). *Symptomatic seizures* refer to those for which a cause has been identified: a stroke, head injury, tumor, infection, scar tissue following a penetrating head injury or surgery to the brain, or any other damage to the brain.

Partial seizures begin at a focal point in the brain and can be simple or complex. In *simple partial seizures* there is generally no change in level of consciousness, and the person will experience motor movements (called *Jacksonian seizures*) or sensory sensations (called *sensory seizures*) depending on the focus of the seizure. *Complex partial seizures* (also called *psychomotor* or *temporal lobe seizures*) include interference to higher-level cerebral functioning and a disturbance of consciousness. The victim may experience an "aura" preceding the seizure (e.g., an unpleasant smell, a feeling of fear, a visual hallucination) and during the seizure may perform purposeless movements such as lip smacking or picking at clothing. They may experience hallucinations or perceptual distortions, alterations of mood, or obsessional thinking. Complex partial seizures usually arise in the temporal lobe, in particular in the hippocampus underlying the temporal lobe.

Generalized seizures are caused by bilateral electrical activity that is usually symmetrical from the outset but that in some cases can develop following a partial seizure. There is always a loss of consciousness. Included are generalized tonic-clonic seizures, absence attacks, complex absences, and myoclonic and akinetic seizures. In *generalized tonic-clonic seizures* (sometimes called *grand mal seizures*) the victim often cries out and is overtaken by tonic muscular contractions in which the limbs are rigidly extended for about a minute, followed by a clonic phase in which the muscles stiffen and relax, causing the limbs to jerk rapidly at first, and then more slowly. During the convulsions, which usually last 2–5 minutes, breathing stops or becomes shallow, the victim froths at the mouth, and there may be a loss of bladder or bowel control. The victim is not able to be aroused for a short time and, on regaining consciousness, is usually confused with no memory of the seizure. Generalized tonic-clonic seizures are often followed by a period of deep sleep, and the sufferer may later suffer from nausea, headache, and vomiting. *Absence seizures* (or *petit mal seizures*) involve a sudden transient lapse of consciousness, often barely perceptible to an observer. Absence seizures tend to be restricted to the childhood years, and if frequent they can result in significant learning difficulties at school. *Complex absences* also include movements such as chewing or lip smacking and tend to be of longer duration than *simple absences*. *Akinetic seizures* (or *drop attacks*) involve a sudden loss of postural tone so that the person slumps or falls to the floor. *Myoclonic seizures* result in jerking movements for a very brief period.

Medication to Reduce Seizures

Drug therapy is the most common form of treatment for epilepsy, and the seizures of many persons are completely or almost completely controlled as a result of taking the right drug at the correct dosage level for them. Successfully medicating people with epilepsy is not always a simple task, however. First, the types of seizures the individual has must be carefully assessed so that the correct medication for that type of seizure can be prescribed. The amount of antiepileptic drug in the bloodstream must be carefully monitored to ensure that the level is high enough to prevent seizures but not so high that side effects of drowsiness or even toxicity occur. Whereas some people seem to require more than one type of antiepileptic drug, experts recommend that one drug only (*monotherapy*) should be used if possible. Systematic studies of the effects of antiepileptics on cognition are beginning to emerge, but the conclusions across studies about specific drugs are not always consistent. Nevertheless, enough evidence has now accumulated to state with some certainty that many of the existing antiepileptics have some adverse effects on cognition, although these side effects may be relatively mild when used in monotherapy. New antiepileptic drugs with fewer side effects are continually being researched and released onto the market.

Occupation and life stage can also influence the drug regimen, and subtle side effects of the drugs should be monitored in the context of the person's lifestyle. For example, a slight lowering of alertness may not be a major problem for a person who is retired or in an undemanding job, but it may be a major problem to someone whose job requires quick reaction times or long hours of concentration or study. Some drugs are considered inadvisable or too dangerous to be taken in the early stages of pregnancy; thus, the doctor must be alert to the possibility that a woman may conceive, either by design or accident. Many side effects of the drugs are idiosyncratic; that is, one person may find a drug highly satisfactory, but another may have many debilitating side effects from the same drug. Individual sensitivity to side effects may also vary across time. Finally, the issue of compliance is important in that erratically taken drugs may result in a higher level of seizure activity or drug toxicity.

Surgical Management of Epilepsy

In cases in which a brain lesion (e.g., scar tissue, a benign tumor) is clearly the focus of the seizure for people with partial seizures, the lesion can often be removed with a good chance of reducing or curing the seizures. In the common situation where seizures clearly arise from one circumscribed area only (usually the temporal lobe and underlying hippocampus or the frontal lobe) and the epilepsy is *idiopathic* (i.e., no evidence of an underlying lesion or structural abnormality), surgery to remove (or *resect*) the brain tissue where the focus lies can be highly successful in curing or reducing the seizures. Candidates for surgery are carefully assessed to ascertain their suitability for this rather drastic procedure, and only people whose seizures cannot be satisfactorily controlled by medication or who suffer severe side effects from anti-epileptic drugs are considered (Milner 1975).

Before surgery, extensive electroencephalographic (EEG) studies are carried out to pinpoint the location of the focus and to ensure there are no epileptic foci in other areas of the brain. Also, MRI is often used to determine whether there are subtle changes in the brain tissue that may be associated with the epilepsy. For example, the MRI scan can be used to measure the volume of both hippocampi and may demonstrate that the hippocampus on the side of the epileptic focus is smaller than the hippocampus of the other hemisphere.

Neuropsychological tests are carried out to determine which hemisphere is dominant for language and to make sure that any cognitive impairments the person has are consistent with the area from which the epileptic discharge emanates. For people with complex partial seizures originating in a temporal lobe, memory and language functions are of particular importance. A person who has both verbal and visual memory impairments may have dysfunction of both temporal lobes, not only of the lobe where the epileptic focus lies, meaning that if an extensive temporal lobe and hippocampal removal is performed on the epileptic side, this patient may be left with one dysfunctional temporal lobe and, as a result, sustain severe memory deficits. The case of H.M. (Chapter 3), who became amnesic after he had both hippocampi removed to cure his epilepsy, alerted neurosurgeons and neuropsychologists to the dangers of removing one temporal lobe without first ensuring the integrity of the other (Penfield and Milner 1958).

As a more direct check, the patient may undergo a special procedure called the Wada test, named for the man who developed it (Jones-Gotman 1987; Wada and Rasmussen 1960). In this test a drug, sodium amytal, is injected into the internal carotid artery of one hemisphere of the brain while the patient is awake. This anesthetizes that hemisphere for about 5 minutes, causing the patient to become paralyzed on the opposite side of the body. Before the sodium amytal is injected, the neuropsychologist gives the patient a number of baseline tests of speech, object naming, and memory. While the hemisphere is anesthetized, the neuropsychologist tests the other, awake hemisphere to assess how well it copes with speech, naming, and memory.

The specific tests and details of the Wada procedure vary from center to center, but a description of the Montreal Neurological Institute technique will provide a general overview of the types of tests given and how the results are used to provide the neurosurgeon with important information. The memory tests are considered particularly important, and the patient is usually shown five simple items to remember that use both verbal and visual memory (two pictures of objects, a real object, a sentence, and a word). When the anesthetic wears off, the patient is asked to recall or recognize among a number of distractor items the five items shown when only one hemisphere was awake. If most of these items cannot be remembered, the temporal lobe and hippocampus that remained awake cannot mediate memory. If this is the temporal lobe that has the epileptic focus and is going to be removed, then this does not pose a problem, as this lobe was already known to be dysfunctional. However, if the awake hemisphere was not the one with the epileptic focus, removing the other epileptic temporal lobe and its underlying hippocampus may result in amnesia. The neurosurgeon may then decide the operation cannot go ahead or, more commonly, will excise a much smaller section of the temporal lobe and leave the hippocampus intact. These less extensive operations are less likely to cure the epilepsy, but there is some chance that the seizure frequency will be reduced, and when the hippocampus is left intact, memory functions do not seem to worsen significantly.

In some cases functional MRI (fMRI) studies will provide useful information, and where this technology is readily available it is increasingly taking the place of the much more invasive and less reliable Wada test. Studies using fMRI can be used to directly visualize the origin of the seizures (Archer, Briellmann, Abbott, Syngeniotis, and Jackson 2001; Jackson, Connelly, Cross, Gordan, and Gadian 1994) or to detect blood flow changes in the brain associated with cognitive, sensory, or motor activity (Binder et al. 1996; Wood, Saling, Abbott, and Jackson 2001). Sometimes the seizure focus is very close to the motor or sensory strip, and in such a case fMRI can allow the motor or sensory cortex to be mapped so that the surgeon knows which parts of the cortex can safely be removed without causing a paralysis or a loss of sensation in a body part that would be more disabling than the seizures the surgery was designed to cure. The lateralization of language can readily be assessed very safely and reliably using fMRI (Binder et al. 1996). An example might be a person who is strongly left-handed and who comes from a family of left-handers. If the epileptic focus is located in the temporal lobe of the left hemisphere, but the fMRI studies show that the right hemisphere is the active one during speech tasks, then resecting a part of the left temporal lobe will be less risky, and the surgeon might decide to resect a larger area.

Major neurosurgery may appear to be a rather extreme measure for a healthy person to contemplate simply because of focal seizures, but for people who suffer from frequent debilitating seizures despite trying various antiepileptic drugs, the chance of a permanent cure of their epilepsy makes even such nonreversible measures worthwhile. In fact, the Wada procedure and temporal lobectomy do not carry a significant risk, and it is uncommon for patients to suffer significant long-term problems as a result of these procedures. For some, the chance to have this operation becomes the most important aspect of their lives, and when the operation is successful (as in the vast majority of cases), many view it almost as a miracle. With ever-improving and safer assessment techniques (e.g., fMRI), along with more accurate and safer microsurgical techniques, surgical intervention for epilepsy is becoming more attractive. As research studies find out more about possible long-term negative as well as positive outcomes from surgery and weigh these outcomes against the negatives and positives of drug therapy for focal seizures, it may well be that in the future, surgery becomes the best option even for those people for whom drug therapy works reasonably well. A lifetime on drugs may come to be viewed as more expensive and result in more medical, psychological, and cognitive problems than a one-off surgical resection on an area of cortex that is assessed as functionally not essential for the patient.

Psychological Methods to Reduce Seizures

Psychoeducation about epilepsy and antiepileptics is a first step in assisting an individual who wishes to cope better with his seizures and usually improves compliance with medication regimens; knowledge usually reduces the anxiety and stress of having epilepsy. In turn, the seizure frequency or severity in some cases may decrease. Education about self-care strategies may also reduce seizure frequency. Simple guidelines, such as limiting or avoiding caffeine, nonprescription drugs, excessive stress and fatigue, hydration, hypoglycemia, and extreme temperatures may be helpful for some people.

Behavioral modification and cognitive–behavioral programs have been tried with some success in selected cases. Such programs require a careful assessment of the context in which the seizures occur to determine whether any patterns emerge regarding the antecedents of seizures and the events (consequences) that follow seizures (Parsonson and Smith 1986). For example, if seizures are frequently preceded by a stressful event, a program might be set up to assist the patient in reducing the stressful events in her life, either by changing her circumstances (e.g., changing to a less stressful job or leaving a stressful relationship) or learning more effective ways to reduce the emotional effects of the stressful event (e.g., by learning relaxation methods or exploring psychological and cognitive ways to combat stress, worry, and anxiety).

If careful assessment shows that having a seizure may in some way be rewarding (e.g., increased attention and concern expressed by parents or a reason not to go to work or school for a day or two), a program could be set up to remove these consequences and provide the same rewards at other times so that they are clearly not associated with having seizures. For example, the parents could be instructed to do only what is necessary for the safety and comfort of their child following a seizure, but no more, and to give the child increased attention and concern at other times, either unrelated to any specific behaviors or related to behaviors they would like the child to increase (e.g., attention to the good things about the child's schooling and concern about areas of unhappiness with the purpose of working out ways with the child to overcome these problems).

In selected cases, biofeedback training has been used with some success to change or augment EEG patterns, based on the idea that epileptiform discharges are incompatible with certain frequency bands in the EEG (Kogeorges and Scoot 1981). A confounding factor is that the biofeedback situation is conducive to relaxation, and it may be this relaxation that is instrumental in the seizure reduction. Indeed, training the client to relax when cued by the earliest sign of a seizure onset is sometimes effective in controlling seizures (Wells, Turner, Bellack, and Hersen 1978).

There are, of course, many sufferers of seizures who have little or no specific control over them and whose pattern of seizures makes no sense in terms of consistent antecedents or consequences. Even in these cases, it may be worth looking in detail at common sense self-care strategies (e.g., a sensible program of sleep, exercise, relaxation, and food and beverage intake) to ensure the sufferers are minimizing factors possibly associated with seizure activity.

Neuropsychological Aspects of Epilepsy

Neuropsychological impairments in people with epilepsy may be a result of the brain dysfunction or lesion that also causes the epilepsy, a result of the epileptic activity or brain damage caused by the epileptiform activity itself, or a result of antiepileptic medication. Indeed, all of these organic factors may contribute to neuropsychological impairment, and it may be difficult, if not impossible, to tease apart the relative effects of each variable. In addition, other psychosocial factors related to the seizure disorder may cause or exacerbate neuropsychological impairment. For example, children with epilepsy may have poor school attendance and, even when they are in class, may have poor concentration as a result of subclinical epileptiform activity or because of poorly controlled seizure activity. Some children who suffer frequent absence seizures may not be diagnosed correctly and may be viewed as children with a poor attention span. Worry, stress, anxiety, embarrassment, low levels of confidence and self-esteem, and depression are all understandable emotional consequences of epilepsy, and all of these feelings can impact cognitive efficiency.

Extreme care must therefore be taken when hypothesizing about the causes of poor performances at school, at work, and on neuropsychological tests. In some cases, cause and effect are a little clearer than in other cases. For example, a person who suffers focal seizures might be expected to have cognitive deficits congruent with dysfunction or damage to the specific area of the brain where the seizures begin but to have none of the significant deficits usually associated with damage to other areas of the brain. Thus, a person with complex partial seizures that on EEG clearly begin in the left temporal lobe might well have impairments on tests of new verbal learning but is less likely to have impairments on tests of new nonverbal, visuospatial learning. If, however, that same person demonstrates a general slowing of responses across a range of verbal, visual, and psychomotor tests, it is often impossible to say whether this slowing is from the epileptiform activity, the antiepileptic drugs, or anxiety and depression.

Without losing sight of the complexity of assessing neuropsychological performance in people with epilepsy, many studies have demonstrated that certain patterns of deficit are more commonly associated with particular types of epilepsy than with other types. Overall, it has been shown that many of the subtests that make up an IQ battery such as the Wechsler Intelligence Scales are not sensitive to the subtle impairments found in some people with epilepsy. As a consequence, various test batteries have been devised that include tests sensitive to the deficits most frequently associated with epilepsy and with the use of antiepileptic drugs (e.g., Dodrill 1982). Such batteries include measures of attention, manual speed, speed and accuracy of perceptual registration, new verbal and visual learning and memory, aphasia screening tests, and tests of frontal-lobe functions such as changing mental set and decision making. Loiseau et al. (1980) assessed the memory skills of 100 people with epilepsy and 100 controls matched for age, sex, social status, and education; the epilepsy group showed impairments in remembering lists of words and geometric patterns.

Some researchers have suggested that attention deficits are more common in people with generalized seizures than in those with focal seizures, and there has been some experimental evidence for this in both adults (Kimura 1964; Mirsky, Primac, Marsan, Rosvold, and Stevens 1960) and children (Fedio and Mirsky 1969). Perceptuomotor impairments, often seen as clumsiness, have also been found to be more common in children with various forms of epilepsy than in groups of control children (Schwarz and Dennerll 1970). Speed of mental processing and reaction and response times can affect a wide range of abilities, and people with epilepsy are impaired compared with controls (Bruhn and Parsons 1977). Poor mathematical skills (Green and Hartlage 1971) and reading difficulties (Long and Moore 1979) have been found in significant numbers of children with epilepsy compared with nonepileptic children of the same age. This finding holds true even when the epileptic students are at an appropriate academic level in other areas of schooling.

Group studies such as this, however, tell us very little that is meaningful about the individual patient with epilepsy. The most useful studies have been those that have studied the deficits associated with epilepsy arising from a particular focus. Temporal lobe epilepsy has attracted more neuropsychological study than other forms of epilepsy. Most studies have concentrated on people who are candidates for a temporal lobectomy to cure or reduce their complex partial seizures. It has been consistently found that people whose seizures arise in the temporal lobe or hippocampus of the hemisphere dominant for language (usually the left) tend to demonstrate impaired functioning on tests of new verbal learning and memory, but relatively normal functioning on tests of visual, nonverbal memory. Although not as marked, the reverse pattern is not uncommon for people with seizures beginning in the nondominant temporal lobe. These patterns of results are clearer postoperatively (Milner 1954, 1975), which is hardly surprising given that 6–8 cm of the temporal lobe and the underlying hippocampus is removed on one side. A few studies have demonstrated the same pattern in people with temporal lobe epilepsy who have not had surgery (Delaney, Rosen, Mattson, and Novelly 1980; Dennerll 1964).

Psychosocial Consequences of Seizures and Neurosurgery

Many people with debilitating epilepsy experience understandable psychological consequences of their epilepsy (Rosenbaum and Palmon 1984). For some, the embarrassment that accompanies having a major seizure in a public place is one of the most
devastating consequences of this group of disorders. The fear of being out of control,
a fear of dying during a seizure, and a belief that the seizures either indicate brain
damage or cause brain damage are also common and understandable consequences of
epilepsy, especially if education about seizures in general and that individual's seizure
disorder in particular is lacking.

The level of understanding about seizures has certainly improved over the years,
at least to the extent that most people in Western societies no longer believe that a
person who has a seizure is controlled by demons, is crazy, or is necessarily brain
damaged. Nevertheless, many people are still frightened when they observe someone
actually having a grand mal seizure, and many employers still feel reluctant to hire
someone with epilepsy, even if the epilepsy is well controlled and the job is safe for
a person with epilepsy (e.g., does not involve dangerous machinery or driving the
public). Epilepsy still carries with it a heavy burden of social stigma (Schneider and
Conrad 1980), although some studies have shown that the perceptions of the epilepsy
sufferer about the social stigma attached to epilepsy are unrealistically high. That is,
some people with epilepsy believe others will see them as brain damaged or less
employable, when in fact they find little or no basis for this belief when they look
carefully at their lives. Findings like these clearly have implications for psychological
interventions aimed at assisting people with epilepsy to "examine their real-life experiences" as a step toward increasing their self-confidence and self-esteem.

With surgical interventions for focal epilepsy becoming more common it has become apparent that not everyone who has a successful outcome, whether a partial or
a complete cure of their seizures, lives happily ever after. For many people who have
had epilepsy for most of their lives, a major adjustment is called for when they find
themselves seizure-free. An obvious example is that of driving. Before their surgery
they may not have been able to drive, which in turn may have curtailed various social
activities as well as occupational choices. If following surgery they remain seizure-
free for 1–2 years, they will need to make the decision about whether to take up
driving and all that means. No longer will their inability to drive or their seizures act
as a convenient excuse not to go to a party, if they have always found social interaction
with strangers stressful. Family members who may have structured many of their
activities around the constraints of their relative's epilepsy may also have to readjust
their lives and their ways of thinking about their relative. This may be enormously
positive and liberating for many families, but for others it can be quite threatening.

Sarah Wilson and her colleagues from Melbourne have called the negative psychosocial consequences of successful epilepsy surgery the "burden of normality" (Wilson, Bladin, and Saling 2001), and their studies have resulted in a number of important
recommendations. Before deciding whether an individual is an appropriate surgical

candidate, psychosocial assessments that tap into those aspects of personality and family systems that are associated with good or poor ability to adjust to a new seizure- and sickness-free life should be added to the more traditional neuropsychological and seizure-focus assessments. In addition, it is of utmost importance to prepare prospective surgical candidates carefully for all the possible outcomes of surgery. For some people, only a complete cure will satisfy them, and disappointment and even depression may follow if seizures, even at a much reduced frequency, continue. Others may be delighted by a partial reduction of seizures such that medication can now control them satisfactorily.

Of course, few patients believe that becoming seizure-free might also cause problems and result in psychological distress, but they need to be alerted to this possibility as well. Knowing about the many possible reactions to the loss of seizures "normalizes" those reactions and makes it more likely that an affected individual (or a family member) will be aware of what is happening and seek help. Surgical programs for epilepsy treatment thus need to ensure that long-term medical, cognitive, and psychological follow-up is in place for all their patients, whatever the outcome of the surgery on their epilepsy.

Psychological Interventions and Therapies

Therapy can be helpful both for people who might benefit from strategies to cope with their epilepsy and its consequences, and for those who are readjusting to a seizure-free life following successful surgery. There are as many ways to do this as there are psychological therapies, and different approaches will be helpful for different people. Straightforward cognitive therapy techniques (Beck, Emery, and Greenberg 1985; Kendall and Hollon 1979, 1981; Scott, Williams, and Beck 1989), such as replacing internalized self-deprecating statements with positive statements, learning how to be assertive when attending job interviews, and practicing ways to tell others about the epilepsy so that they will understand realistically how it does and does not affect the sufferer, will be the most useful and least threatening techniques for some people. Individuals who become depressed or anxious may also benefit from cognitive therapy. Others may gain more from a systemic or solution-focused style of therapy (Lipchik 1988; Lipchik and de Shazer 1986; White 1986), in which situations in the past and present when the client coped and felt confident are rediscovered, called *unique outcomes* by White (1986). The client decides whether she wants to pursue this alternative "coping and confident" life story or script or stay with the "unconfident, epileptic" script she currently perceives as guiding her behaviors and feelings.

Yet another group of therapies employs psychodynamic techniques to assist clients to understand and express their emotions and make connections between the ways they feel now and how they felt in earlier stages of their lives. For example, psychodynamic techniques may help an adult who perceives himself as a "useless epileptic" to reexperience the devastating feelings of rejection and isolation he felt as a small boy when his peers taunted him about his epilepsy, and when he was forbidden by his parents to play football or swim with his friends in case these activities "brought on a fit." He can be helped to make connections between those understandable feelings from childhood and the feelings of "uselessness" and "not belonging" he still experiences as an adult. An exploration of his adult life shows him that his epilepsy is well controlled, he is successful at his job, and he has many good friends. He may now be able to empathize with the small boy he once was, put behind him the distressing emotions he experienced then but that no longer serve any useful purpose, and move on to a happier, more confident state.

Combinations of various psychological techniques can also be used to advantage with the same client. This eclectic approach to therapy is becoming increasingly acceptable as evidence accumulates that no particular therapeutic method is consistently more effective than any other. What is more important is that the therapist is empathetic toward the client and skilled in the therapies used and that the client has confidence in the therapist and is comfortable with the therapy technique (which does not imply that she will be comfortable while participating in the therapy process). It is also important that the client at all times has control over what she will participate in and has clear strategies she can put into practice to enable her to terminate at will and without penalty any therapeutic process or situation.

Finally, encouraging people with seizures and their families to establish or become involved in support groups for people with epilepsy is often beneficial. In the early stages, the sufferer and her family can receive emotional and practical support and education about epilepsy and can be relieved of the common belief that they are the only one suffering in a particular way. Later, as established members of such a group, they can give support to others and join in educating the public and making political statements about the rights of people with epilepsy. These activities are not only important to all sufferers of epilepsy but are often personally empowering and of themselves a way to combat the psychosocial consequences experienced by individual patients.

Case Presentation

Background

Rangi grew up within a large extended Maori family in a rural community north of New Zealand's largest city, Auckland. He remembers his childhood as a happy, carefree time until his seizures began when he was about 14 years old. At the time, he was unaware that the sensations he was experiencing were seizures. He describes a seizure as feeling a great fear entering his body, and goosebumps breaking out on his skin. The feeling lasts about 2 minutes and then subsides, leaving him feeling shaky and on edge. Although he can talk through them and understand what people are saying, and can even continue moving in a normal way, his usual response is to stop what he is doing and almost freeze in fear. As a teenager, these "turns," later diagnosed as complex partial seizures, occurred in flurries of three or four seizures an hour or two apart about once every 2 weeks. No one else in the family had ever had seizures of any kind, and when Rangi attempted to describe these feelings to his mother, she understandably had no reason to suspect they were seizures or in any way had an organic basis.

By the time Rangi left school when he was 17, the fear episodes were occurring almost daily, and Rangi's life was ruled by them. On days when they were particularly frequent, at the end of the day he would be left feeling on edge, jumpy, and with the potential to overreact. For example, he would lash out with his fists if anyone "got in his way" or made a remark he perceived as critical or rude. Fortunately, he was able to talk with his great uncle, a man of considerable wisdom, who understood his problems as spiritually based and advised him to take his problems to a *tohunga* (Maori medical man). Following Rangi's consultations with the tohunga, the fear attacks decreased in frequency, and even when they did occur, he was better able to recover from them. He began to spend more time at his tribal *marae* (Maori meetinghouse), his violent outbursts decreased, and he began to feel in control again.

After a year in his hometown, earning a minimal wage as a gas pump attendant, Rangi decided to move to Auckland, live with some of his cousins, and seek an apprenticeship as an automobile mechanic. This he achieved remarkably successfully, and he was quickly able to fit into a supportive family network as well as learn the ways of the city. Although he was still experiencing fear attacks once or twice a week, Rangi did not tell any of his Auckland family or friends about them, but he made sure he went back up north to his home marae at least every other weekend to "ground himself." About 10 months after beginning his mechanics apprenticeship, when Rangi was 19, he had his first generalized seizure. He was at work when it happened; he recalls the fear entering his body, and the next thing he remembers is being questioned by a doctor in a white coat in Auckland Hospital. He remained in the hospital for a week, during which time he had a second generalized seizure, and his fear attacks increased to 10 or more a day. A CT brain scan was normal, but when he was connected to the EEG machine while being videoed for 12 hours, it became clear that the onset of each fear attack was correlated with epileptiform activity arising from the vicinity of the right temporal lobe.

Rangi's fear attacks were diagnosed as "complex partial seizures with secondary generalization," and his new life of antiepileptic medication and frequent visits to *pakeha* (white New Zealander) medical doctors began. Over the next 8 years, Rangi's neurologist tried different medication regimens but was never able to reduce the fear seizures significantly. Their frequency varied; and occasionally Rangi would experience none for as long as 2 weeks, but more often he had from three to 10 a day. The medication did appear to control the generalized seizures, as the only times Rangi had one was when he forgot his medication.

Psychosocial Consequences

Following his first generalized seizure, Rangi felt embarrassed on returning to his apprenticeship and in retrospect thinks his boss at the garage was uncomfortable in his presence and kept him away from the more interesting and difficult jobs. Rangi left the apprenticeship within months of being discharged from hospital, relieved on doing so as he felt he could now keep his secret. He told only his parents, one brother, one sister, and his closest friend (a cousin) that he had epilepsy, but he downplayed the number of fear seizures he had. After a period on unemployment benefit, he managed to obtain a job as a builder's laborer. He was constantly worried that his boss would find out he had epilepsy and fire him on the grounds that it was dangerous for an epileptic to work near machinery and up ladders. He did not, in fact, work with dangerous machinery, and he was very careful to take his medication regularly to avoid a generalized seizure and to return north to ground himself at his home marae as often as he could.

When he was 21 he meet Anne through a friend, and they were married when Rangi was 23. Anne first realized the severity of Rangi's epilepsy when he had a generalized seizure at their engagement party. Many years later, as part of a therapy session, she recorded her recollections of that occasion and how it affected her.

> The first time I saw Rangi fitting, I was terrified. It was at our engagement party and absolutely all our friends were there as well as our families. Even though he had told me he had epilepsy, and I had seen someone at school years ago having a convulsion, I just wasn't prepared for my boyfriend to look like that, like he was crazy almost. I felt so embarrassed for him—and me too I suppose—with everyone crowding around while he was so totally out of control, and then wetting himself. Everyone pretended they didn't notice that he had wet himself and were all very sympathetic when he came around. No one at the party other than my family ever talked to me about it, but even now, years later, I still feel hot when I remember that party. I hadn't told my family or friends that Rangi had epilepsy, and Rangi had told only one really close friend and his family. Most of Rangi's fits were not really noticeable to anyone else, and he hardly ever had major seizures, probably because of his medication. We figured out later that with all the excitement of our engagement party, he forgot to take his pills.
>
> I didn't tell Rangi for years how I really felt about that occasion. He was embarrassed enough knowing he had a fit without being told how awful it was. I told him later that it only lasted a minute or two, and hardly anyone was in the room. I had a really difficult time after that wondering if I had done the right thing getting engaged to someone with that sort of problem, and I think it was guilt more than anything that kept me in the relationship. It took months before I felt the same about Rangi again, and only then because he didn't have another major fit. Now that I know so much more about epilepsy, I feel ashamed that I felt like that and feel really strongly about the importance of education and support groups for people like Rangi and me and education generally for the public.

Anne's words will probably resonate with many epilepsy sufferers and their families. Although Anne was sympathetic to his need to retain close ties with his *whanau* (extended family), she was not aware of the importance of Rangi's visits north in helping him cope with his fear attacks. Two years after their marriage, while on holiday with Anne's family, Rangi had another generalized seizure (again because he had forgotten to take his medication), and although he was not hospitalized, this crisis resulted in a discussion between Rangi, Anne, and her parents. As a pakeha family they were able to understand the medical diagnosis and treatment of epilepsy, but they were unable to comprehend Rangi's spiritual understanding of the fear attacks that overtook him and his need to return to his home after a particularly bad week to feel grounded.

Over the next few years, Rangi and Anne tried many ways, both Maori and pakeha, to help Rangi and their marriage. Anne became more involved with Rangi's whanau, and gradually her involvement in and understanding of Maori ways and beliefs expanded. In Auckland, Anne and Rangi began to attend support groups run by the local branch of the National Epilepsy Society, and their knowledge about seizures and how to cope with them increased dramatically. As Rangi commented, however, all the knowledge in the world did not help when one of his fear seizures came on. He was always on edge and sometimes felt depressed for days. His seizures undermined his confidence and self-esteem and contributed to a poor ability to make decisions. To help himself, Rangi enrolled in various men's groups to work on his self-esteem and assertiveness. He found that although these groups helped him at the time, a bad day of fear seizures would undermine any progress he had made.

In addition, both Rangi and Anne noticed that Rangi was having increasing problems with his memory. For example, he seemed to have difficulty remembering the route to friends' houses unless he had been there many times, and he was always forgetting where he left his car or his car keys. He would sometimes have difficulty remembering he had met someone before. The face would seem familiar, but he was often unsure whether he had met that person or someone resembling that person. He frequently forgot names and had to keep a diary to remember the dates and times of appointments or social occasions. He also felt he had much less energy than before starting on his medication and said he felt less able to cope with learning new skills. He remained a builder's laborer, even though it "bores me to tears" because he believed he would not be able to cope with learning a new trade.

Anne and Rangi's marriage survived. When Rangi was 26, they had their first child. Before this, they had talked about the possibility of neurosurgery to help Rangi and had been encouraged by observing how successful this operation had been in two members of their epilepsy support group. The neurologist was unsure about how useful the operation would be for Rangi, however, given that he had generalized seizures in addition to his complex partial seizures. After their child was born, Rangi felt he must do something to reduce his seizures if he was to be a good father to his son. After discussions with his neurologist, he was put on the waiting list for a workup to see whether he would be a suitable candidate for a temporal lobectomy.

Rangi was booked for a neuropsychological assessment and admission to the hospital for EEG monitoring in 6 weeks. He and Anne then went north to discuss the situation with his whanau. The details of what occurred within Rangi's whanau and in their consultations with the tohunga were never discussed with the pakeha professionals in the hospital system, but the outcome was that the tohunga strongly advised Rangi to stay away from the hospital and the surgeon's scalpel and to stop taking his medications so that he could be healed the Maori way. In many instances, Maori healing has had results far superior to those of western medicine for Maori people, especially in cases where Maori experience difficulties that would be viewed as psychological or psychiatric disorders by western medicine and society (Durie 1977; Sachdev 1989; Woolford 1990).

Unfortunately, this did not hold for Rangi, and 3 weeks after his return north, he had a generalized seizure that did not stop spontaneously but continued into *status epilepticus* (continual convulsing). He was rushed by ambulance to the nearest hospital, where the seizure was finally terminated after more than an hour of convulsing by an intravenous injection of Valium. Rangi was then flown to Auckland Hospital, and with his and his wife's permission, his antiepileptic medication was recommenced. He had four more generalized seizures over the next week before he finally stabilized and was able to be discharged, suffering as before about 10 fear seizures a day. While he was in the hospital, his parents and siblings traveled to Auckland, and a meeting was held with them, the Auckland members of the same *iwi* (tribe), the Maori medical staff who were co-opted to assist with the process, and the epilepsy team. Rangi, with the support of his whanau, decided to remain on his medication but to postpone the surgery until his iwi up north were able to reach a decision. Four months later, Rangi returned to the neurologist and said he had decided to proceed with the operation and had whanau and iwi support for this decision.

Temporal Lobectomy and Its Outcome

To undergo a full workup for surgery, Rangi had a neuropsychological assessment as an outpatient and was then admitted to the neurology ward for a week. He was gradually weaned off his medication over 3 days and then underwent continual EEG monitoring while being videoed each day from 9:00 AM until 5:00 PM. The result was some excellent recordings of epileptiform activity contained in the right temporal lobe/ hippocampal area occurring simultaneously with fear seizures. Rangi had one generalized seizure, which began as a fear seizure with epileptiform activity in the right temporal area and then rapidly spread to the rest of the cortex of both cerebral hemispheres. Otherwise, there was no indication of abnormal EEG activity arising from any region other than the right temporal/hippocampal area.

Rangi's neuropsychological assessment showed a man of average intelligence. He had an excellent immediate memory span of eight digits forward and was also able to repeat seven digits backward, attesting to a normal attention and concentration span and good working memory. He had no impairment of verbal memory on tests involving learning word lists and recognizing previously seen words (the Recognition Memory Test), although he did have lowered scores on a memory test involving the recall of short stories. New Zealand studies have demonstrated that healthy Maori men of Rangi's age and educational background score poorly on these Wechsler Memory Scale memory passages, presumably as a result of inherent cultural bias. Like Rangi, however, the Maori men scored in the "high average" range on list learning, perhaps because of the oral tradition of the Maori and their ability to learn extensive genealogies (Ogden, Cooper, and Dudley 2003; Ogden and McFarlane-Nathan 1997). Rangi's performance on nonverbal memory tests, such as the Rey Complex Figure, fell below the 25th percentile, demonstrating a true impairment for him given that young Maori men as a group perform at the same or higher levels than pakeha men on this test (Ogden and McFarlane-Nathan 1997). His performance in recognizing faces on the Recognition Memory Test fell one standard deviation (SD) below average (based on English norms). On tests of psychomotor speed (the Digit Symbol test of the revised Wechsler Adult Intelligence Scale WAIS-R), his performance fell 1 SD below average and below his average scores on the other WAIS-R Performance sub-tests. This psychomotor slowing may have been a result of his medication.

Thus, Rangi's neuropsychological performance was consistent with an epileptic focus in the temporal lobe or hippocampus, mediating nonverbal, visuospatial memory. There was no evidence of any dysfunction of the temporal lobe dominant for verbal memory. Rangi was strongly left-handed, however, as was his mother. Although estimates vary, about 70% of left-handers and 96%of right handers are left-hemisphere dominant for language (Milner 1975); thus, it was unlikely that Rangi had language functions predominantly in his right hemisphere. If he did, however, his left temporal lobe rather than the right might mediate nonverbal memory and was therefore dysfunctional according to neuropsychological tests. Thus, removal of his right temporal lobe and hippocampus (to remove the epileptic focus as demonstrated on EEG) might result in severe generalized new learning and memory problems and possibly cause some language impairment. Rangi was therefore given a Wada test before the final decision was made regarding his suitability for surgery. Rangi's understandable anxiety about the Wada was somewhat allayed by giving him a careful explanation of the procedure and the neuropsychological tests that would be given as part of it. The Wada went well, and the results were good, demonstrating that Rangi was left dominant for language. On recovering from the effects of the sodium amytal, he could remember four of the five items he had been shown while his right hemisphere was anesthetized.

Rangi now felt confident that his best hope lay in Western medicine and was cautiously optimistic that the surgery would cure his seizures. He was well informed about the risks as well as the benefits of temporal lobectomy. He was aware that although the most people undergoing the operation were "cured" of their epilepsy or experienced a significant reduction in their seizure frequency with or without ongoing medication, in some cases surgery made no difference in the epilepsy or even made it worse. He was also aware that the final outcome of the surgery might not be known for a year afterward because of the possibility that the surgery itself and the disruption caused by it could cause seizures for a time, while the brain regained stability. He knew he would remain on medication for at least a year even if he had no further seizures.

Rangi never faltered in his determination to have the operation, as he was now feeling quite depressed about his frequent and debilitating fear attacks, his belief that the drugs he had to take impaired his cognitive functioning and alertness, and his fear that his generalized seizures would increase. He believed that if he continued in his present state of low self-esteem and bouts of depression that resulted from his numerous fear attacks, sooner or later Anne would leave him, and because of his epilepsy, he believed he might lose custody of their child.

Rangi returned to the hospital 3 weeks after his neuropsychological assessment for his operation. The neurosurgeon removed 8 cm from the pole of his right temporal lobe and 4 cm of the underlying hippocampus. The operation took 4 hours from beginning to end and was uneventful. Rangi's recovery was marked by severe headaches for 3 days immediately after the surgery, and he was upset when he experienced a flurry of fear seizures 2 days after surgery. He was able to overcome his disappointment when he was reminded that he could have seizures for some months while his brain recovered from the surgery. Bedside memory testing demonstrated that his memory abilities were grossly unimpaired. After discharge from the hospital, he continued to have fear seizures for several weeks despite being on medication. Within 3 months postoperatively, however, the seizures had stopped altogether, and 1 year after his surgery he was weaned off his medication. Five years later, he had remained free of seizures and medication and had moved back up north with his family. He worked as a Maori craftsman (carving bone and greenstone pendants) and did seasonal farm work. Although glad to be free of Western medicine, he remained grateful to the epilepsy team at the hospital for curing his seizures.

Two years after his surgery, Rangi returned to the hospital for a follow-up neuropsychological assessment. A comprehensive assessment soon after surgery is not recommended because it can take many months for memory functions to reach presurgery levels. In some cases memory and cognitive functions may even improve in the years after successful surgery, presumably because the patient's attention span and concentration improve when seizures and subclinical epileptiform activity no longer interfere and interrupt the learning process, and antiepileptic medication no longer decreases alertness and speed of response; this is particularly pertinent to school-aged children.

Rangi demonstrated scores similar to his presurgery scores on the subtests of the WAIS-R, with the exception of the Digit Symbol subtest. Here his score had increased, demonstrating an improvement in psychomotor speed. He also demonstrated slightly improved scores on the verbal memory tests. In contrast, his recall of the Rey Complex Figure now fell at the 10th percentile, a significant drop from his presurgery scores. His ability to recognize faces on the Recognition Memory Test also decreased, although he still performed well above chance. This further impairment on nonverbal memory tests is consistent with his right temporal and hippocampal resection and indicates that before removal these were mediating some nonverbal memory functions, albeit imperfectly.

Rangi had learned not to rely on his visual memory and made sure he verbalized as well as possible any visual material he wanted to remember. He did not find it at all disabling, particularly as his visuospatial perceptual and constructional skills were excellent. His beautiful, intricately carved pendants were proof of this.

Discussion

Epilepsy is a debilitating disorder, and in carefully selected cases a temporal lobectomy can dramatically change the lives of the victims. At the other extreme are the many people who must suffer epilepsy for life or take medication that may decrease their alertness while it reduces their seizures. Only focal seizures can be helped by removing a section of cortex, and people who suffer generalized seizures are unlikely to benefit from surgery unless, like Rangi, their seizures begin as focal seizures. In a very small number of people with intractable generalized seizures, the large commissure that connects the two hemispheres (the corpus callosum) is partially or completely split to prevent the spread of seizures (Bogen, Sperry, and Vogel 1969; Sperry 1974; see Chapter 18).

Much has been learned about the roles of the temporal lobes and hippocampi by studying the cognitive and memory abilities of people who have had temporal lobectomies. Some large neurosurgical centers, such as the Montreal Neurological Institute, specialize in this operation. Since Wilder Penfield carried out his pioneering unilateral temporal lobe resections in the 1950s (Penfield and Milner 1958; Penfield and Roberts 1959), many important discoveries have been made by neuropsychologist Brenda Milner and her many colleagues and students in their elegant studies of groups of right and left temporal lobectomy patients (Milner 1975). The major criticism of all studies on neurosurgical patients who had severe and intractable epilepsy before their surgery is that they may have abnormal brains as a result of their epilepsy; thus, the results of studies on these groups cannot validly be generalized to normal brains. This criticism may be true, but the impairments demonstrated by healthy, nonepileptic people who have sustained sudden focal damage to one or other temporal lobe as a result of an accident, stroke, or tumor are consistent with the impairments found after temporal lobectomies, suggesting that the brains of most people who suffer complex partial seizures are not markedly abnormal.

The particular case of Rangi raises issues about the importance of cultural sensitivity and appropriateness both in assessment and when discussing illness and potential treatments with the patient. In Maori culture, which has many similarities to the culture of the American Indian, decisions of the family and tribe often take precedence over individual decisions (Durie 1984). In Rangi's case, the failure of the Western system to respond appropriately and sensitively to cultural differences from the very beginning of the process nearly resulted in catastrophe. The head is *tapu* (sacred) to many Maori tribes (Sachdev 1989), and thus the prospect of neurosurgery requires deep discussion among members of the family, guided by the knowledge of the elders, the spirit of their ancestors, and the counsel of the Maori tohunga. When clear information was given to the Rangi's family, they were able to integrate Western knowledge with their own and make a decision that they could support and live with.

Every culture has different beliefs and its own reality, and it behooves clinicians and scientists to respect these beliefs and to be humble in light of the knowledge embodied by the culture of the people they are trying to help. Western technology may often be able to perform physical cures, but if the patient loses self-respect and the support and respect of his people, the "cure" will be hollow indeed (Sachdev 1989; Woolford 1990).

Two years after his operation, I asked Rangi whether the long workup to the operation, the upset it caused his people, the operation and painful recovery, the months of worrying after the surgery when he continued to have seizures, and his further impairment of nonverbal memory was worthwhile. His answering smile said it all, but he eloquently expressed his feelings with words as well.

> I'm a whole man now, and my evil spirits have fled. For every day that goes by and I have come through with no fear and my head held high, I bless you. Every day when I drive my kids to school without thinking I might be overtaken by a seizure and put their lives at risk, I give thanks for you fellas down here in the city. Mostly, I figure my people's ways of healing are best for my people, but I've got to hand it to you, some of your knowledge is good, and my people are grateful for what you have done for me. It wasn't too much fun at the time, but once our people decided to go with it, I never doubted it would work. I tell you, we would do it all again without a second thought if we had to. If you have any more Maori fellas in my situation, you just call on us to talk to them.

More recently, over the past 6 or so years, I have on occasion spoken with Rangi, usually in connection with his ongoing volunteer work with the Epilepsy Society. The most salient demonstration of Rangi's increasing well-being occurred about 2 years ago, when I heard an interview with him on National Radio in which he was speaking out for the rights of Maori people. Throughout Rangi's fluent and impassioned arguments, epilepsy was never mentioned, even when he spoke of the problems inherent in applying a Western model of health to Maori health and well-being. Clearly epilepsy no longer ruled Rangi's life.

5

The Breakdown of Language
Case Studies of Aphasia

I have a poignant, vivid visual memory of Luke from the first time I met him. A powerfully built Maori man with a mane of tangled black hair and tattoos on both arms and bare chest, he was sitting upright in his hospital bed in the sunny hospital ward. His left hand was hovering over a large board covered with letters and numbers, and as I approached his bed he looked up at me. It was the image of fear distorting his strong face and shadowing his dark eyes that struck me so forcibly and remains with me still.

Luke had collapsed at a party the evening before. At first his friends thought he was drunk, but when he awoke from his semicomatose state the next day, unable to speak and weak down his right side, they realized this was more than the usual hangover and took him to the accident and emergency department at Auckland Hospital. A computed tomography (CT) brain scan revealed that Luke had suffered a *cerebrovascular accident* (CVA), a general term that refers to a stroke or brain hemorrhage as a result of a blockage or rupture of an artery or vein. In Luke's case the CVA was a collection of blood within the brain substance of the inferior posterior region of the left frontal lobe.

He was transferred to the neurosurgery ward, and when I saw him only a few hours later, he was desperately trying to spell the words that his lips refused to form, using a communication board of letters and numbers given to him by the speech pathologist. His three friends were sitting around his bed and looked as frightened as he did. With much hesitation, Luke managed to spell out "V-O-C-E G-O-M-N H-E-P M-E." This we translated as "Voice gone, help me."

After the age of about 4 years, most of us take for granted our easy ability to produce and understand complex and structured strings of words to communicate with others who speak the same language. When this ability is without warning suddenly taken from us, it is hardly surprising that our overriding emotion is often fear. For Luke and his friends, their fear did not spring from knowledge about the relationship between language deficits and left brain damage but was rather the fear of the unknown. In their experience, only very old people suffered strokes that led to speech problems. Luke was only 28, and although they were aware that motorbike and car crashes could result in head injuries, causing speech problems and limb weaknesses, he and his friends had never before experienced a drinking binge that had such a devastating result.

After careful assessment, it was decided that Luke was suffering from expressive, or Broca's, aphasia; that is, his most severe difficulties were in verbal expression. His ability to comprehend language, although by no means normal, was relatively unimpaired. The cause of his aphasia was a sudden hemorrhage into the cortical area mediating expressive language (i.e., speech and spontaneous writing). This type of hemorrhage into the brain usually affects a defined or focal area of cortex and is called an *intracerebral hematoma*. Luke's excessive drinking may have been a factor in precipitating his hemorrhage, but this is a rare consequence of excessive alcohol consumption. Often an intracerebral hematoma occurs spontaneously in people who suffer from high blood pressure (*hypertension*), but it can sometimes occur with no obvious cause in healthy people of any age.

Beth, the second person with aphasia I describe in this chapter, differs from Luke in a number of ways. Beth's language impairments resulted from a much more common type of CVA, in which the blood supply is cut off from a region of the cortex, causing *ischemia* (a loss of oxygen), which can result in an area of dysfunctional or dead brain (called a *stroke* or *infarction*). Typically, these types of strokes occur in people over the age of 60 years and are often the result of the gradual buildup of deposited material (*atheroma*) on the inside of the arteries supplying the brain. Atheroma buildup can be caused by excessive cholesterol and smoking. The atheroma finally blocks off the artery altogether, and if that artery is the sole supplier of blood and oxygen to an essential part of the brain, a thrombotic stroke, causing impairment of the functions mediated by that part of the brain, will result. On occasion, this type of stroke results not from the gradual blocking of an artery but from a fragment of the atheroma (called an embolus) that escapes from an artery in some other part of the body and is carried in the bloodstream and lodges in an artery in the brain. An embolic stroke can result. Emboli can break off from arteries leaving the heart or even following operations or damage to arteries in other parts of the body.

Beth, the 62-year-old woman whose story will be told here, suffered a large left temporoparietal stroke as the result of a thrombotic blockage of her left middle cerebral artery. Beth had lived on a sheep farm all her life and was a large consumer of sheep meat as well as rich dairy products. In addition, she had been treated in the past for hypertension and had been a heavy smoker since the age of 16 years. Too much cholesterol in the diet, hypertension, and a history of smoking are all risk factors for stroke.

Beth's language problems were classified as receptive, or Wernicke's aphasia. Her ability to comprehend spoken or written language was severely impaired, but her spoken language was fluent and, if not attended to closely, sounded almost normal. Anyone attempting to understand Beth's speech, however, quickly realized that her sentences were often nonsensical. At first, Beth did not appear particularly concerned, perhaps because she was unable to comprehend that her speech was muddled and confused. Her family was, however, very upset by her sudden loss of ability to communicate with them. As Beth's condition improved somewhat, her frustration with making herself understood did surface from time to time. More detailed descriptions of Luke and Beth's impairments and outcomes follow a section providing some background to the classification of aphasia.

Theoretical Background

Classification of Aphasia

Broca's aphasia and Wernicke's aphasia are perhaps the best described acquired language disorders, but a number of other aphasia types are characterized by a mixture of features that do not fit comfortably with either Broca's or Wernicke's aphasia. Indeed, many patients do not fit all the parameters of any of the traditional aphasia classifications but fall somewhere between two classifications or perhaps have an aphasia that includes all the components of two or more classifications (Caplan 2003). This variety across patients is hardly surprising given that brain lesions are rarely confined to identical areas across patients. In addition, individual differences in the exact localization of many language functions have been demonstrated during the electrical stimulation of the brains of awake humans during some types of surgery for epilepsy (Ojemann 1979, 1980).

There is an increasing trend for clinicians involved in the assessment and rehabilitation of people with aphasia simply to describe the pattern of impaired and intact language abilities the patient demonstrates and to dispense with the academic, often misleading notion of classification by aphasia type. A broad understanding of the main ways aphasia has been classified can, however, aid our basic understanding of the breakdown of language and clarify how different language components relate, in a general sense, to specific areas of the cortex.

Major Aphasia Classifications

Broca's aphasia   This syndrome, also known as expressive, nonfluent, or motor aphasia, is named for neurologist Paul Broca, who first described it in 1861. His patient, Leborgne (commonly referred to as "Tan" because that was the only utterance he could make), was found at postmortem to have a lesion of the third *frontal gyrus*, which he postulated to be the seat of motor-speech memories. This area is now known as *Broca's area* and remains the area most frequently associated with expressive aphasia (see Fig. 5-1). The other most important area is the *precentral gyrus*, immediately adjacent to Broca's area, which contains the motor neurons for the tongue and lips. Lesions deep to Broca's area, but sparing the cortex, have also been shown to produce expressive aphasia (Levine and Sweet 1983).

The major feature of Broca's aphasia is a severe nonfluency of speech, which may

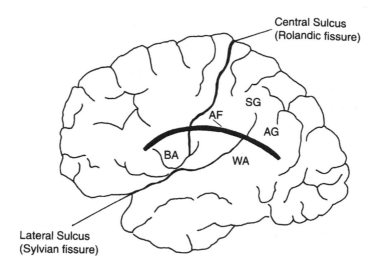

Figure 5-1 A simplified diagram of a lateral view of the left hemisphere of the human brain, showing the language areas. BA, Broca's area; WA, Wernicke's area; SG, supramarginal gyrus; AG, angular gyrus; AF, arcuate fasciculus.

be so extreme as to render the patient mute. More often, speech is limited to a few stereotyped expressions or expletives. Less severely affected patients may be able to provide sensible one-word answers to questions and even produce short, agrammatical "sentences" with many hesitations. Nouns and verbs are more likely to be preserved, in contrast to grammatical modifiers and prepositions, resulting in unmelodic speech. Familiar concrete objects are easier to articulate than common grammatical terms such as *or, if, but,* and *where.* For example, a Broca's aphasic may answer the question, "What is wrong with you?" by saying in an effortful and staccato manner, "Peech gone, can't palk, talk." Nearly every sound requires a fresh start, and many words are incorrectly pronounced. Words beginning with letters like *p, b,* or *m,* which are formed at the front of the mouth, are easier to say than letters like *s* and *t;* so "speech" sounds like "peech," and "talk" is articulated as "palk." Verbs usually appear in their simplest form; so the patient says, "Me go" rather than "I am going."

The right hand is often paralyzed because the lesion that causes Broca's aphasia may also encroach on the motor strip for the hand. Writing with the nonparalyzed left hand is nonfluent, like the patient's speech. Copying may be better than writing spontaneously or to dictation. Words are misspelled, correct letters are poorly formed, grammatical words are left out entirely, and perseveration of letters may occur.

Some patients have difficulty swallowing food and saliva, although this usually fully recovers over days to weeks, and many patients with Broca's aphasia also suffer from oral apraxia. Apraxia refers to a difficulty miming or performing learned motor skills on command. Thus, patients severely affected with oral apraxia may be unable to poke out their tongue or whistle on verbal command or in imitation of the examiner.

The degree of speech loss is highly correlated with the degree of oral apraxia (De Renzi, Pieczuro, and Vignolo 1966).

Language comprehension is usually impaired to some degree. Simple requests are often understood, but severe Broca's aphasics are unlikely to be able to understand a three-step command, even if each step is simple. Even when only a "yes" or "no" response is required, some patients may have difficulty comprehending more complex language input. Often the comprehension of numbers and symbols is also impaired.

In general, Broca's aphasics are alert and appear to interact with their caregivers and family in an intelligent, unconfused manner. Their nonverbal memory is good, they have no difficulty recognizing doctors and other caregivers, and they can follow a simple daily schedule. They are often emotionally fragile and easily angered or reduced to tears. Most Broca's aphasics have a weakness (*hemiparesis*) or paralysis of the right arm, which may recover along with the recovery of speech. If speech does not recover, the arm weakness usually persists. When the lesion encroaches into the parietal lobe, some right-sided sensory loss may be apparent. Because of the anterior focus of the lesion, a visual-field defect is rare; if present (perhaps because of transient swelling extending posteriorly), it usually resolves quite quickly.

Wernicke's aphasia   In an article published in 1874, neurologist Carl Wernicke described 10 aphasic patients whose main difficulty was an inability to comprehend speech. He had autopsy data on four patients, and each had a lesion that damaged the left temporal lobe. Later studies confirmed that this type of aphasia, known as sensory, receptive, or fluent aphasia as well as *Wernicke's aphasia*, was commonly associated with damage to the left posterior superior temporal lobe (see Fig. 5-1).

The main hallmarks of Wernicke's aphasia include a severe comprehension deficit that affects the understanding of both spoken and written language, as well as fluent, grammatically correct, but nonsensical speech and writing. Because the patient is unable to understand what is said, repetition is also impaired. The fluent speech (or writing) is full of phonemic and semantic paraphasias; for example, *bell* might be substituted with *dell* (a phonemic paraphasia) or with *ring, ring* (a semantic paraphasia). Nonexistent words (*neologisms*) may also occur. Syntax is largely preserved, giving the speech a normal, melodic sound. With close attention and knowledge of the speaker, it is often possible for the listener to gain some meaning from the conversation.

The patient may seem unconcerned or even unaware of these problems. Often confusion and an apparent loss of intelligent behavior are present although difficult to assess given the patient's comprehension deficit. If able to be assessed, verbal memory would presumably be impaired, especially if the temporal lobe lesion was extensive or encroached medially into the hippocampus. There is usually no limb weakness, although where the lesion is very large and extends forward to the postcentral strip, there may be some loss of tactile sensation. A visual-field defect affecting the upper right quadrant, and sometimes the whole right field (a *homonymous hemianopia*), is almost always present.

Other Types of Aphasia

Conduction aphasia results when Broca's area is separated from Wernicke's area. The lesion can damage the supramarginal gyrus, which lies above and around the posterior end of the sylvian fissure and the white matter tracts that connect the two speech areas (the *arcuate fasciculus*), or the lesion surrounds the posterior end of the sylvian fissure. Verbal output is fluent, with many phonemic paraphasias. Comprehension of language is relatively well preserved, but repetition is extremely impaired. Reading aloud is also impaired, in contrast with reading silently for comprehension, which is preserved. Writing is somewhat disturbed by spelling errors, omission of words, and word sequence changes. Sometimes conduction aphasia is accompanied by a motor or sensory loss or a visual-field defect on the side opposite the lesion. Apraxia on verbal command and imitation may also be present.

Global aphasia is produced by a large lesion that damages both Broca's and Wernicke's areas. Speech is nonfluent, and comprehension, repetition, and naming are severely impaired. The patient cannot read or write. Most patients have a right hemiplegia.

Transcortical motor aphasia (TMA) is characterized by halting, nonfluent speech, but unimpaired, fluent repetition of sentences. Comprehension of speech and reading aloud and for comprehension are also unimpaired. Naming and writing are often impaired. A right hemiplegia is usually apparent, and a right sensory loss or visual-field defect sometimes occur. The lesions associated with TMA are in the language-dominant frontal lobe, often directly superior or anterior to Broca's area, and their primary features seems to be that they separate Broca's area from nearby cortical areas that are necessary for normal speech.

Transcortical sensory aphasia (TSA) resembles Wernicke's aphasia except the patient can repeat spoken language (although is unable to comprehend it). The responsible lesions often lie in the angular gyrus superior, anterior, or posterior to Wernicke's area.

Anomic aphasia is the most common form of aphasia, and in its pure form, the patient is frequently unable to find the correct word. Speech is fluent, and repetition and comprehension of spoken and written language are preserved. The lesion can be almost anywhere in the language-dominant hemisphere, and anomic aphasia is the most common form of aphasia seen after head injury or in dementia of Alzheimer's type.

Reading and Writing Deficits

Acquired alexia or *dyslexia* refer to an inability to read following brain damage (Coslett 2003); *agraphia* refers to an inability to write (Roeltgen). The two deficits can occur together or in isolation. For example, patients with alexia without agraphia often have lesions of the posterior part of the corpus callosum (the *splenium*) and the left occipital lobe (causing a right visual-field defect). They cannot read because the words they see in their intact left visual field are projected to the nonverbal right hemisphere and cannot be transferred back across the damaged splenium for comprehension by the verbal left hemisphere. This is called a *disconnection syndrome*. Spontaneous writing remains unimpaired as the left-hemispheric language areas, the anterior part of the corpus callosum, and the hand motor areas are intact. Agraphia without alexia sometimes results from left-hemispheric angular gyrus lesions, often as one symptom of Gerstmann's syndrome (see Chapter 6).

Case Presentations

Case 1: Luke

Background   Luke grew up in a large family in a poor area of Auckland. He never enjoyed school and left when he was 15. From then until his admission to hospital at the age of 28, he had a few labor jobs but more often than not relied financially on unemployment benefits. He passed his time riding motorbikes with his mates, petty thieving, playing snooker, smoking marijuana, and consuming large quantities of alcohol. His friends recalled that he had suffered at least three minor head injuries over the past few years from fights and minor motorbike accidents. He had no history of serious head injury. For some years before his hemorrhage, Luke had been living with his friends in a rundown house, although he visited his family frequently.

Luke remained in the hospital for 10 days, during which time his ability to speak improved a little, as did the weakness of his right arm and hand. A second CT scan performed 8 days after his admission CT demonstrated that the area of hemorrhage around Broca's area had reduced considerably. This reduction occurs as the hematoma is reabsorbed. The cortex and underlying white matter can be permanently damaged by the hemorrhage, but in Luke's case the cortex did not appear to have been extensively damaged. He was transferred to a live-in rehabilitation unit, where he had daily physiotherapy and speech therapy.

Short-term neuropsychological and psychosocial outcome   During the first week after his stroke, Luke was unable to utter more than single words, but he was able to use his communication board to spell out nongrammatical and misspelled sentences of three or four words. He would become quickly frustrated and angry when he was unable to make himself understood, and the words exploding from his mouth were often swear words, a common occurrence with Broca's aphasia. It has been suggested that emotionally motivated expletives can be produced by the right hemisphere. On one occasion, he became so angry that he threw the communication board at the speech pathologist and then swept his water jug and glass off his bedside table with his left arm. He appeared to comprehend the lecture he subsequently received from the speech pathologist and the doctor, and their threat to tie his arms to the bed did not have to be put into practice.

Assessment of Luke's language functions demonstrated reasonable comprehension of spoken and simple written English. He had difficulty comprehending syntactic function words, however; for example, he could not demonstrate comprehension of the sentence, "The cat is under the chair." When asked to point to the picture that best described the sentence, he was just as likely to point to a picture of a cat on a chair as a cat under a chair. According to Luke's mother, his reading had been poor before his hemorrhage; it was therefore difficult to assess his comprehension of more difficult written passages.

Luke also demonstrated apraxia of the left arm. When asked, "Show me how you brush your teeth," he made large circling movements in the air. His comprehension of the command was intact, however; he could nod in confirmation when I performed the correct movement, although he could not copy my movement correctly. He could use a real toothbrush correctly. He also had oral apraxia and was unable to pretend to whistle, blow a kiss, or sip through a straw.

By the 10th day following his hemorrhage, when Luke was transferred to the rehabilitation unit, he could articulate short sentences with few function words, such as "Phone Mum. Clothes, umm . . . (patting his arm) . . ."coat, . . . black, umm" (at this point, the psychologist suggested the word "leather") "Yes, yes, leather coat, jacket, jeans peease, please." His speech sounded strained and had impaired prosody; that is, the normal intonations and melody of speech were sometimes lost. Luke's ability to repeat simple sentences had improved, although he became muddled if the sentences were more than about five words long or syntactically complex or deviant. For example, Luke could repeat "Auckland is in New Zealand," but he had difficulty with "Wellington is above Christchurch and below Auckland" and "The boy eats the food."

Once Luke was settled at the rehabilitation unit, the speech pathologist began twice-daily sessions with him. She found that his ability to repeat sentences improved if she sang the sentence with a strong intonation pattern. She would begin by asking Luke to sing after her a sentence he knew well, such as "Mary had a little lamb" and then, using the same melodic line, she would sing, "I would like some orange juice." Once Luke had the melody and rhythm of the sentence, he then copied the therapist as she said the sentence with the same strong intonations. He then graduated to more difficult sentences. This activity uses the principle behind a type of therapy called melodic intonation (MI) therapy, first developed by Albert, Sparks, and Helm (1973), based on the observation that some aphasic patients are still able to produce words while singing, contrasting with severe impairment of their normal speech. This observation led to the idea that combining slower speech with intoned patterns with a precise rhythm and distinct stresses on words would assist the patient in expressing longer, more complex sentences.

Some, but not all, aphasics are helped by MI therapy. The best candidates seem to be those with good auditory comprehension skills relative to their expressive ability and repetition ability and those who possess good self-monitoring skills (Shewan and Bandur 1986). Gradually, MI therapy takes the patient through a series of exercises, from repetition to spontaneous production of intoned sentences, and from melodic intonation to normal speech prosody. Luke appeared to respond well to MI therapy, although the speech pathologist used other forms of speech therapy with him as well. In addition, spontaneous recovery was probably also occurring, making it impossible to say with certainty exactly what was responsible for Luke's improvement.

This difficulty highlights one of the common problems in assessing the usefulness of rehabilitation methods in aphasia and other cognitive and motor problems following brain damage. To assess the effect of a particular therapy strategy, strict adherence to a carefully designed program that allows the influence of the therapy on the problem to be discriminated from various other recovery variables is necessary. One way to do this is to design an experiment using the patient as his own control and take baseline measures of various aspects of language and other deficits, such as apraxia, before commencing a therapy strategy aimed at improving one aspect of the patient's disorder. If the therapy is effective, monitoring of all aspects of the disorder will demonstrate faster improvement in the targeted aspect of language than in other areas. If the therapy is stopped after a short time, the patient's improvement in that particular aspect of language should stop or slide backward but improve again when the therapy recommences.

This type of single-subject design methodology (Barlow and Hersen 1984) has its origins in operant or behavioral psychology. It is often more practical and ethical than assessing a therapy strategy via group methodology, wherein a group of patients with aphasia and therapy is compared with a group of patients with aphasia who do not have therapy. Even so, in a busy rehabilitation unit, it is difficult to use single case designs stringently, particularly given the attraction of approaching the patient's many problems from as many therapeutic angles as possible over the same period. There are ways to assess multiple therapies within the same single case study design by using multiple baselines of different behaviors and staggered implementation of each type of therapy for each behavioral deficit. The practicalities of carrying out such complex experimentation with every patient unfortunately work against its regular implementation.

Usually, when such programs are put in place, it is the psychologist who designs and oversees them. The entire program, however, is a team effort. The speech pathologist is involved in deciding which therapy is needed to treat which aspect of the aphasia and carrying out the daily intervention. Similarly, the physical therapist may be involved in an intervention to increase arm movements, which may be included in a multiple baseline design. Finally, the patient must be highly motivated if the program is to proceed satisfactorily. At every stage, he will receive feedback about his progress, often in the form of simple graphs. If two different aspects of his aphasia are improving at an equal rate, despite the fact that the therapy is aimed at only one aspect, either spontaneous recovery is occurring (and will thus continue even if therapy is stopped) or the therapy program has generalized to other aspects of the aphasia (thus, stopping the therapy will result in stopping the progress in more than one aspect of the aphasia). A third possibility is that some other variable is having a general effect on the aphasia. For example, if the attention the patient receives from the rehabilitation staff has resulted in the patient feeling less depressed and more optimistic about his prognosis, as a result he may be motivated to try harder.

Luke's therapy program was multidimensional, and the efficacies of individual interventions were not assessed. He received not only speech and physical therapy but also individual and family psychological counseling, which appeared especially helpful in enabling him to cope with the cessation of his alcohol consumption, forced on him by his confinement in the rehabilitation unit. In the first 2 weeks there, he "escaped" three times and was found in a nearby hotel. No doubt the other drinkers thought that his strained and staccato speech was a result of intoxication. It was made clear to Luke that his escapades would not be tolerated, and if they continued, he would be discharged from the unit.

A close watch was kept on Luke for the next month, and during this period he became quite depressed and apathetic and would participate in speech and physical therapy sessions only if he was continually encouraged. Counseling sessions with Luke and his family and friends seemed to help Luke, and his mood and motivation gradually improved. He found that keeping active helped him to fight his need for alcohol; as he gained control over his desire to drink, he began to feel justifiably proud of this achievement.

Another helpful intervention was suggested by Luke's friends. They took turns spending the day at the rehabilitation unit, going to every therapy session with Luke. Their participation in speech and physical therapy not only encouraged Luke but often added a much-needed humorous touch to the sessions, as they would often "crack up" (laugh) at Luke's attempts to express himself orally or to perform some physical exercise. This interaction seemed to alleviate Luke's frustration with his slow progress and cause him in turn to "crack up" at his friends' attempts to copy him. He would then cheerfully try again. The presence of jovial friends at therapy sessions may well have a negative effect on progress for some people; clearly, the details of a rehabilitation program must be tailored to fit the individual. Luke's friends were there for him between therapy sessions when he wanted to relax; they were sensitive to his moods and knew when to leave him, when to cheer him up, and when to listen to him express his feelings. They became skilled at understanding Luke's nonverbal communications and at times were able to relieve him of the weary task of trying to communicate important ideas to staff verbally.

Billiards became a regular feature of Luke's day, at first with a friend helping him push the billiard cue, but gradually gaining the strength and coordination to manipulate the cue himself. His friends agreed to cut down on their smoking habits to encourage Luke to do likewise. The knowledge that Luke's hemorrhage may well have been in part a result of his heavy smoking had, of course, been a salutary experience for them.

Long-term neuropsychological and psychosocial outcome   Luke was discharged to live with his parents 3 months after his hemorrhage. He continued to attend speech and physical therapy as an outpatient twice a week for a further three months. An assessment of his language functions 6 months posthemorrhage demonstrated that his ability to speak spontaneously and with normal intonation was almost back to normal levels. He still occasionally missed function words and at times had trouble finding the right word, although when cued by the first letter he could normally produce it. His repetition was now good, as was his comprehension of auditory and written material. He had completely recovered from his apraxia and had regained reasonable strength in his right arm.

At this point, Luke was given a full neuropsychological assessment, which demonstrated that his nonverbal, visuospatial abilities were average and his verbal abilities were low average. His level of verbal ability may have been in part a result of his left frontal damage and aphasia but was also almost certainly a reflection of poorer verbal skills before his hemorrhage. He had always been a poor reader and as a Maori had struggled with the European-style schooling system. In addition, many of the neuropsychological tests available to assess him at that time were probably culturally inappropriate, the visuospatial tests less so than the verbal tests. This problem highlights the importance of developing appropriate tests with appropriate normative data for the various different cultures and subcultures the neuropsychologist assesses (Ogden 2001a; Ogden, Cooper, and Dudley 2003; Ogden and McFarlane-Nathan 1997).

Luke did well on all the memory tests he was given, but he performed poorly on a test of word fluency. Word fluency frequently remains impaired following recovery from Broca's aphasia, suggesting that it is not entirely a test of language but may also be a test of initiation and the use of strategies for performing a task. This idea is supported by the finding that people who suffer left frontal lesions but no aphasia also have problems with word fluency tasks.

Following his 6-month assessment, Luke and his therapists had a meeting and decided that his recovery had plateaued at near-normal levels and that further improvement would occur slowly as he proceeded with as normal a life as possible. Luke shifted from his parents' house into a house with his friends. With the help of the rehabilitation unit, he was able to obtain a part-time job doing light work weeding and planting in a plant nursery. A year later, he was working at the nursery full time, had a steady partner, and was driving a car (although he no longer rode motorbikes). He reported that he drank alcohol no more than once a week, and even then he kept his alcohol consumption to moderate levels; also, he had given up smoking. He said he felt that his speech had improved even further and gave him trouble only when he was tired or had had a couple of drinks. He said this was a good reason to cut down on his alcohol consumption; everyone thought he was drunk long before he really was.

Luke declined the offer of a final follow-up assessment, but his comments provided a much more appropriate outcome measure:

> I reckon that the important thing is me getting on okay, and it doesn't matter too much what all them tests show. Seems to me I might do better not to know how you fellas think I'm doin' and just get on with my life. Don't take it personal, I've got you lot to thank for my job, and giving up all those bad habits like drinking and

smoking and others I won't mention in your presence! The only thing I'm really sorry about is giving up the bikes. I just might get another bike now I know I'm okay again. I think that hemorrhage put some sense into my nut, so I'll be the guy in the slow lane from now on!

Case 2: Beth

Background   Beth lived an active life in a rural community from the time of her marriage to a farmer at the age of 21 until she awoke one morning confused and muddled in her speech. The previous day she had celebrated her 62nd birthday with her husband and her three adult children and their families. She had retired to bed in the early evening, well before the festivities were over, complaining that she felt very tired. Her husband later recalled that he had noticed that her speech had become a little jumbled after dinner, but he had attributed this to the excitement of the day and her fatigue. In retrospect, Beth may have been suffering from a *transient ischemic attack (TIA)* caused by spasm and narrowing of her left middle cerebral artery and a decrease in the blood flow and oxygen supply to the posterior part of her left hemisphere. During the night this developed into a full stroke.

In the morning her doctor visited Beth and, after diagnosing a stroke, called an ambulance to transport her the 80 km to Auckland Hospital. A CT scan of her brain some 15 hours or longer after her suspected stroke showed an area of low density in the region of her left temporoparietal cortex, and an angiogram demonstrated a complete blockage of the inferior division of her left middle cerebral artery. She was started on warfarin, a drug that causes thinning of the blood and thus sometimes allows blood to pass through a narrowed vessel, reversing a thrombotic stroke. Unfortunately, the medication did not improve Beth's condition. That area of her cortex had been deprived of oxygen for too long and a nonreversible infarction had resulted.

Beth's speech was fluent and reasonably melodic but often almost incomprehensible. She frequently seemed to have an understanding of the general meaning of what was said to her, although this was sometimes difficult to assess because of her jumbled speech, punctuated with many phonemic paraphasias. She seemed unable to repeat words or sentences, although repetition was difficult to assess properly because of her poor ability to understand instructions. When she was shown a page of writing, she attempted to read it aloud, but again her words often came out as paraphasias, although she occasionally read single words correctly. She was given a paper and pencil and asked to write her name. She managed this, although when she got to the *t* of "Beth," she wrote it four times before writing the *h*.

Beth did not seem particularly upset or frustrated by her difficulties, and she happily chatted to her family whenever there was a gap in their conversation. She almost certainly had a right visual-field defect, given the location of her infarct, although this was difficult to test accurately because of her inability to follow verbal instructions. She had no limb weakness, but she could not feel light touch on her right arm (as a result of damage to the primary sensory cortex).

The following transcript of a conversation I had with Beth about 2 weeks following her stroke provides a good illustration of her fluent but confused oral language and impaired comprehension, typical of jargon or Wernicke's aphasia.

JAO: Do you like to be called Elizabeth or Beth?

Beth: (Laughing) Oh no, I've got to be called Beth.

JAO: Do you know where you are now?

Beth: Oh yes, its 200 and just a 150 millibits from Where the hell am I now . . . from down here.

JAO: So where do you live?

Beth: I live away down from up here.

JAO: What is it called, do you remember? Can you say the name of the place?

Beth: This is W————. . . and you go up to O————. . . and you keep on up to there to W————. . . and that's 200 kiraneekers, and that's my plin. (Beth's pronunciation of the Maori place names was correct or almost correct).

JAO: Is it by the sea?

Beth: No, its about, about 3 minutes from here, and then it comes out. (Laughs) Can you fix that one up?

JAO: Can I understand that? Not all of it.

Beth: No.

JAO: Do you know what you're saying inside your head?

Beth: Oh yes, (laughs) oh yes, I don't know that alright.

JAO: What does it sound like to you when it comes out?

Beth: Well he's . . . umm . . . well he's never been, you see, you can't, you can't fill the nimbufill (laughs) sillo.

JAO: It must be very frustrating.

Beth: I know what I sing, oh yes, I know the truth. The sillo banger. I don't say nothing that's frivo, 'cause I think it's impilivariver, and it's what you fancy with you can care a little bit of patrinta. You get the next one, and you come and get the ne-e-xt one, and you can't get that one.

JAO: And you can't get that word. Oh, it must be really frustrating.

My translation of Beth's last statement goes something like this. "I know what I sound like, oh yes I know the truth. The silly bits? I don't say anything that's frivolous, 'cause I think it's important, and it's what you fancy you can do with care and a little bit of patience. You get the next one (word), and you come to the next one, and you can't get that one." Occasional comments would be said strongly and fluently and almost sounded as if they were coming from another person with completely normal language. For example, Beth interrupted her own comments when trying to answer my question about where she was, with the question "Where the hell am I now?" said in a totally normal tone, as if to remind herself of the question she was meant to be answering. One hypothesis is that these spontaneous comments come from the right hemisphere, which is thought to possess some capacity to express exclamations and expletives.

Beth remained in the hospital for 3 weeks; although she had speech therapy daily, no improvement was noted in either her speech or comprehension. At the end of the second week, she began to demonstrate some frustration at times, as illustrated by the following.

> Speech Pathologist: (Pointing to a cup) What is this?
> Beth: (Shaking her head vigorously from side to side) Go away, take it over, go away, go away, no, not me, not it again, go away.

Long-term neuropsychological and psychosocial outcome   Beth was transferred to a private nursing home, where she remained until her death from a second, much more extensive, stroke 4 years later. During those 4 years, her speech and comprehension did not improve. At first, when she was settled in the lounge of the nursing home with the other patients, she would chatter happily at them, although they could not understand most of what she was saying. After a number of weeks, she became increasingly withdrawn and would often sit passively in front of the television for hours on end. The occupational therapist made an attempt to interest her in knitting, which she had been skilled at in the past, but Beth seemed unable to coordinate her hands, possibly because of a mild sensory loss in her right hand. She would sometimes get up from her chair and wander aimlessly about the nursing home and would have to be led back to her room. Beth required full nursing care and was often incontinent if not taken to the toilet regularly. She usually ate whatever was put in front of her but never asked for more food or drink. One possibility is that Beth sustained numerous small hypertensive strokes while in the nursing home, and her deterioration may have been caused by the accumulation of brain damage from these small strokes, resulting in vascular dementia (see Chapter 17).

Her family visited her regularly but found their visits distressing because Beth rarely seemed to recognize them and only once showed visible emotion, which was when Beth's youngest daughter brought her new baby to see Beth. She placed the baby in Beth's arms, and when she took the baby back and bent to kiss Beth goodbye, she was distressed to see tears welling up in Beth's eyes and rolling unheeded down her cheeks. Usually, however, Beth gave no outward signs of feeling upset when her family left or if they did not visit.

Beth spent the last 4 years of her life in a world where she could not communicate effectively with other humans. What her thoughts and feelings were over this period remains unknown and raises the question of whether we can reason if we have lost "inner speech" along with loss of the ability to construct and understand coherent verbal language. If we cannot think and reason verbally, can we experience emotions fully? This question is addressed further in terms of the right, nonverbal hemisphere's capacity for self-awareness in split-brain subjects (see Chapter 18). Beth's occasional signs of frustration and the one instance of emotional response to her infant granddaughter suggest that she did have the capacity to reason and feel emotions and that her increasingly passive and withdrawn behaviors were an understandable psychological response to her inability to communicate.

Discussion

The ability to communicate with others is clearly one of the most valued functions we possess. Verbal language is generally considered the most important communication medium for humans, although there are cases of humans who are unable to communicate verbally but can do so successfully in other nonverbal ways. Often, however, even these nonverbal means of communicating are essentially a language. The sign language of the deaf, for example, uses the fingers to produce letters and words and the visual or tactile system to receive the language rather than the tongue and mouth to produce the language and the auditory system to receive it. If Beth had been skilled at sign language before her stroke, it is likely that she would have lost the ability to communicate in this medium as well as losing the ability to communicate using speech.

True nonverbal communication involves the expression and comprehension of gestures that cannot easily be expressed in words or with symbols and that have the same meaning for the communicator and the receiver. When tears welled up in Beth's eyes, her daughter felt distressed because Beth was communicating her sadness. The expression and understanding of emotions add richness to our relationships and communications, but our ability to use emotional, nonverbal communications to succeed, and sometimes simply to survive, in our complex human world is severely limited. Presumably, the evolution of verbal language went hand in hand with the increasing ability of the human species to reason and think abstractly. Humans were thus able to increase the complexity of their world. Modern humans could not survive in the world they have constructed without the ability to think and communicate with symbols and words. Emotions and other forms of nonverbal expression, although often communicating subtleties of meaning that words could never fully communicate, are nevertheless not specific enough to allow us to go about our daily activities easily and successfully.

The breakdown of language is devastating for the patient and distressing for everyone with whom the patient tries to communicate. Losing the ability to comprehend language appears, for a number of reasons, to be more disabling than losing the ability to express language while retaining the ability to comprehend it. When comprehension is severely impaired, expressed language becomes incomprehensible. When comprehension is reasonably intact, most individuals who have expressive impairments can find other, nonverbal ways to express themselves. In addition, if they can comprehend, it is likely that they have "inner speech" and can think and reason in words. Thus, their inability to speak and write, although extremely frustrating and debilitating, is less likely to impinge on their sense of self, their intellect, and their personality.

Beth and Luke provide examples of two common forms of aphasia, but the complexity of the brain–behavior relations in language and the rich anatomical and functional connections between the expressive and receptive language areas make categorization of aphasia a tricky task for the clinician. Other types of aphasia, such as transcortical motor and sensory aphasia, were described earlier in this chapter, and many other combinations can occur (Caplan 2003). Whereas it is of theoretical interest to examine a CT or MRI scan of the brain in an attempt to delineate the lesion the patient has suffered and to try and understand how that lesion might relate to the pattern of language impairment and sparing the patient demonstrates, in many cases it may not be possible to slot the patient into any of the traditional aphasia categories. In practical terms, it is usually more useful (from the rehabilitation point of view) simply to describe all the patient's impairments without labeling the aphasia type and to plan a rehabilitation program that addresses each impaired aspect of language in a way that is appropriate for that particular individual. Concurrently, as with all rehabilitation programs that focus on neuropsychological impairments, it is important to address the psychosocial problems that result from the patient's changed status and to work actively toward preventing long-term psychosocial problems from developing in the future.

Luke and Beth differ considerably not only in the type of aphasia they have but also in their *etiology* (cause of the disorder) and *prognosis* (probable course the disorder will take). Luke's brain damage was caused by a hemorrhage into the brain tissue, and as the blood was reabsorbed, many of the neurons that had been rendered dysfunctional by the CVA began functioning again, although others were probably permanently damaged. In some cases, an intracerebral hematoma can occur during a different type of hemorrhage, called a *subarachnoid hemorrhage* (SAH), in which blood is expelled at high pressure from a weak point on an artery, dispersing blood around the outside of the brain within the subarachnoid space (see Chapter 12). Sometimes the blood is also expelled at high pressure into the brain tissue, causing a localized hematoma. If Luke had suffered an SAH, however, a CT scan probably would have shown blood around the brain, and a lumbar puncture would have shown red blood cells in his cerebrospinal fluid.

Luke's youth may well have contributed to his ability to recover, both in terms of the plasticity of his brain (i.e., perhaps other neurons were able to take on the functions of the damaged neurons) and because his health was generally good. Also, his energy levels and motivation to recover were high.

In contrast, Beth's lesion was caused by blockage of an artery, resulting in the death of the neurons in a large area of cortex. Fiber tracts may also have been permanently damaged. Even so, had Beth been younger, healthier, and more motivated to get well, she might have shown some improvement over time and with a lot of hard work. If substantial improvement had occurred, it might have been because some pockets of neurons were transiently damaged but not destroyed by the stroke or because other cortical areas were able to take over some functions.

The type of aphasia is related not to the etiology of the lesion, but to the location of the lesion. The pattern of recovery or the rate at which the language deficits worsen are, however, related to the etiology of the lesion. If Luke's lesion had resulted from an infarction, he may not have recovered his speech to the same extent, and if Beth's aphasia had been caused by an intracerebral hematoma, she may have had a better prognosis.

6

A Body in the Mind

A Case of Autotopagnosia

One of the most exciting aspects of working in the area of clinical neuropsychology is the ever-present possibility that a patient will present with behaviors you have never seen before and at first find almost unbelievable. Even when your case is very unusual, a literature search will probably turn up a few other cases with similar symptoms. These cases will provide you with some background knowledge and assist you in your choice of tests with which to begin assessing and comparing your patient with previous cases. Nevertheless, it is likely that the case will not be exactly the same as other published cases, and you may need to use all your creativity to design new tests that will enable you to gradually narrow down the possible underlying causes of your patient's deficits. If the patient has a stable brain lesion, you will be able to take your time and not only read the literature carefully but also analyze one set of test results before embarking on the design of follow-up tests. Michael, the man with visual agnosia and prosopagnosia, is an example of such a case (Chapter 8). His lesion is stable, and his deficits have remained relatively unchanged over many years, allowing thoughtful and ongoing assessment of his deficits to test new hypotheses about brain–behavior relations.

A different type of challenge arises when your patient has a transient lesion, such as a blood clot in the brain tissue (*intracerebral hematoma*), that may resolve along with any deficits as the blood is reabsorbed. At the other end of the spectrum are rapidly changing lesions, such as malignant tumors. These tumors are often treated with steroids to reduce the swelling around them, which often results in a speedy resolution of the unusual symptoms you were interested in assessing. Alternatively, the tumor may grow rapidly, causing your patient to become increasingly confused or producing new symptoms that render the patient untestable.

Julian, the man featured in this chapter, falls into this latter category.[1] He had a sudden onset of dramatic symptoms as a consequence of a malignant tumor growing

---

1. This chapter is based on Ogden (1985c), and further details about Julian (under the initials J.P.B.) can be found in that paper.

in his left hemisphere. When he was first admitted to the hospital and it was realized how unusual some of his symptoms were, I decided to design a series of tests that would allow me to test the various hypotheses put forward in the literature. While awaiting the results of his tumor biopsy from the neuropathology laboratory, Julian was happy to participate in many hours of assessment. He became almost as intrigued as I by his strange deficits and remarked that he would rather be occupied with games and tests than worrying about what his tumor might prove to be.

Theoretical Background

Although the left hemisphere is clearly associated with language abilities, it is also important to many other cognitive functions. It is something of a paradox that some cognitive functions cannot be "observed" in people with normal brains but, rather, must be inferred following brain damage and consequent dysfunctions. Some of the dysfunctions Julian displayed are quite rare, and it is possible that this is because in many other patients with apparently similarly situated left brain lesions, these dysfunctions are masked by the more obvious language deficits that are common following left-hemispheric damage. This situation points up a variable that neuropsychologists must always take into account when observing brain–behavior relations: No two brains are exactly alike in terms of higher cognitive functions and their relationship to anatomical (or perhaps neurotransmitter) systems. Julian could not write or spell lucidly (*agraphia*), and he had a very mild word-finding difficulty (*anomia*); otherwise, his verbal abilities seemed largely spared. He could read and had no difficulty understanding speech, and his own speech was fluent and correct. Why his verbal abilities were relatively unaffected is unclear, but presumably this was a consequence of the detailed localization of language systems peculiar to his brain and the boundaries of the damage caused by his tumor. Whatever the reason, his excellent ability to understand instructions and to respond verbally made his other left-hemispheric deficits easy to assess. A brief theoretical description of each of these deficits follows.

Apraxia

Apraxia is an inability to carry out learned skilled movements (e.g., waving, brushing one's hair) despite good comprehension, full cooperation, and intact motor and sensory systems. It was first described by Jackson (1878) and Liepmann (1900, 1905), but the term is now rather loosely used to describe a range of disorders, such as dressing apraxia and constructional apraxia (see Chapter 7) as well as the more traditional apraxias such as ideomotor apraxia (or motor apraxia) and ideational apraxia.

The patient with *ideomotor apraxia* fails to carry out a motor action on verbal command but is easily able to perform it spontaneously. For example, the patient cannot poke out his tongue on command but licks his lips spontaneously. This condition is often but not always associated with certain types of aphasia, and when specific forms are present, they can provide useful language-oriented brain-localization information. One explanation postulated by Geshwind (1965) to explain ideomotor apraxia is that it is a result of a disconnection between the cortical area, which understands the spoken command, and the motor area, which produces the activity. For example, if the *arcuate fasciculus* (the fiber tract linking the receptive and expressive language areas) is damaged, it might disconnect the area for speech comprehension from the premotor area that mediates the speech action. Ideational apraxia appears to be rarer and has been defined in various, rather confusing ways. De Renzi, Pieczuro, and Vignolo (1968) describe it as an inability to handle real objects, although the use of the object can be pantomimed. The two types of apraxia overlap and are often observed in a mixed form in Alzheimer's patients.

Gerstmann's Syndrome

This constellation of four deficits—agraphia, acalculia, right-left disorientation, and finger agnosia—was first described by Gerstmann (1930, 1927) and further detailed by Critchley (1953). A recent review of the various disorders that make up Gerstmann's syndrome can be found in Denburg and Tranel (2003). There is considerable controversy over whether Gerstmann's syndrome exists at all. It has been argued that this group of symptoms may occasionally be found simply because they are each mediated by anatomical systems that are physically close to one another, not because they are intrinsically or functionally bound together, perhaps because all the symptoms have some cognitive subcomponents in common (Caplan 2003; Critchley 1966). When some symptoms are present without the others, one argument in support of Gerstmann's syndrome states that this may be because certain symptoms require more severe damage to the underlying system than others, or because the part of the system common to all the symptoms has been spared. The more parsimonious explanation is that the symptoms are indeed entirely independent of one another and that calling it a *syndrome* is misleading. This dilemma regarding syndromes is not uncommon (Caplan 2003) and can be easily resolved if syndromes are simply viewed as descriptive terms without the necessity for explanations as to why those symptoms tend to occur together. When the four Gerstmann symptoms coexist, the lesion is almost always in the posterior left parietal lobe, often involving the parieto-occipital junction region.

Agraphia refers to difficulties with writing (Roeltgen 2003). Because writing is a complex skill requiring the cooperation of a number of abilities, agraphia can result from lesions in many parts of the brain and a range of different deficits. For example, patients with right parietal lesions often repeat elements when writing (see Chapter 7); this is called visuospatial agraphia. The agraphia usually associated with Gerstmann's syndrome results in writing or printing that is well formed, but spelling and word order are often incorrect and omissions are frequent (Kinsbourne and Rosenfield 1974). *Alexia* (a reading impairment) is not present; therefore, the patient can read his poorly written sentences and often see that they are incorrect.

Finger agnosia simply refers to not knowing (agnosia) the fingers; that is, the person cannot name the fingers (e.g., index finger) or point or move a finger when the name is given. Also, he may not recognize which finger has been touched by the examiner. Obviously this disorder cannot be readily assessed in patients who are aphasic or who have sensory loss in their fingers.

Right-left disorientation refers to confusion in discriminating a rightward direction from a leftward direction. It is often assessed by asking the patient to point to left and right body parts on themselves or on a picture of the front or back view of a person; or the patient may be asked to find her way through a street map by following verbal commands to turn left or right. Although this can be viewed as a spatial disorder, it is almost always consequent on a posterior left (or dominant) hemispheric lesion.

Acalculia is a deficit in calculating (Denburg and Tranel 2003). Calculation is another example of a very complex function that can be disturbed by lesions in many areas, including right parietal lesions that result in a difficulty with manipulating the spatial positions of figures. Patients with left-hemispheric lesions are more likely to have difficulties with the logical-grammatical relationships involved in, for example, "take away 6 from 10." The problem seems to arise from not being able to interpret the meaning of "take away," and these patients are as likely to add the two numbers together as to subtract them. Thus, this may be a subtle type of comprehension impairment, even in a patient who generally appears to have normal language comprehension.

Autotopagnosia

This rare disorder is associated either with generalized brain damage (Pick 1922) or with lesions of the left parietal lobe (De Renzi 1982; Ogden 1985c). The main symptom is an inability to point on verbal command to human body parts, either one's own or those on another person (or doll or picture of a human). Patients with this disorder vary with regard to the exact symptomology they display. For example, Dennis (1976) described a patient who had a word-naming deficit that was specific to naming parts of the body, and De Renzi and Scotti (1970) reported a case of a patient who had difficulty pointing to parts of inanimate objects on command in addition to an inability to point to body parts.

The varying symptoms of patients with an inability to point to body parts have stimulated a range of hypotheses about the underlying cognitive deficits causing the disorder (Denburg and Tranel 2003). One hypothesis postulates that it is a language-related problem (e.g., a category-specific comprehension deficit; McCarthy and Warrington 1990); this hypothesis fits well with the association of the disorder with a lesion in the posterior left (language) hemisphere. A second hypothesis suggests that it is the result of a more generalized difficulty with pointing to the parts of any object (De Renzi and Scotti 1970). This hypothesis has a visuospatial aspect and, as such, fits well with the location of the causative lesion in the (visuospatial) parietal lobe. The third hypothesis postulates that the inability to point to human body parts is the result of a disruption of a discrete body image that is mediated by systems in the region of the left parietal lobe (Ogden 1985c). Although intriguing, this concept is more difficult to link to the type of abilities we usually associate with either the left hemisphere or the parietal lobe.

Careful and creative assessment of the patterns of ability and disability of single cases that demonstrate autotopagnosia enable the examination and refinement of various theories about the complex cognitive functions underlying the disorder. Of course, as with all higher cognitive disorders, it is clear that a complex disability such as autotopagnosia could occur for more than one underlying reason. A subtle disruption of language comprehension, for example, or an inability to analyze complex wholes into parts may cause the disorder. When patients who fit each of these hypotheses have been described, it is important that all these possibilities are carefully explored in new cases. If they can be ruled out as explanations for the new case, then new hypotheses that are perhaps more specific to the disorder can be tested. Julian's case provides an excellent illustration of this type of neuropsychological hypothesis testing. Frequently, despite the experimenter's best efforts to test the new hypothesis fully, sooner or later another researcher will come up with yet another possible explanation for the disorder that the assessment has not ruled out. Often, depending on the type of brain lesion and the degree of recovery or deterioration, it is not possible to return to the patient later to carry out further testing.

Such hypothesis testing using single cases (also see Chapters 3 and 8) is an exciting aspect of clinical neuropsychology that draws on clinical skills and knowledge as well as knowledge of experimental single case methodology and cognitive psychology (Carramazza and McCloskey 1988). Some rare disorders are of limited duration, especially in patients with traumatic or rapidly progressive lesions.

The challenge is considerable for the neuropsychologist, who must obtain informed consent for the proposed research from the patient, read the relevant literature, devise the appropriate tests and assessment procedures, and assess the patient, adapting and creating new tests where necessary. All this must occur before clinical treatment, such as steroid medication, reduces brain swelling and the symptoms of interest along with it, or spontaneous recovery occurs. In some situations, the patient's cognitive state worsens, masking the disorder of interest, or a deteriorating medical condition renders further assessment impossible or unethical. Obviously, from the experimental point of view, it is better to study cognition in patients who have stable lesions, such as infarctions (e.g., Michael in Chapter 8), but when a patient with a very rare disorder, such as autotopagnosia, comes along, it is important to seize the opportunity to find out more if, of course, the patient is clearly willing.

Case Presentation

Background

Until his admission to Auckland Hospital at the age of 59, Julian lived a contented life with his wife, Anne, in a small seaside town in the sunny far north of New

Zealand. He worked as an automobile and boat mechanic and spent his spare time fishing and "messing about in boats." The first sign that all was not well was the gradual onset of a weakness of Julian's right arm after a long weekend sailing trip, which Julian put down to tiredness and advancing age. Soon after, Anne's concern grew when she noticed he was having difficulty writing, and he had two minor car accidents when he veered to the right. Within 3 months a right-arm weakness spread to his right leg until he was unable to stand alone. He was also becoming increasingly confused. After seeing his local doctor, Julian was flown to Auckland and admitted to the Auckland Hospital neurology ward. On neurological examination, he demonstrated a right visual-field cut (*homonymous hemianopia*) to confrontation, mild weakness of his right arm and leg, and preserved tactile sensation on his right side but right-sided tactile extinction on double simultaneous stimulation (see Chapter 7). When blindfolded, he was unable to name objects placed in his right hand, but he could name them when placed in his left hand. His comprehension seemed unimpaired and his speech was fluent and normal.

A computed tomography (CT) scan of his brain (Fig. 6-1) revealed a large, well-

Figure 6-1 A computed tomography scan with contrast of Julian's brain showing a large metastatic carcinoma in the posterior left parietal lobe. The left hemisphere is on the left side of the scan. The most inferior or lowest cut through the brain is in the top left corner of the figure, and the most superior or upper cut is in the bottom right corner. (From Ogden 1985c, p. 1011, by permission of Oxford University Press.)

defined cystic mass with surrounding edema in the left parietal region of his brain, causing a slight midline shift from left to right. Julian responded rapidly to steroid medication, regaining strength in his right limbs and becoming fully alert, orientated, and in his own words, able to "think clearly" again. He underwent a biopsy of the mass 7 days after admission to the hospital, and a week later he and Anne were given the disturbing results. The mass had proved to be an unusually large metastatic carcinoma, and further tests revealed a primary tumor in his lung. Metastatic brain tumors are highly malignant, with a survival rate after diagnosis often a matter of months. The large size of this tumor and the 3-month history of symptoms suggested that it had grown to this size very rapidly and that Julian's condition would probably deteriorate quickly, even with the reduction of edema afforded by the steroids.

Julian was in the hospital for 2 weeks before the results of his biopsy were known, and throughout this period he remained optimistic about his future. Six days after admission he was alert, fully orientated, and cooperative, and he was keen to "have a go" at various neuropsychological tests. Throughout 8 days of extensive testing, he remained jovial but appropriate and demonstrated excellent insight into his performance. I kept him and Anne informed about my reasons for carrying out the various experimental tests, and he frequently expressed amazement at his own dramatic impairments. As always, when assessing neuropsychological disorders, especially in single case studies, it is often instructive to observe and note the patient's behavior and comments carefully. If the patient agrees, it is helpful to film the assessment for later analysis, which was done in Julian's case.

Neuropsychological Assessment

Overall verbal, visuospatial, and memory abilities   Julian was strongly right-handed, as were both of his parents, his three siblings, and one of his two children. As his wife was left-handed, it is likely that their left-handed child inherited his handedness from her. It was reasonable, therefore, to assume that Julian was left-hemisphere dominant for language.

An aphasia assessment demonstrated that his conversation was intelligent, clear, and fluent, and he showed a readiness to initiate conversation. On tests of oral language comprehension, he scored easily within normal range, and his comprehension was also good when it was assessed by asking him questions about a passage he had just read. He scored in the normal range when asked to tell a story about a complex picture, to read single words and complex paragraphs aloud, and to match written words with pictures and vice versa. When asked to pick specific objects from an array of objects, he did so without hesitation or error. On naming tasks, he occasionally struggled to find the correct word, but he could describe the function or shape of the thing he was trying to name. On an oral word-fluency task, he performed at the lower end of average range. He had writing difficulties, which will be described later.

On the WAIS (given before later versions of the Wechsler Adult Intelligence Scales were available on our service), he scored in the average to high-average range on all the verbal subtests except arithmetic, with which he had great difficulty. On the Performance scale, he scored poorly on most of the tests and found the Digit Symbol and Block Design tests almost impossible. Further assessment of his visuospatial construction skills demonstrated that although he could not put patterns together, he usually knew when his attempts were incorrect. This result suggested that his difficulties may have been related more to a difficulty with construction than the result of a pure visuospatial deficit. On the Wechsler Memory Scale, Julian demonstrated severe deficits on the verbal learning tests, although his score for the simple nonverbal memory test, Visual Reproduction, was normal.

Apraxias   *Dressing apraxia*: On admission, Julian demonstrated great difficulty in putting the correct arms and legs into his pajamas, even when these were held in place for him. He was fully aware of his confusion. By the eleventh day, he was able to dress himself correctly.

Ideomotor apraxia: During the first 8 days, Julian could not wave, salute, or pantomime stirring a cup of coffee, brushing his teeth, or hammering a nail into wood with either hand on verbal command, although he could accurately identify these actions when performed by the examiner. He was often aware of his difficulties and made comments such as "How stupid I am. That is not a salute!" His ability to imitate these actions was slightly better but still clumsy. He also had oral apraxia demonstrated by his inability to poke out his tongue, blow, or pretend to sip through a straw on verbal command, despite having normal spontaneous movements of his mouth and tongue.

Ideational apraxia: Occasionally, Julian demonstrated elements of ideational apraxia when using real objects. For example, when asked to pick up a toothbrush from an array of objects in front of him and to brush his teeth, he picked up the toothbrush and began shaving with it. The conversation then proceeded as follows:

> Examiner: What are you doing?
>   Julian: Well I'm shaving, aren't I?
> Examiner: What's that in your hand?
>   Julian: A toothbrush.
> Examiner: What do you normally do with a toothbrush?
>   Julian: Brush my teeth, of course!
> Examiner: Where are your teeth?
>   Julian: Where are my teeth? (laughing) Well, my teeth are in my mouth presumably!
> Examiner: Show me how you would brush your teeth.

At this point, Julian once again began to shave with the toothbrush. He realized he was not doing it correctly and said, "Damn, I can't seem to do it."

Gerstmann's syndrome   Julian had clear evidence of all the symptoms of Gerstmann's syndrome, and these persisted throughout his stay in the hospital.

Agraphia: At first Julian was unable to hold a pencil in his right hand, but on the sixth day he demonstrated severe agraphia for both spontaneous writing and copying a printed sentence when using his left nondominant hand. He had difficulty forming letters and would, for example, form a *B* instead of a *J* and a *c* instead of an *a*. He would often exclaim, "That is not what I wanted to write. I wanted a *J*, not a *B*." By the tenth day, he was able to hold a pencil in his right hand but made similar mistakes as with his left hand. When asked to print the sentence, "I will be very pleased when I can go home," he printed in capitals "I WILL BE EVEY LLEASED WENW I CAN GO HOEM." In contrast, his oral spelling was good, and he spelled 18 of 20 words correctly. These included regular as well as irregularly spelled words, such as *debt, rogue, mortgage*, and *subtle*. His reading was also correct and fluent, if rather slow. That is, he had agraphia without alexia (reading impairment).

Right-left confusion: Julian confused right and left frequently and was unaware of his errors. This confusion persisted even when his other deficits improved.

Acalculia: Although Julian could read numbers and understood their value (e.g., "2 is a very small number, 22 is much larger, and 100 is very large"), he was unable to carry out even simple calculations other than addition. For example, he could not subtract 6 from 10 and tended to add the two numbers together. He was also unable to multiply or divide. When given a string of numbers and asked to repeat them backwards (Digit Span), he was never able to get more than three digits backward and usually only made it to two. He commented that he could not understand how to go about saying them backward. He also sometimes had problems with simple logical-grammatical relationships, such as responding to the command "Place the pencil under the book." He was equally likely to put the pencil on top of the book as under it, which suggests that his acalculia may also be a problem related to logical-grammatical relationships such as "take away" or subtract.

Finger agnosia: Julian could not name or number his fingers on either hand (or someone else's fingers) when I touched them, whether or not he was looking at them. He was also given a "nonnaming" test of finger agnosia by being asked, while blind-folded, to say how many fingers lay between two fingers being touched by me. He failed this as well.

Autotopagnosia   On the sixth day after admission, Julian was able to name quickly and accurately any body part I pointed to, whether it was his own body, a doll's body, or a photograph of a man's naked body. In stark contrast, he made numerous errors when I named a body part and asked him to point to it. His strategy seemed to be to search the body until his eyes rested on the body part for which he was searching. His search usually commenced somewhere on the upper part of the body, and if he did not happen on the body part, he seemed unaware that he should look lower down, below the waist. When I asked him to point to specific parts below the waist, he would often look puzzled and comment, "I can't reach that," or "That part seems to have disappeared." On one occasion I was sitting directly in front of him with my hands on my knees and asked him to point to my hand. He looked all over my upper half, exclaiming, "Where's it gone?" At one point, he accidentally touched my hand with his. He clearly realized he should have been able to locate body parts and often laughed at his own inability to find them. For body parts above the waist, he would sometimes indicate correctly, apparently as a result of his eyes falling on the body part during his search, but even in these cases he often expressed uncertainty. He would often indicate the wrong part; for example, the wrist for the elbow, or he would touch the shoulder (on command to point to the elbow) and then gradually move his hand along the arm until he reached the elbow and say, "It's about here."

On days 10 to 12 after admission, Julian was formally tested on his ability to name body parts I pointed to on himself, myself, three dolls, and a photograph of a naked man. In total 78 body parts were pointed to, and his naming responses were correct on all of them. He was then asked to point to named body parts on the same bodies (124 commands in all). He was also blindfolded and asked to point to named body parts on himself (30 commands in total). Throughout testing he was asked to use his right hand for half the responses and his left hand for the other half. He made an approximately equal number of errors with each hand. His results on these tests of pointing to body parts on verbal command demonstrated a greater inability to locate body parts on other people's bodies (mine or a photograph) than on his own body, whether sighted or blindfolded, and if his numerous right-left errors were ignored. Strangely, when Julian was asked to point to items of named clothing on himself or me (nine commands), he was quick and accurate, although he still demonstrated left-right confusion (e.g., for left shirt cuff he pointed to right shirt cuff).

When Julian was presented with an array of pictures of isolated body parts and asked to point to specific parts on verbal command, he responded without difficulty, demonstrating that his comprehension of body-part names was normal. He was also given a nonverbal test of locating body parts to ensure that his difficulty was not related to a language comprehension deficit. He was shown pictures of the front and back of a naked man with numbers on different body parts. He was then asked to point to the part on his body that corresponded to specific numbered parts on the drawing. He demonstrated that he was able to point to the numbers correctly, but in 12 responses he made six errors when pointing to the corresponding body part on himself (excluding left-right errors). Thus, he still demonstrated autotopagnosia even when comprehension of body-part names was not required.

The qualitative data obtained throughout Julian's assessment often proved instructive in understanding his deficits. For example, when I asked Julian to point to the doll's stomach, he looked puzzled and moved his finger up and down the doll saying, "Where has the stomach gone to? It seems to have disappeared. How silly!" Later, when asked to point to the doll's elbow, he pointed to its stomach and said, "Here is her elbow; it is probably a bit further up." When asked to point to his own eyebrow, he pointed to his eye and said, "It is about here; the eyebrow might be a bit further up." On being asked to point to the doll's armpit, he pointed to its groin. When I pointed out his error and asked him to tell me why he thought he went wrong, he said, "I start at the bottom and then seem to get lost in space from where I am." Julian's comments and methods of finding body parts seemed to indicate that he had difficulty remembering exactly where they should be in relation to the body.

When asked to draw a stick figure of a man, Julian's drawing looked reasonably accurate. I then asked him where the foot would go and he pointed to the arm, drew a stick at the end of it, and said, "It would go here on the end of the leg." I then asked him where the hand would go and he pointed to the "foot" he had just drawn on the end of the arm and said, "His hand would go here on the end of the foot—no, that's not right, the hand goes on the arm." Julian was shown a model of a face with removable features that slotted into holes on the face. I removed the parts while he watched and then asked him to put them back. He named each part correctly as he picked it up but put the ears where the eyes should go, the eyes where the ears should go, the mouth on top of the head where a hat was meant to slot in, and the nose in the correct place. He then went to put the spectacles on and said, "They won't fit, the ears are in the way!" He then attempted to put the hat on top of the head and found the mouth was in the way. He then realized there was something wrong. A few days later, when I asked him to do it again, he got it correct; but when I asked him if he remembered how he had done it previously, he was greatly amused and said, "I had things everywhere! The mouth on top of the head and the eyes and ears mixed up!"

Julian's problem was not caused by his perception and identification of body parts in isolation. When his attention was drawn to a particular part on a body, or when he was given a picture or model of an isolated body part, he could always name it accurately. He also knew the function of the parts, but when he was asked to describe the location of body parts, he had some difficulties. For example, when asked what a mouth was for, he replied it was for eating, drinking, and talking. When asked what a foot was for, he replied there were two of them and they were to stand on and walk with. When he was asked where his left foot was however, he replied, "My left foot is down underneath my left boot. At the end of my left leg." For "right thigh" he answered, "Opposite side to my left thigh. It is a thick and heavy piece, around my middle." His description of the location of his right elbow was, "About the middle of my body. Just below my right elbow bone." He said his ear was "underneath my eyebrow," and his mouth was "in the middle of my face—between my two nostrils, underneath my eyes."

His deficit was not part of a more generalized inability to analyze wholes into parts: In contrast to his difficulties in locating body parts, his ability to locate parts of objects and animals was normal. For example, on a toy truck he pointed quickly and accurately on verbal command to the driver's seat, front wheels, flashing light, steering wheel, headlights, engine, passenger's seat, and door to the driver's seat. On a real vase of flowers, he pointed on command to a petal, leaf, the vase, water, and a stem, and on a picture of an elephant, he pointed to the mouth, eye, toes on the foreleg, tusk, tail, back leg, and ear. He could also put labels with the names of New Zealand towns in the correct places on an outline map of New Zealand, and he put the parts of a story ("Little Red Riding Hood") into the correct sequence.

Personal and Social Consequences

Although Julian's symptoms had been causing him difficulties for some months before his admission to hospital, he had not allowed them to influence his life much. In part, this may have been the result of a psychological denial mechanism sometimes observed in patients with a relatively slow onset of symptoms. Fear of a serious illness can underlie a delay in seeking medical help for both sufferers and families, and it is not particularly uncommon for patients to suffer a debilitating leg weakness or an inability to use an arm for several months before they see a doctor. In some cases this apparently unconcerned attitude may in itself be a result of brain dysfunction (especially following right parietal or bilateral frontal lobe damage; see Chapters 7 and 9), but in Julian's case, a psychological explanation seems more plausible. A delay in diagnosis and treatment can have serious consequences in the case of a progressive lesion such as a malignant tumor. If the tumor has grown too large by the time it is diagnosed, the chance of successful treatment (by surgical removal, radiotherapy, or chemotherapy) may be significantly reduced.

In Julian's case his tumor had grown unusually large by the time it was diagnosed. After a biopsy was taken, the diagnosis of a secondary metastasis (with a primary later found in the lung) was a shock to Julian and his family. Julian was offered radiotherapy, but he made a lucid and understandable decision to decline any further treatment other than steroids. This decision was based partially on his dislike of Auckland and a yearning to return to his quiet and beautiful seaside village to spend the remaining months of his life among his family and friends. On returning home, he continued to "mess about in boats" until he became too disabled to walk at all. His ability to speak and understand speech began to deteriorate 6 weeks after his discharge from hospital, and he died 3 months later.

Given the very high malignancy and size of Julian's tumor, it is debatable whether his life would have been prolonged significantly if he had remained in Auckland a further 4–6 weeks for radiotherapy. There seems little doubt that the quality of life he was able to enjoy for a few more weeks was vastly superior to the quality of life he would have had to endure by remaining within the hospital system away from the people and environment he loved.

Feeling comfortable with a patient's decision to refuse treatment is often difficult for medical professionals and therapists, perhaps because they believe it is their duty to provide the patient with every reasonable option for survival. The knowledge that in rare cases the growth of even malignant tumors such as Julian's can be significantly slowed by aggressive treatment, thus adding quality time to the patient's life span, no doubt puts pressure on many doctors to encourage treatment. It is impossible to predict how an individual patient will react on being diagnosed with a terminal illness. Some continue to fight for their lives long past the time the medical profession has given up; others continue to deny their terminal condition, and that nothing more can be done for them, even when they are totally dependent on others for their care and their quality of life seems abysmal to others. Others, like Julian, seem able to make a clear decision to live what remains of their life as well as they can, without looking for miracle cures. The important lesson for the doctor or therapist is that, wherever possible, the final decision should lie with the patient. In such a case, the most valuable contribution the medical professional can make is to give the patient as much information as possible about the prognosis and the pros and cons of available treatments both to fight the illness and to relieve the symptoms. Counseling can be offered to assist the patient in making these decisions and to facilitate coping with issues of grief, loss, and dying. At that point, the professional's role is over, and all that remains is to feel at ease with the patient or the family's decision.

Discussion

Julian was unusual in that he demonstrated a number of the relatively uncommon deficits that can follow damage to the left parietal lobe. Gerstmann's syndrome, ideomotor and ideational apraxia, and autotopagnosia are rare disorders, partly perhaps because many patients with left parietal lesions have language deficits that may mask more subtle disorders or make the assessment of other deficits difficult or impossible. Julian's autotopagnosia differed in some interesting ways from other cases of autotopagnosia in the literature. His problem was clearly not one of analyzing whole objects into their components (cf. De Renzi and Faglioni 1963; De Renzi and Scotti 1970), as he had no difficulty pointing to the parts of objects that were not human bodies. Nor did it appear to be related to a category-specific comprehension difficulty (cf. McKenna and Warrington 1978), as he could accurately point to and give the function of isolated body parts when they were presented in a random array. Julian's case provides support for the existence of a discrete body image that can be disrupted by a lesion of the left parietal lobe. His difficulty can be defined as a problem in finding the exact location of various body parts in relation to the whole body. This deficit can be explained if we assume that we rely on a mental image of the body for our knowledge of how the various body parts are related to one another. If Julian lost the ability to evoke a body image, then he will have also lost the template that tells him where to locate a body part relative to the rest of the body.

The importance of building a series of similar cases is demonstrated when Julian's case is viewed alongside other cases. Although he had Gerstmann's syndrome and apraxia, other patients with autotopagnosia have been described who do not have these deficits. Instead, they have problems with analyzing whole objects into parts or comprehending body-part names, which Julian did not have, which suggests that autotopagnosia is independent of the various symptoms that make up Gerstmann's syndrome, apraxia, and a generalized deficit of analyzing wholes into parts. As all these deficits can follow left parietal lesions in various combinations, it is likely that the cortical and subcortical substrates that mediate these different functions are anatomically close to one another. Another possibility is that these functions rely on a number of interrelated anatomical circuits and that, depending on which circuits are disconnected and where, different disorders and combinations of disorders result. If every case reported with autotopagnosia had all the other symptoms mentioned above, a more likely hypothesis would be that the same cognitive subcomponent underlies all the symptoms.

Given the very large metastasis that Julian had, it was surprising that he did not have significant language problems and that he showed little generalized mental deterioration. This case provides the neuropsychologist with a lesson in individual differences. Group studies of brain–behavior relations are useful in that they allow us to predict with some degree of confidence that a lesion to a particular area of the brain is likely to produce certain symptoms. The fact that every brain is also unique in subtle ways (analogous perhaps to faces), however, means that when we are presented with a particular individual, we cannot take for granted the pattern of his or her abilities and disabilities, even given detailed and accurate imaging of the patient's brain and lesion. An assessment that begins with a range of tests that will expose expected deficits often needs to be followed by carefully selected tests that will allow the definition of less common patterns of functioning. It is this variability in brain–behavior relations that makes neuropsychological assessment and research a continual challenge.

7

■

Out of Mind, Out of Sight

A Case of Hemineglect

Bed rounds on neurosurgical wards can be depressing affairs, and this one was no exception; that is, until we reached Janet's bed. She was a middle-aged woman and sat propped up by pillows with her left leg hanging rather awkwardly over the side of the bed. She was wearing an attractive pink nightgown and matching bed jacket, but when dressing she had apparently been unable to put her left arm into the left sleeves of the garments, leaving her shoulder exposed. The nurse touched her bare shoulder and asked her to put her arm into the sleeves. "No thank you," replied Janet. "I'd rather leave it like it is if you don't mind." "It looks rather uncomfortable" replied the nurse, "and whatever will your visitors think?" "Well," replied Janet, "I'm starting a new off-the-shoulder fashion. I would think it might cheer the visitors up." The nurse, trying to keep a straight face, offered to help Janet get her arm into the sleeve as it might be awkward for her to do it by herself. Janet was laughing by this stage, and said firmly, "Perhaps I will do it later, but I think I will leave it like this for now, if it is all the same to you doctors and nurses!"

Janet was displaying signs of the neurological disorder variously known as hemineglect, hemispatial neglect, unilateral spatial neglect, and unilateral inattention. This spatial impairment quite commonly follows focal damage to one hemisphere of the brain in humans (and also in monkeys and cats). The main symptom is an apparent unawareness or unresponsiveness to stimuli in the side of space opposite the brain damage. The stimuli may be in any modality, but in humans neglect of visual stimuli seems to be the most common form of the disorder. Neglect of the limbs opposite the brain-damaged side is also quite common, which can result in difficulties with rehabilitation (e.g., teaching a patient to walk on the "neglected" leg, or to use the "neglected" arm.) Although neglect can occur following both left-and right-hemispheric damage (Ogden 1985a, 1987a), the more severe and lasting cases of neglect usually follow right-hemispheric lesions (Heilman, Watson, and Valenstein 1993, 2003).

In the course of my doctoral research, I examined 48 patients with hemineglect (Ogden 1985a, 1985b, 1987a), and since then I have seen many more patients with this fascinating disorder (Maguire and Ogden 2002; Ogden 1987b, 1988b, 2002).

Many of these patients would make excellent subjects for this chapter, but I decided to tell Janet's story both because she demonstrated so vividly many of the classic symptoms of neglect and because of her delightful sense of humor. Often Janet's sense of humor seemed to lighten the tragic situation in which she found herself, not only for others but apparently for herself as well.

Working with neurological patients is stressful at the best of times, and patients who can on occasion laugh at themselves possibly experience a better quality of life than those who find their disorder and its consequences continuously depressing. Curiously, patients with left-sided neglect from a right-hemispheric lesion not uncommonly joke about their problems, and in cases where this is extreme or clearly inappropriate, it suggests a lack of awareness about the seriousness of their condition (labeled *indifference*) that itself seems to be the result of the right-hemispheric lesion (Gainotti 1972; Heilman, Watson, and Bowers 1983). Certainly some researchers have tentatively suggested that the right hemisphere is the "depressive" hemisphere and the left hemisphere the "happy" hemisphere (Tucker 1981). When the left hemisphere is damaged, the healthy right hemisphere may dominate emotional expression, resulting in the "catastrophic" depressive reaction sometimes seen following left-hemispheric damage. When the right hemisphere is damaged, as in Janet's case, the patient may appear indifferent or even amused by her disorder, perhaps because her emotional response is unable to be appropriately moderated by the damaged right hemisphere. In the case of patients with hemineglect following a right-hemispheric lesion, another possibility is that their comments are attempts to rationalize their strange behaviors and are not intended to be amusing. Nevertheless, the patients themselves often seem amused by their own comments.

The verbal comments made by some patients to explain their neglect or to enable them to avoid responding to stimuli in their neglected hemispace can provide some insights into the psychology of neglect. Therefore, although this study focuses on Janet's case, throughout I also draw on the behaviors and comments of other similar patients to highlight particular aspects of this class of disorders.

Theoretical Background

Descriptions and Definitions

In 1876 John Hughlings Jackson reported a patient who tried to read by starting at the lower right-hand corner of the page and proceeding backward. Among other symptoms, she also had difficulty dressing and finding her way around. At autopsy she was found to have a glioma of the right posterior hemisphere. Jackson dubbed this disorder *imperception*. Today some of her spatial difficulties would probably be considered to arise from her neglect of the left hemispace. Although a smattering of articles on spatial disorders following right-hemispheric lesions appeared in the late nineteenth century and the early twentieth century, hemineglect did not reach prominence in the neurological literature until the mid-twentieth century, probably as a result of an article published by Brain in 1941. He reported three cases of patients with large right parieto-occipital lesions whom he suggested suffered from a deficit of "spatial orientation . . . inattention to or neglect of the left half of external space" (p. 253).

Since this time the number of studies devoted to the various hemineglect/inattention disorders has steadily increased, and since the mid-1980s there has been an explosion of research papers in the area. Now it is becoming difficult to find an issue of any one of the numerous scientific journals devoted to neuropsychological study that does not contain at least one article on some aspect of hemineglect.

There are a number of reasons for the popularity of these disorders. Hemineglect is common acutely following unilateral brain lesions, and experimental subjects can be readily found in neurology wards and rehabilitation and stroke units. Research on how to improve rehabilitation methods for these patients is seen as important and increasingly well funded. Perhaps most important of all is the fascination these disorders have for scientists who are interested in what the study of impaired brain function can tell us about normal brain function. Cognitive neuropsychologists are carrying out increasingly elegant experimental manipulations in an attempt to tease apart the components of hemineglect. Although we now know a great deal about these disorders and the neuroanatomical circuits implicated in their different aspects, we are still looking for the answer to the basic question: How is it that patients do not respond overtly to the stimuli or their own limbs in their neglected hemispace, yet at another level demonstrate in various indirect ways that they are aware of their presence in that hemispace?

Hemispace refers to the *extracorporeal* (outside the body) space to the left or right of the body and head midline. It is distinct from the visual field and from the hand or ear receiving sensory input. For example, if a person places her right arm across her body, her right hand will now be in her left hemispace. Only in the situation where a person aligns body and head and visually fixates directly ahead do the left and right visual fields and left and right hemispaces coincide. If the head or eyes are moved to the left or right, the visual fields are displaced accordingly. The hemispaces are not, however, tied to eye movements, and they therefore will no longer coincide with the visual fields.

Hemineglect can occur in one or more modalities in the same patient. A patient with a right-hemispheric lesion and left-sided neglect often fails to complete the left side of drawings he is asked to copy (see Fig. 7-1), misses the words on the left side of a page he is reading, ignores people standing on his left, collides with the wall on his left when walking down a corridor, and in severe cases, eats only the dinner on the right side of his plate and then complains that he is hungry! Some patients with left-hemispheric lesions demonstrate the same types of neglect, but on the right side of space (see Fig. 7-1). Visual extinction is a less dramatic disorder that often occurs in patients with visual neglect but that has been shown to be independent of it. The patient responds to a visual stimulus seen in isolation in either the right or left visual

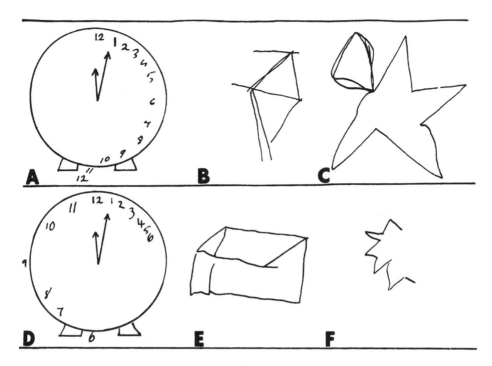

Figure 7-1 Drawing tests of hemineglect. Patients are asked to put the numbers on the clock face and to copy a cube and a five-pointed star. A–C are the drawings of three different patients with right hemispheric lesions and left visuospatial neglect. Clock A was drawn by Janet. D–F are the drawings of three different patients with left hemispheric lesions and right visuospatial neglect. (From Ogden 1985a, p. 63, by permission of Academic Press.)

fields, but when bilateral visual stimuli are presented, response is only to the stimulus in the field on the same side as the lesion. Extinction is equally frequent after right- and left-sided brain damage.

The other common form of hemineglect is neglect of the side of the body opposite the lesion, sometimes termed *motor neglect*, or *intentional neglect* (Heilman et al. 2003) because it results in a paucity of motor movements of the limbs on the affected side. For example, patients with right parietal lesions may demonstrate an apparent lack of interest in the left side of their bodies and be unwilling to incorporate it into their activities. For example, Janet was reluctant to dress the left side of her body, and she allowed her left leg to hang over the edge of the bed. Such patients often appear hemiplegic because their left arm hangs motionless or is held stiffly against the body. In some cases the patient does have a weak arm because of damage to the motor strip, but in others much of the weakness is the result of neglect rather than to a motor loss; for example, if the patient can move her arm with concentrated effort, or sometimes unconsciously moves the neglected arm to brush a fly from her face. Motor extinction is said to occur when the patient can raise either the right or left arm to command but when asked to raise both together raises only the right arm.

Less common forms of hemineglect include neglect of sounds in the hemispace opposite the lesion (*auditory neglect*) and neglect of tactile stimulation on the limbs opposite to the lesion (*tactile neglect*). Auditory and tactile extinction to the contralesional (i.e., opposite the lesion) stimulus when bilateral stimuli are presented simultaneously are more commonly demonstrated than auditory and tactile neglect.

The other fascinating group of behaviors related to hemineglect involves an unawareness or denial of hemiplegia or sensory loss, which may take the form of the patient denying that a hemiplegic limb belongs to him (*anosognosia*), or of him calling the limb unpleasant names (*misoplegia*). Some patients deny that they have lost movement or sensation in a limb or deny that they have a visual field loss. More commonly, the patient will agree that he has a hemiplegia or sensory loss but will appear quite unconcerned about it (*anosodiaphoria*).

Neuropathology

The neuroanatomical correlates of the different forms of hemineglect are complex. Even after intensive research by many neuroscientists, they are by no means well understood. In the past it was thought that lesions to the right posterior parietal lobe, especially the cortex around the temporoparietal junction, were most frequently associated with hemineglect. More recent studies using magnetic resonance imaging (MRI) brain scans have enabled detailed topographical mapping of the lesions of patients with hemineglect, and these scans show that the lesions of patients who have persisting hemineglect are large and usually encroach on two or more cortical or subcortical brain areas, the most common being the posterior parietal lobe (especially the angular gyrus), superior temporal gyrus, medial temporal lobe, frontal lobe, and the basal ganglia (Karnath, Ferber, and Himmelbach 2001; Karnath, Himmelbach, and Rorden 2002; Maguire and Ogden 2002; Mort et al. 2003). The cingulate gyrus and thalamus can also result in neglect, but this is a relatively infrequent consequence of damage to these areas (Damasio, Damasio, and Chang Chui 1980; Heilman and Valenstein 1972; Ogden 1985a; Watson and Heilman 1979). Lesions in all the same areas in the left hemisphere can also result in hemineglect of the right hemispace or limbs (Gainotti, Messerli, and Tissot 1972; Maguire and Ogden 2002; Ogden 1985a), but the symptoms tend to be much less severe and recovery more rapid (Ogden 1987a). Most patients who require rehabilitation to overcome their neglect are therefore patients with right-hemispheric damage and left-sided neglect.

Neglect is usually at its most dramatic immediately after the brain damage occurs (e.g., immediately following a stroke) or when the brain lesion is a very aggressive, highly malignant tumor (e.g., a glioma or astrocytoma growing rapidly within the brain tissue and causing surrounding swelling, or *edema*). A very large, slow-growing, benign tumor (e.g., a *meningioma*, which grows from the meninges on the surface of the brain, gradually increasing the pressure on the underlying brain) can also cause a buildup of increasingly severe neglect symptoms. The acute, dramatic symptoms of neglect frequently resolve spontaneously over a number of days to weeks. The patients in whom the most rapid resolution is seen tend to be those with large meningiomas. Such patients often come to the notice of a neurologist because they are frequently colliding with objects on one side; on examination, a meningioma is discovered. On removal of the meningioma, the neglect symptoms often resolve almost immediately, presumably because the pressure on the brain is removed. In the case of aggressive tumors, patients are often medicated with steroids in an attempt to reduce the edema that surrounds the tumor. This treatment serves to reduce the area of the dysfunctional brain tissue, and a decrease in the severity of neglect may follow. In these cases, the neglect may increase in severity again as the tumor grows.

Patients who suffer a hemorrhagic stroke (i.e., a bleed into the brain tissue) may demonstrate immediate symptoms of hemineglect, but these symptoms often resolve as reabsorption of the blood occurs, allowing some of the neurons affected by the blood to become functional again. The most common type of stroke is caused by a reduction of blood and oxygen to an area of the brain, resulting in an area of dead brain matter called an *infarction* (see Chapter 5). Patients who suffer neglect following this type of stroke, particularly when it is a large stroke occurring in the middle cerebral artery territory of the right hemisphere, are less likely to undergo a complete recovery of their neglect because the infarcted area is unable to recover. Even so, the proportion of patients who demonstrate persisting hemineglect (i.e., longer than 3 months) is very small compared to the high number who demonstrate hemineglect immediately following their stroke (Maguire and Ogden 2002).

Stroke victims whose static lesion means they are unlikely to get worse, and who also often show spontaneous recovery to a lesser or greater extent, are those most likely to benefit from rehabilitation methods aimed at teaching them to be more generally alert and more aware of their neglect and to make a conscious effort to overcome it (e.g., Robertson and Cashman 1991; Robertson and Hawkins 1999; Robertson, North, and Geggie 1992). As most people who suffer from this common type of stroke are elderly, age may be a confounding factor in the speed of recovery from neglect. Theories of neglect have proven to be useful in informing the development of promising rehabilitation methods, and theories and rehabilitation will be covered briefly in the next two sections.

Theories of Neglect

As yet, no definitive theory has been put forward to explain all the aspects and forms of neglect. Most theories tend to fall into one of two categories, attentional and representational. There are a number of attentional theories that seek to explain the neglect phenomenon as well as the finding that right-hemisphere lesions result in neglect more often than left-hemisphere lesions. Some rely on evidence that points to the right hemisphere dominating attention to both sides of space, whereas the left hemisphere attends mainly to the right side of space (e.g., De Renzi, Faglioni, and Scotti 1970). Heilman et al. (1993) view attention as a result of physiological arousal or activation. They postulate that when the right hemisphere is damaged, it is underaroused and less able to attend to both sides of space. Thus, the left side of space is relatively neglected, but the right side of space can be attended to by the intact left hemisphere. In contrast, when the left hemisphere is damaged, the intact right hemisphere can attend to the left hemispace but can also attend to the right hemispace.

Kinsbourne's (e.g., 1977) attentional hypothesis does not rely on right-hemispheric dominance for bilateral attention but postulates that both hemispheres attend to both sides of space and that each attends more to the opposite side of space. The right hemisphere influences leftward movements, and the left hemisphere influences rightward movements. Following a lesion to the right hemisphere, the nonlesioned left hemisphere can generate unopposed orienting responses toward the right side of space, biasing attention toward the right in both hemispaces. Thus, neglect is a directional phenomenon resulting in a gradient of inattention (and neglect) that is most pronounced in the far left of the left hemispace, less pronounced in the right of the left hemispace, and so on, so that attention to the far right of the right hemispace is normal (Kinsbourne 1993).

Kinsbourne (1994) also hypothesizes that there are many lateral opponent processors in the brain that mediate directional attention, and the type of neglect that results will depend on which processors are damaged. For example, this allows for the finding that some patients will neglect the contralesional side of the whole environment (*environment-centered* or *space-centered neglect*), whereas others will neglect the contralesional sides of a number of objects within the environment (*object-centered neglect*). To explain the greater severity of neglect following right-hemispheric lesions, Kinsbourne suggested that the left hemisphere is activated by the verbal interaction of the patient with the examiner, which results in attention being drawn to the right. This activation compounds the inattention to the left hemispace following a right-hemispheric lesion and compensates for the inattention to the right following a left-hemispheric lesion. The left hemisphere could also be activated by right arm and hand movement in a right-handed person carrying out paper-and-pencil neglect tasks.

Studies by Posner, Cohen, and Rafal (1982) and Posner, Walker, Friedrich, and Rafal (1984) have suggested that the reason patients with neglect have difficulty in overcoming their tendency to attend to the side of space opposite their intact hemisphere is not difficulty with moving their attention to the neglected side of space but, rather, difficulty in disengaging their attention from the nonneglected side of space. These studies showed that subjects with visual neglect, when given a visual cue that indicated where the stimulus might appear before it was presented, showed an improved ability to detect stimuli in their neglected hemispace. When the cue was on the nonneglected side but the stimulus then appeared on the neglected side, however, the subjects were more likely to miss the stimulus than under noncue conditions. That is, once they focused their attention on their nonneglected side, it seemed they had difficulty disengaging their attention.

Mesulam (1981, 1983) took account of the different areas that, if damaged, may result in neglect by postulating a cortical network for directed attention and unilateral neglect. He suggested that damage to the inferior parietal cortex would disrupt the sensory template of the extrapersonal world; that damage to the frontal cortex, including the frontal eyefields, may disrupt a motor map for the distribution of scanning, orienting, and exploration of the extrapersonal world; and that damage to the cingulate cortex and surrounding areas may disrupt a motivational map for the distribution of interest and expectancy. The arousal level of each of these areas is regulated by input from the reticular formation. If any one area is damaged, or the connections between the areas are disrupted, contralateral neglect may result. Damage to a particular area may result in a particular clinical form of neglect. For example, parietal damage may be more likely to result in sensory neglect (visual, auditory, or tactile), and a frontal lesion may be more likely to result in motor neglect. (See Ogden 1988b for a possible example of a dissociation between these two types of neglect in a single patient.) Unfortunately, given that most patients with persisting neglect have large lesions that often encroach on the frontal, parietal, temporal, and basal ganglia areas of the brain (Maguire and Ogden 2002), it has proven extremely difficult to test the hypothesis that different forms of neglect are the consequence of lesions in different brain regions or circuits.

Robertson and colleagues (Robertson, Mattingley, Rorden, and Driver 1998) have shown that patients with left neglect also have a nonlateralized problem with sustaining attention and have demonstrated that neglect can be decreased by increasing general alertness (e.g., with a loud sound).

Halligan and Marshall (1994b) have proposed a global–local processing theory to help explain left visuospatial neglect. There is evidence that the undamaged right hemisphere guides global, or holistic, processing of stimuli and directs focal attention to the spatial locations that can then be analyzed further for detail. The left hemisphere is better at attending to detail. Following a right-hemisphere lesion, the left-hemisphere processing system of the patient amplifies local-level information, and this local-level detail captures the attention of the patient in the right hemispace. The impaired global level processor has difficulty directing the patient's attention toward the left, although the patient may be able to overcome this if prompted or motivated in some way (Marshall and Halligan 1994a).

The other main theoretical approach to neglect was first suggested by De Renzi, Faglioni, and Scotti (1970). They postulated that neglect symptoms are a reflection of an underlying "mutilated representation of space." These authors suggested that patients with right-hemispheric lesions who could not find a marble when it was in the left-side corner of a tactile finger maze appeared unaware that the left side of space even existed. This idea has been supported by Bisiach and colleagues, who found that patients with left-sided visuospatial neglect neglected the left sides of images retrieved from long-term memory. In a fascinating study, Bisiach and Luzzatti (1978) asked their patients with left-sided visuospatial neglect to name from memory the buildings in the Piazza del Duoma (a square in Milan) as though they were viewing the square from the door of the cathedral at one end. They were then asked to name the buildings while imagining viewing the square from a vantage point at the end of the square opposite the cathedral and looking toward it. On each trial they named the buildings that would be on their right from their imagined viewpoint and omitted the buildings that would be on their left; that is, on each trial they named different buildings.

In another study, Bisiach, Luzzatti, and Perani (1979) asked patients to decide whether pairs of sequentially presented random shapes that were visible only when they were moving past a small centrally positioned slit in a display were the same or different. Some pairs were the same, some differed on the right, and some differed on the left. To make this judgment, the subject had to construct a mental image of each shape because only partial information was available in central vision at any one time. Patients with left visuospatial neglect made more errors of "same" when the shapes differed on the left than when they differed on the right. I performed a similar experiment with patients who had either left- or right-hemispheric lesions, and found evidence that both categories of patients made more errors of "same" when the shapes differed on the side opposite to their lesion (Ogden 1985b).

These ideas, which implicate representational space in visuospatial neglect, suggest that there are anatomic structures in the brain that are used for both visual perception and visual imagery. When these structures are damaged on one side of the brain, visual perception may be disrupted on the opposite side of external space, and visual imagery may be disrupted on the opposite side of imagined space.

Rehabilitation of Neglect

In recent years there have been considerable advances in the understanding of the multiplicity of the impairments underlying neglect, and rehabilitation programs have been developed to address those specific impairments. This type of rehabilitation research is an excellent example of the way in which practitioners can use theories that have been supported by scientific evidence to inform the development of rehabilitation strategies (for reviews see Aimola Davies 2004; and Manly, Hawkins, Evans, Woldt, and Robertson 2002). The effectiveness of these rehabilitation strategies then needs to be assessed in clinical populations, using carefully designed research studies.

It is clear that most patients with neglect have a difficulty with directional attention. Early rehabilitation ideas utilized methods intended to cue the patient to visually scan the left side of space (e.g., putting a large red marker on the left side of the page of a book and telling the patient to look at the marker every time they completed a sentence, telling them to look toward their left arm used as an "anchor" and placed on the left side of the page, or putting jingling bracelets on the left arm in the hope that the noise would remind the patient to look over in that direction. Training patients over numerous trials to look voluntarily to the left proved extremely time consuming, and even if some small success was achieved for some patients, this success was transitory and did not generalize to tasks other than the task used in the training sessions.

Ian Robertson and his colleagues from the United Kingdom have carried out many excellent theory-driven studies on the rehabilitation of neglect. One series of studies utilized visuoperceptual cueing by means of moving the contralesional arm on the left of the task being carried out. The arm was moved either passively (i.e., by the experimenter) or actively (i.e., by the patient, on command or to turn off a buzzer than sounded if the arm was not moved). So far it appears that the most effective strategy in decreasing neglect on a paper and pencil cancellation test is the active movement of the contralesional arm. This effectiveness remained when the arm was hidden from view, but if the arm was placed in the ipsilesional hemispace, the neglect did not decrease. If the ipsilesional arm was moved in the contralesional hemispace, it did not have the same effect, and if both arms were moved simultaneously, each in their own hemispace, the effect was abolished. Robertson and colleagues (Robertson and Hawkins 1999; Robertson, Hogg, and McMillan 1998; Robertson and North 1994) hypothesized that movements of the contralesional limb in the contralesional hemispace may result in sufficient activation of the lesioned right hemisphere to reduce the inhibitory competition from the nonlesioned left hemisphere. This was more effective if both the movement of the arm and the postural placement of the arm in the contralesional space worked together. As Aimola-Davies (2004) points out, this fits with another theory proposed by Rizzolatti and Gallese (1988), who postulated that interconnected circuits control any one sector of space, and activation of more than one of these is required to overcome the neglect behaviors. A few studies have now demonstrated that for some patients as few as 8–9 hours of contralesional limb activation treatment can generalize to more movement of the contralesional limbs over a period of 18 months or longer (Robertson, McMillan, MacLeod, Edgeworth, and Brock 2002).

Another interesting technique has been devised to redirect the attention of neglect patients. It has been shown that neurologically normal people who are asked to point to objects while wearing optical prisms that distort their view 10 degrees to the right adapt their pointing accordingly (Mattingley 2002). There is a brief after-effect such that once the prisms are removed, when asked to point straight ahead in the dark, the individual points to the left of straight ahead. As a patient with left neglect points to the right when asked to point straight ahead, it was hypothesized that the prism adaptation after-effect might result in more accurate straight-ahead pointing. Studies so far have been promising, even after only 50 pointing responses while wearing the prisms. A reduction in errors in pointing ahead, and a reduction of neglect on paper and pencil neglect tests (e.g., line bisection, line cancellation, drawing) lasted at least 2 hours after prism removal (Rossetti et al. 1998). These findings of reduced neglect on a range of neglect tests implicate changes in the representation of space at higher cognitive levels, and not just a recalibration of visuomotor coordination as demonstrated by the adapted pointing behavior. Further studies using more sessions of prism adaptation over a 2-week period demonstrated improvements in neglect on both tests and everyday behaviors for 5–17 weeks (Frassinetti, Angeli, Meneghello, Avanzi, and Lavadas 2002).

It has been shown that to effectively rehabilitate a patient, that patient must be able to sustain attention on the task. Patients with right-hemispheric lesions tend to be more impaired on measures of sustained (nondirectional) attention than are those with left-hemispheric lesions. Thus, assisting the patient to increase their general level of alertness and to be able to maintain this alertness it is likely to be especially important for patients with left neglect. Strategies such as a loud alerting noise at regular intervals during training on rehabilitation for neglect tasks is therefore recommended. The patient can be gradually trained to self-alert, for example by telling themselves to "attend" (e.g., Robertson, Ridgeway, Greenfield, and Parr 1997; Robertson, Tegner, Tham, Lo, and Nimmo-Smith 1995).

The impairment of global processing that some neglect patients demonstrate was overcome in a study by Seron, Coyette, and Bruyer (1989), and later by Maguire (2000). These studies demonstrated that some patients with left visuospatial neglect could be motivated to attend to the left side of drawings of objects only if they could not identify an object from the information on the right side of the drawing. For example, when shown a picture of a symmetrical object like a desk, they identified it correctly, but of course they could do this from the details on the right only. When shown a picture of a toothbrush with the handle on the right side of the picture, they also identified it correctly, showing that they must have also attended to the brush on the left side of the picture. However, when they wcre shown a picture of a car colliding with a tree that was on the left side of the picture, they identified it only as a car and neglected to comment on the fact that it had crashed into a tree. It seemed as if their global processor was not forced to scan to the left of the picture because an object was able to be identified by the details on the right only.

Overall, these rehabilitation study results point to the importance of carefully assessing individual patients with hemineglect to see which of the many impairments they may have that may cause or exacerbate their neglect (Robertson and Murre 1999). These impairments commonly include a difficulty in sustaining attention generally, a difficulty directing attention toward the contralesional side, and a difficulty with global processing. A rehabilitation program can then be designed to address each of the patient's difficulties. First, a program aimed at regularly alerting the patient and increasing the ability to sustain attention might be put in place, followed by a program of contralesional limb activation treatment, and later a prism adaptation intervention program. Ideally, each intervention should be assessed for effectiveness, using a single case design, before the next intervention is begun. Each intervention may build on the previous one, or one intervention may be more effective for some neglect behaviors and others for different neglect behaviors.

If these interventions are begun in the early postacute stage, spontaneous recovery may very well make it difficult to establish the effectiveness of the interventions. There is, however, a view that rehabilitation should begin early to ensure that the patient receives training that will stimulate appropriate synaptic reconnections and lessen the possibility of the patient developing behaviors and movements that foster faulty connections (Robertson and Murre 1999). In reality, in most cases of neglect spontaneous recovery is rapid, occurring within days to a month of the stroke. Therefore, patients who still demonstrate neglect at 1 month postlesion would probably benefit from rehabilitation, which might at least enhance any further spontaneous recovery.

In the following case study, rehabilitation was not particularly effective, in part because some of the newer and more theory-driven rehabilitation strategies had not yet been developed, and in part because Janet's lesion was not a static stroke, but a malignant tumor. Thus, as her tumor regrew following surgery, her neglect reemerged.

Case Presentation

Background

Janet's friends described her as an energetic, intelligent woman with a great sense of humor. She had left school at the age of 17 years and worked as a typist before marriage. She had two children, and during their school years she was an active member of various community groups. She enjoyed amateur landscape painting and pottery. At the age of 45, Janet enrolled in a part-time course in business management at the local polytechnical institution and completed the course with excellent grades 2 years later. She then obtained a position as the administrative secretary for a company that manufactured art supplies.

On her 50th birthday, after driving home from work, she collided with the left side of the garage doorway. She and her husband attributed this collision to a lapse of attention because she was thinking about birthday celebrations the family were having in her honor that night. Her birthday was a great success, and her sense of humor was apparent when she blew out the 50 birthday candles on her large birthday cake and managed to blow all the candles out on the right side, leaving those on the far left still burning. According to her husband, she seemed unaware of this, and when he pointed to the burning candles, she remarked that they looked so pretty it seemed a shame to blow them out. She did so, however, when her husband said she would not be able to cut the cake.

Two days later, Janet was admitted to the neurology ward after her husband heard thumping sounds in the bathroom and found Janet lying on the bathroom floor, dazed, disoriented, and incontinent. She was unable to describe what had happened, but it seemed likely that she had suffered a generalized seizure. Neurological examination revealed sensory loss in the left arm, a visual-field cut in the left field (a homonymous hemianopia), and marked visuospatial and motor neglect. Computed tomography (CT) scan showed a large mass with surrounding edema in the right parietal lobe (see Fig. 7-2). A biopsy of this mass was done, and histology confirmed a grade 2 astrocytoma (malignant tumor). Janet was medicated with steroids to reduce the swelling, and 5 days later the neurosurgeon "debulked" the tumor mass before starting radiotherapy treatment. A follow-up CT scan 5 days postoperation showed that the mass was much smaller and the edema much reduced.

Janet began rehabilitation therapy before her radiotherapy began and continued for

Figure 7-2 A computed tomography scan of Janet's brain showing a large glioma in the right posterior parietal lobe.

another 3 months after its completion. She was able to return part-time to her job 5 months after her operation, but 18 months later, the onset of hemiplegia and a return of her neglect symptoms forced her to take an early retirement. A CT scan at this time showed that the tumor had increased in size again and was now larger than it was originally. Other than taking steroid medication, Janet refused any further treatment but attended physiotherapy three times a week in an attempt to delay the debilitating physical effects of the tumor. She remained optimistic to the point of being unrealistic until her death 4 years after her initial diagnosis.

Throughout her illness, Janet displayed a range of neglect symptoms that varied in severity, depending on the size of her tumor and the amount of edema surrounding it. The severity of her symptoms had spontaneously reduced by the time she had completed her course of radiotherapy, and rehabilitation therapy specifically aimed at teaching her to be aware of her left side and her neglect appeared to decrease her neglect even further and enabled her to return to work. When her symptoms returned, forcing her to retire, attempts by her physical therapist to help her overcome her neglect were largely unsuccessful. The various types of neglect Janet displayed and the stages she went through are described in some detail, with additional illustrations from other patients.

Neuropsychological Outcome

General intellectual and memory abilities   Three days after Janet's first admission to the hospital, and the day before her surgery, assessments on the Verbal subtests of the Wechsler Adult Intelligence Scale-Revised (WAIS-R) and on the National Adult Reading Test (NART), a test designed to produce an estimate of premorbid IQ, demonstrated that she fell easily within the "superior" Verbal IQ range. Her score on Similarities, a test of verbal abstraction, was particularly impressive, with only one incorrect answer, indicating that her frontal lobes were not obviously affected by her tumor, which was supported by a superior score on a test of oral word fluency. On this test, the patient is asked to give as many words beginning with a particular letter as possible in one minute. Patients with frontal-lobe dysfunction tend to score poorly on this test.

Only two of the Verbal subtest scores fell below average: those on Arithmetic and Digit Span, neither of which is a true test of verbal ability. An exploration of why she did relatively poorly on Arithmetic suggested at least two factors as the cause. First, Janet had not received a good education in mathematics at school (a relatively common finding at that time in a woman of her age), and she had avoided working with numbers since, even in her current job as an administrative secretary. In addition, she demonstrated marked difficulty with the spatial manipulation of figures, which became apparent when she was asked to perform on paper simple additions that involved carrying figures from one column to the next (e.g., 128 + 194). She would place the number to be carried under the right-hand column and had difficulty adding the figures in the left-hand column. Such difficulties are symptoms of visuospatial neglect. She also had a relatively poor Digit Span score of repeating five digits forward and only two digits backward. This problem could have been a reflection of poor concentration and decreased ability to sustain attention, a common problem for neglect patients; however, given her excellent attention to other verbal tests, this seems unlikely. Another possibility is that when asked to repeat a series of digits backward, she was able to hold a sequence of five numbers in her mind, but when mentally tracking backward, she neglected the numbers on the left. Indeed, she always repeated the last two numbers correctly but refused to give any more. Most people attempting to give a sequence of digits backwards will not refuse to give numbers of which they are unsure but will make a guess, often getting the correct digits but in the wrong order. Perhaps Janet was neglecting to "see" the digits on the left of her mental representation. The hypothesis that Janet neglected mental images was explored later.

On the Performance subtests of the WAIS-R, all of Janet's scores were average or lower. On some of these tests, it was clear that Janet was neglecting the left side of the task (e.g., on Digit Symbol, Picture Arrangement, and Block Design). In addition to her neglect, she seemed completely unable to copy the more complex Block Design patterns; for example, in one 3 × 3 pattern, she placed eight blocks in two vertical rows and did not even use the ninth block. When asked if her design looked like the picture, she replied, "It seems near enough to me." Her impaired perception of her poor ability was particularly striking considering her past hobbies of landscape painting and pottery. Her score on Object Assembly, which involves putting together jigsaw pieces of objects without knowing what they are, was equally poor, and she was again unconcerned about her abysmal productions. Her performance therefore showed symptoms of both neglect and a generalized visuospatial problem, which is common following parietal lesions of either hemisphere, but more pronounced after right parietal lesions.

On an early edition of the Wechsler Memory Scale (WMS), Janet's scores were impressive, and her overall Memory Quotient fell in the superior range. Her scores on the two verbal memory subtests were excellent, but on Visual Reproduction her score was only average, as she missed the figure on the left of the third design. This early edition of the WMS is heavily biased toward verbal ability and does not assess nonverbal memory well because even the simple designs to be remembered in the Visual Reproduction subtest can be verbally labeled. More recent editions of the Wechsler Memory Scales have included more and better subtests of nonverbal memory functions, although these functions remain difficult to define and assess.

Tests of hemineglect   *Visual hemineglect*: Janet was given a book to read aloud, and she proceeded to read fluently but missed two or three words on the left of every line. When the passage clearly did not make sense, she would occasionally insert a word that was not on the page. A year later, her daughter said she would receive letters from her mother written down the right side of the page. Her writing was also difficult to read because of her tendency to repeat some letters. For example, when writing *Janet* she would reiterate the curves of the *n* three or four times, and when writing *hospital* she would repeat the *i* a number of times. Although this could be viewed as *perseveration* (i.e., repeating the same behavior), which is commonly associated with frontal-lobe pathology, the reiteration of letters in cursive writing is also found following right parietal lesions. In these patients, it is categorized as a type of *spatial agraphia*.

Janet was asked to put the numbers in on a clock face (Fig. 7-1A) and to copy a necker cube, a star, and a scene (see Fig. 7-3 and the middle line in Fig. 7-4.) It is interesting that when patients with visuospatial hemineglect are asked to copy this collection of drawings and to complete the clock face they are often inconsistent with respect to the objects on which they will demonstrate neglect.

One patient will draw in the clock figures carefully and accurately but completely neglect one half of the other drawings. Another will put numbers on one half of the clock, draw a complete star, and make a reasonable attempt at the cube, showing some neglect by drawing the neglected side more carelessly than the nonneglected side. Indeed, the same patient will neglect the left side of the cube one day and copy the star quite well and the next day draw both sides of the cube and neglect the left side of the star. These idiosyncrasies and the comments the patients make suggest that hemineglect is not a simple sensory or perceptual deficit but a "higher" cognitive disorder. It is almost as though the patient is aware at some level that the left side of the object exists but deliberately chooses not to respond to that side.

Janet's response when asked to copy the scene of the house, fence, and trees provides an example of this "meta-awareness." She dutifully copied the tree on the right and the house; then she put her pencil down, saying she had finished. I pointed to each item in the model of the scene and asked her to name them. She did so

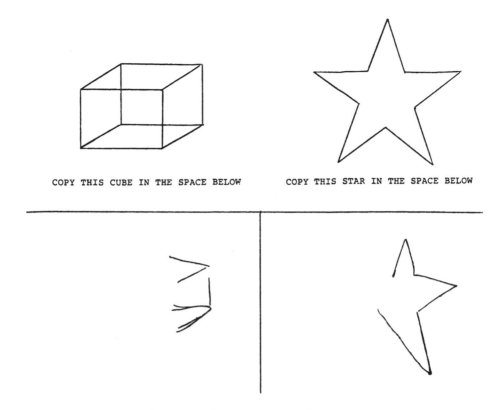

COPY THIS CUBE IN THE SPACE BELOW   COPY THIS STAR IN THE SPACE BELOW

Figure 7-3 Janet's copies (bottom row) of a cube and a star.

correctly. I then asked her if she would draw in the fence. She did so, saying, "Well I will if you really want me to, but it will probably blow down in the next wind!" I then asked her to draw the rest. "That really is all I can draw," she said. I pointed to the tree on the left. "That tree? I can't draw trees," she replied, and I could not induce her to draw it. Another patient, when encouraged to draw in the fence, remarked, "That will blow down before the night is out!"

Janet was presented with a page covered in lines about 2 cm long, and she was asked to draw lines across each one (Albert 1973). She crossed the 16 lines on the right of the page and neglected the 22 lines on the left. The page was then shifted completely to her right side so that her left visual field cut would be less likely to restrict her vision. She was asked to look carefully across the page and cross out any lines she had missed. She responded by crossing the same lines again, saying, "I think I've crossed out some of these before." She continued to neglect the lines on the left, demonstrating an interesting aspect of neglect. Some patients do not simply neglect stimuli on the left side of their body (and therefore in their left hemispace relative to their body); rather, they seem to divide whatever they are looking at into right and left sides and then neglect the left side. Another example is shown in the bottom line of Figure 7-4. This patient, asked to copy the scene, neglected the left sides of both the tree and the house on the right of the drawing as well as the fence and tree to the left of the house. It is as if she looked at the right tree and then the house as separate entities, divided each in half, and drew the right half. She then looked at the whole scene and neglected the fence and the left-sided tree completely. Only a few patients display this type of neglect behavior, and even then they may not demonstrate it consistently. The phenomenon of neglecting the contralesional half of each object in a display has been termed *object-centered neglect*, whereas the more usual neglect behavior of neglecting the contralesional half of the whole display, or environment, has been called *environment-centered neglect*.

Figure 7-4 In the top row is the "scene" the patient is asked to copy. In the middle row is Janet's copy of the scene showing left neglect. In the bottom row is the copy by another patient with a right basal ganglion lesion, showing neglect of individual items in the drawing as well as neglect of the drawing as a whole.

In everyday life, visual hemineglect causes difficulties because the patient may neglect the wall on her left, the cars on her left, the people on her left, and sometimes even the food on the left of her plate. People who have a left visual field cut but do not have neglect quickly learn to compensate for their loss of vision by moving their eyes or head to the left. Patients with neglect do not compensate for their field cut, and thus the visual loss exacerbates their neglect and makes rehabilitation more difficult.

Janet did not ignore people standing on the left of her bed, as do some patients with neglect. One man I assessed would either completely ignore his visitors if they stood on his left side, or he would swear at them. As soon as they came around to his right side, he would greet them warmly. On one occasion, I made the mistake of sitting down on his left side to test him. I managed to get his attention, but when I asked if he would cross out lines on a page (he had done this before), he snarled, "I'm not doing any more of your stupid tests, so go away." I asked him if he would like me to sit on his other side, and he replied, "Well, that would certainly be better for me, wouldn't it." I moved around to his right side, and he smiled at me and happily began the line-crossing-out test. He still neglected the lines on the left of the page, but his attitude toward me remained pleasant. According to his family, his "normal" personality was mild and kind, and he never swore.

Neglect of visual images: Janet not only demonstrated neglect when she saw stimuli but she also neglected the left side of visual images. For example, I attempted to test her in a manner similar to that used by Bisiach and Luzzati (1978) when they asked their patients to imagine a square in Milan: I asked Janet to imagine she was standing in Nelson (at the north end of the South Island of New Zealand), looking south to Invercargill (at the south end of the South Island). I asked her to name all the towns and places of interest on her right and then those on her left. I then asked her to imagine she was standing in Invercargill looking north toward Nelson and to perform the same task. In total, she managed to produce the names of most of the towns in the South Island, but each time she gave me a number of towns that would lie to her right from the vantage point she imagined she was at, but only one town on her left. When asked how she did this task, she said she had a picture of a map of New Zealand in her mind's eye and simply read the names of the towns from it. This task demonstrates neglect of an image retrieved from long-term memory.

She was given another task that involved long-term visual memory. With her husband's assistance, I asked Janet to imagine walking through the door of her bedroom and describing the furniture in front of her and on each side of the room. She incorrectly placed the beds, the chest of drawers, a couch, and the shower and toilet cubicles all on her right. When asked what was on her left, she replied, "Nothing much, except I think another door." Her husband then drew the outline of their bedroom and Janet drew the furniture in place. Her husband also drew a picture of the bedroom with its furniture for comparison purposes. Janet incorrectly drew all the furniture on the right side of the bedroom, with none on the left, although this time the furniture was on the right of the picture as she viewed it rather than on the right of the door. Janet also demonstrated neglect of the left sides of the random shapes in the experiment described earlier in which pairs of shapes move past a slit so that the complete shape must be constructed in the imagination. Janet said that pairs of shapes that differed on the left were the same, but that shapes that differed on the right were different. Therefore, it seems that Janet neglected her visual images regardless of whether they were retrieved from long-term memory or whether she constructed them. Neglect of a mental representation does not exclude inattention as a cause for the neglect; it could be that the representation is complete but the individual fails to attend to the contralesional side of the representation.

Motor neglect: Janet had a sensory loss in her left arm when she was admitted to the hospital, and the neurologist had some difficulty assessing whether she had a hemiplegia because of her neglect. It was concluded that she did have a mild weakness of her left arm but that her left leg was probably not weak. To an observer, it appeared that Janet was hemiplegic. She did not use her left arm, and when it was pointed out to her, she called it "that hunk of meat." On one occasion she remarked, "When I get home I will give that hunk of meat a piece of my mind." On another occasion, she asked me if I would remove that arm (pointing to her left arm) from her bed. When I told her it was her arm, she laughed and said, "Well, you could be right I suppose, but it doesn't seem to belong to me!" When asked to raise her left arm, she would sometimes comply, but when she was then asked to raise both arms, she always responded by raising only her right arm.

Janet was sometimes seen walking reasonably well using both legs, but she would often attempt to dress while hopping around on her right leg. She would chuckle loudly whenever she lost her balance and was heard to remark, "It's a good job I used to be an acrobat in a circus, because it helps me put my knickers on when I'm standing on one leg!" When I asked her why she hopped, she queried, "Well how else am I to get around?" As described at the beginning of this chapter, Janet also made excuses for not dressing the left side of her body. These rather childlike attempts to justify her neglect behaviors were in marked contrast to her superior scores on the verbal subtests of the WAIS-R, especially those that indicated an unimpaired verbal abstraction ability. Whether Janet believed we were convinced by her justifications is difficult to say, but as she often laughed at herself when she gave her explanations, I suspect she was aware that we were unlikely to take them seriously. Not all patients make excuses for their neglect, and those who do tend to have right parietal lesions.

Tactile neglect: It was difficult to assess Janet in this regard because of her sensory loss in her left arm and left side of her face, but when asked to say when she was touched on her leg, she was always correct when her right leg was touched but responded only two of 10 times to a touch on her left leg. On both these trials, however, she insisted it was her right leg—not her left leg—that was touched. It made no difference whether the test was carried out with Janet blindfolded or whether she was allowed to watch her legs being touched. This tactile neglect recovered after her operation, but tactile extinction was still apparent. That is, she would respond correctly to touch on either leg alone, but when both legs were touched simultaneously, she would say that only the right leg was touched.

Auditory neglect: Janet did not appear to have auditory neglect in that she responded to a voice and to other sounds coming from either side of her body. Auditory neglect is extremely rare, perhaps because sounds cannot be readily separated into right and left space, as sounds reach both ears. Auditory extinction is much more common and is usually assessed by making sounds close to the patient's ears or over headphones so that the sounds are readily separable in space. Using various dichotic listening tasks where the patient hears, for example, a series of six digits, three to each ear simultaneously, and is asked to repeat all the digits, Janet was able to repeat only the three digits she heard in the right ear. When asked to attend to the digits in one ear only and repeat those, she had no difficulty repeating the right-ear digits; when asked to repeat the left-ear digits, she often repeated only one of them and added two from the right ear. In contrast, when she was presented with three digits in one ear only, she could repeat them back correctly whichever ear was used. That is, she had extinction but not neglect.

Other visuospatial deficits   Janet's general visuospatial difficulty also affected her drawings independent of her neglect. For example, her copy of the scene test seen in Figure 7-4 was confused with lines drawn over the top of other lines. This type of disorder is often called *constructional apraxia* because it involves difficulty in performing the skilled movements (*apraxia*) in constructing something. It is often difficult to assess whether a patient is apraxic, as to do so requires eliminating weakness or sensory loss of the limbs as a cause. Therefore, a better term is *visuoconstructive disability* (Benton and Tranel 1993). Patients with left parietal lesions also frequently have difficulty with visuospatial perception and construction (see Chapter 6), although as with neglect, the problem is usually more severe after right parietal lesions. The problem often manifests in the patient's poor ability to draw and to do the Block Design and Object Assembly tests of the WAIS-R, and in their apparent difficulty in recognizing that their attempts are incorrect. A comparison of Janet's confused attempt at the scene test (Fig. 7-4) with the copy of the patient who also had severe left-sided neglect, whose drawing is shown on the lower line of Figure 7-4, illustrates this problem. The second patient had a right basal ganglion lesion and therefore did not have a general problem with visuospatial perception and construction, as demonstrated by her neat (although neglected) copy. Another patient I assessed with a right parietal lesion made during the surgical removal of a meningioma in the right lateral ventricle, but who did not demonstrate marked visual neglect, had been a carpet layer before his surgery. After surgery he was completely unable to perform his job because he could no longer measure or cut carpets and was unable to fit carpets that had been cut to measure by someone else (Ogden 1984).

Janet's problem with dressing (e.g., leaving her left arm out of her sleeves), although probably related to the neglect of the left side of her body, could also be labeled as *dressing apraxia*; that is, difficulty in performing the skilled movements required to complete the spatial task of dressing. Patients with dressing apraxia are rather like very young children when they first begin to dress themselves. The left arm goes into the right sleeve, trousers are put on back to front, and so on. Again, this problem is generally seen after parietal lesions, both left and right.

Janet also had difficulties reading a map and finding her way. Although some of this difficulty, especially in the early and late stages of her illness, was related to her ignoring turns to the left, her problem was more general than that. Even when she had recovered from many of her neglect symptoms and returned to work, she frequently lost her way when taking messages from one floor to another in her office building. When her husband decided to test her by asking her to direct him while he was driving from their home to her workplace, she got them hopelessly lost, although she had driven the route herself hundreds of times both as driver and, since her illness, as passenger. This disorder is known as *topographical disorientation*, or *topographical memory disorder* (De Renzi 1982).

Recovery of Neglect

Five days after the operation to "debulk" Janet's tumor, and again 3 months later, I repeated some of the visuospatial and neglect tests. She demonstrated a marked reduction of neglect and a small improvement on tests of visuospatial construction, such as the Block Design subtest of the WAIS-R. Her copies of drawings remained confused, but on the scene test at 5 days postoperation, she copied the fence spontaneously. After considerable encouragement, on the crossing-out lines test, she crossed all but three of the lines on the extreme left side. She was still inclined to ignore her left limbs, but she would raise her left arm and walk using both legs if asked to do so. She frequently collided with the left wall or left side of the doorway. She seemed unable to compensate for her visual-field cut. When she began rehabilitation, two bracelets with bells were put on her left arm to see if the noise they made would draw her attention to that arm. She was taught to talk herself through tasks; for example, when walking, she was to say to herself "right leg forward, right heel and toe down, left leg forward, left heel and toe down." When writing or reading, she was encouraged to tie a bright red ribbon around her left wrist and to place her left arm on the table at the side of the paper or book. She was to tell herself to look toward the red ribbon whenever she reached the right side of a line. Janet's family were all instructed in these techniques and told to interact with her from her left side as much as possible.

Janet's neglect certainly resolved significantly over the 3-month period of her rehabilitation, and her awareness of her left limbs improved markedly. As is often the case, it is impossible to say how much of Janet's recovery was to the result of spontaneous recovery (and the debulking and shrinking of her tumor and its surrounding edema by surgery, radiotherapy, and steroids) and how much was the result of active rehabilitation. By the time Janet finally retired from her job, her visual and motor neglect had increased again to a severity that equalled that when she was first admitted to hospital. This time it did not spontaneously recover, and rehabilitation was to no avail.

Personal and Social Consequences

Janet's neglect and other visuospatial problems were caused by a malignant tumor, which although impeded in its growth by surgery and radiotherapy, ultimately caused her death. The 4 years between her first admission to the hospital and her death were dominated by the health system, from surgery in an acute neurosurgery ward, to daily visits as an outpatient for radiotherapy treatment, which made her feel nauseated and continually tired, and then to the physical therapist and occupational therapist three times a week for 3 months for rehabilitation. Five months after her operation, she returned to her job on a part-time basis, but she was unable to function at her previous level. For example, she was no longer able to use the word processor to type memos because her left hand was too clumsy to touch type; when she tried to type with two fingers or her right hand only, she was very slow to find letters on the left side of the keyboard. Although she generally remained optimistic (or unrealistic, as her husband commented to me), she did at times become depressed by what she perceived as the charity her employers were extending to her in allowing her to continue in her job. Nevertheless, she continued at her job for 18 months before being forced to leave because of the relentless increase of weakness in her left arm and leg and a return of severe visual and motor neglect.

She appeared relatively calm when a CT brain scan confirmed that rapid regrowth of the tumor had occurred. Although she refused further medical treatment except steroids to help reduce the swelling around the tumor, she did return to physical therapy for 2 months. It quickly became apparent to the physical therapist that Janet's hemiplegia was progressing too rapidly and that her neglect was too severe to allow any useful rehabilitation, so Janet retired to a semi-invalid state. Her husband took an early retirement to take care of her. She stopped taking steroids, which had caused her face to swell, and she spent her days watching television and talking to family and friends who visited. She became increasingly "inappropriate" as the months wore on, possibly as a result of the tumor encroaching on the frontal lobe. Her speech became slurred (*dysarthric*) as a result of a left-sided facial weakness, but she retained her conversational ability and her somewhat inappropriate sense of humor.

After her death, her husband became quite seriously depressed, partly as a grief reaction to Janet's tragic illness and death and partly because he suddenly found himself with nothing worthwhile to do with his life. He no longer had to care for Janet day and night and had given up his job. After seeing a clinical psychologist for several months, he gradually started socializing again and took up some new hobbies. His life took on meaning again when his daughter asked if he would look after her two children, aged 18 months and 3 years, for 4 days a week while she worked. He said they were easy to care for after Janet, and he quickly became a popular parent-helper at the local play school.

Discussion

Janet's is a classic case of visual, tactile, and motor neglect of the left side following a right parietal lesion. The multimodal nature of her neglect does not necessarily mean that all forms of neglect have the same underlying cause. It may be that different anatomical areas or pathways mediate different types of neglect but that these anatomical areas are physically close to one another. Patients with a large lesion would therefore be more likely to demonstrate a range of neglects. Many patients demonstrate visual hemineglect only and do not appear to neglect their left limbs and respond to their left limbs being touched. I have assessed a few patients who demonstrate motor and tactile neglect but show no signs of visual neglect (Ogden 1983).

Janet's case does not elucidate any particular hypothesis explaining the underlying cause of neglect. Her neglect of visual images supports the idea of De Renzi, Faglioni, and Scotti (1970) and Bisiach and colleagues (1978, 1979) of a mutilated representation of space, but this does not in itself exclude the possibility that she was inattentive to the left side of space or the left side of an object. It may be that when imagining a scene, the entire scene is formed in the mind's eye or visual buffer, but when the image is internally scanned, the left side is neglected. This process would parallel the process in perception of external stimuli, in that the left side is not attended to during the scanning process. It may be that a number of different mechanisms can cause neglect: in some people an attention deficit, in others a deeper mutilation of representational space.

What does seem clear is that many patients with neglect are aware of both sides of space and objects at some level. The study by Seron et al. (1989) demonstrated that left neglect patients would attend to and utilize details on the left side of a picture if the picture could not be identified as something (even if not correct) from the right-side information only. The comments right neglect patients sometimes make about the side they neglect almost suggests that at some level they do perceive the whole object, or all their limbs, but cannot sustain their attention to the left side long enough to respond to what they perceived. When forced to attend to the left side, they may make remarks like those of the patient who said when reluctantly drawing a fence to the left of a house, "That will blow down before the night is out!" Such remarks may be an attempt to rationalize the patient's own experience; that of knowing the left side details are there at some level, but not being fully aware of them (or not being able to sustain attention to the left long enough to be certain of what had been fleetingly perceived).

Neglect is undoubtedly the result of brain damage and is never a purely psychological phenomenon. Thus, if neglect is a conscious behavior at some level, the patient does not necessarily have voluntary control over it. Some patients have anosognosia and are unaware or indifferent to their neglect problems. These patients may be the most difficult to rehabilitate. Even patients who seem to be aware of their own neglect behaviors can nevertheless appear reluctant to moderate them. Rehabilitation does help some patients on specific tasks (Robertson and North 1992; Robertson et al. 1992).

The rapid development of new theory-driven rehabilitation strategies shows promise, and some studies demonstrate generalization from the rehabilitation task to everyday behaviors which, in some cases, lasts for weeks to months (e.g., Frassinetti et al. 2002; Robertson et al. 1995, 1997). It is often difficult to tease apart spontaneous recovery from recovery as a result of rehabilitation, but in clinical practice, perhaps this does not matter.

8

■

VISION WITHOUT KNOWLEDGE
VISUAL OBJECT AGNOSIA AND PROSOPAGNOSIA

I first heard about the man I will call "Michael" when I received a telephone call from a rehabilitation therapist at the Institute for the Blind. She asked for my help in rethinking Michael's rehabilitation program because, as she said, "Something incredible has happened to him and he seems to be getting his sight back, but he still can't see!" She went on to explain that Michael had been classified as totally blind since a head injury nearly 2 years previously, but he had recently begun to see lights at night and movement on the television. She had been trying to improve his sight by showing him various common objects day after day, but he seemed unable to recognize the objects unless he picked them up. Often he would describe the shape of the object in a slow, disjointed manner, but only rarely did this seem to help him recognize the object. At first, she said, he could not read, but practice had brought improvement, and now he could read slowly but quite well.

What the rehabilitation therapist was describing was visual object agnosia,[1] a disorder that has been known to neurologists for more than 100 years. Although certainly uncommon, it is not extremely rare, and numerous accounts have been published in the neuropsychological literature since it was first described by Charcot (1883).[2] It is considered one of the "classic" neuropsychological disorders, and its study tells us a great deal about the complex higher visual processes we humans use without so much as a thought in our everyday lives. Michael's case proved particularly interesting, as it later became apparent that he also had significant memory impairment and a number of other disorders of higher visual cognition, including another "classic" neuropsychological disorder, *prosopagnosia,* or the inability to recognize familiar faces on sight.

This chapter is based on Ogden (1993a), and further details about Michael (under the initials M.H.) can be found in that paper.

1. *Nosia* means to know, and *agnosia* means not to know. Therefore, visual object agnosia means not to know objects by vision.

2. Readers interested in finding out more are referred to two books (Farah 1990; Humphreys and Riddoch 1987).

Following my telephone conversation with Michael's rehabilitation therapist, I arranged for her to bring him to the psychology clinic at the university. Ten minutes before our scheduled meeting, I was having a cup of coffee in the common room when one of my academic colleagues came in. On seeing me he remarked, "I just passed a man in the corridor who, from the look of him, was on his way to see you." When I left the room I saw a tall, well-built young man limping and swaying unsteadily along the corridor, apparently following the person in front of him. His right arm was held at an awkward angle to his body, perhaps in an attempt to steady himself or to protect his body from banging into the wall, and his left arm terminated at his elbow and was finished with a large hook. I greeted his companion (the rehabilitation therapist) and then greeted Michael. He looked at my voice, as blind people tend to do, thrust his right hand out for me to grasp, and with a broad, engaging grin said in a delightful "kiwi" drawl, "Gidday. Am I pleased to meet you!"

So began a friendship and a research relationship between myself and Michael that so far has spanned the last 6 years and that will doubtless continue for many years to come. The reasons for this are many, but paramount is that alongside his unusually rich collection of higher visual disorders is Michael's eagerness to participate in any new experiment I can think up and his interest in his own performance and what it tells us not only about him but also about brain–behavior relations in general. Michael is one of my keenest students, and if it were possible to replace the lost neurons and connections in Michael's brain so that he could function normally again, I would not be surprised if he decided to take up formal neuropsychological studies.

There are, of course, many neurological patients who have disorders almost as interesting as those demonstrated by Michael but who do not become long-term "special" cases. Sometimes this is because they are not interested and willing to participate in ongoing experiments; more often, it is because they have other problems that prevent their involvement. For example, other important attributes that make Michael an excellent research subject are his youth, normal verbal intelligence, excellent attention span, and ability to concentrate for long periods. These are precious commodities in a neuropsychological subject, as often neurological patients have other impairments, such as poor concentration, or difficulty understanding or following instructions, that make them difficult to test. Many patients who would otherwise be good neuropsychological subjects often tire quickly, but in test sessions with Michael, I often tire before him. A final important attribute of this case is the unchanging, stable nature of Michael's brain damage, which resulted from a head injury many years ago. Computed tomography (CT) scans of his brain show that no obvious changes had occurred over a 7-year period.

Special case studies like Michael do not come along too often in the working life span of a clinical neuropsychologist, and when they do, they often become almost "professional" subjects. It is obviously important for researchers to guard against exploiting someone in Michael's position, which in a sense becomes more difficult over time, as a personal bond develops between researcher and subject. The result is that the subject feels reluctant to disappoint the experimenter. One way of trying to balance out this potentially exploitative relationship is for the researcher to use the results of the various investigations in an effort to improve the rehabilitation strategies used with that patient. In this way, the neuropsychologist can become a useful member of the rehabilitation team and perhaps contribute to small improvements in that patient's functioning and quality of life.

Michael's story not only teaches us about some fascinating neuropsychological disorders but also provides lessons in courage, stamina, determination, and an all-important ability to laugh at oneself when all else fails. In Michael's case, these characteristics have enabled him to progress to a reasonably independent lifestyle despite minimal recovery of his visual and memory impairments.

Theoretical Background

The family of cognitive disorders known as the *agnosias* includes a wide range of "not knowing" impairments, many specific to a particular modality. Thus there are not only visual agnosias but also auditory and somatosensory (tactile) agnosias. Within each modality, there are disorders that can be discriminated one from the other. For example, included within the auditory agnosias (i.e., an inability to recognize sounds in spite of adequate hearing) are the disorders of pure word deafness (also termed auditory agnosia for speech, or auditory verbal agnosia) and auditory sound agnosia (also termed auditory agnosia for nonspeech sounds). These disorders are sometimes divided up still further; for example, a number of cases with receptive amusia have been described. In these cases the patient has an inability to appreciate various characteristics of heard music (Piccirilli, Sciarma, and Luzzi 2000). Although most patients with auditory sound agnosia have some level of impairment in their appreciation of music, the description of cases where the patient demonstrates only impairment in recognizing particular characteristics of music, but continues to be able to recognize other sounds (Peretz et al. 1994), implies the possibility of a distinct disorder. Agnosias in the visual modality (many demonstrated by Michael) are more commonly described than the auditory agnosias. The literature on the agnosias is complex and evolving as new cases are discovered and assessed, and new theories and hypotheses are tested and either supported or found wanting (for a recent review of this fascinating area, see Bauer and Demery 2003).

Visual object agnosia is a disorder in which familiar objects can be seen but cannot be recognized. It is "modality specific" in that the object can be recognized via the other senses of touch, sound, or smell. It is not a disorder of naming, as the subject has no difficulty naming the object if it is recognized via touch or another nonvisual sense. At least three broad types of visual agnosia have been hypothesized. The first two types were proposed a hundred years ago by Lissauer (1890). In *apperceptive* visual agnosia, the basic perceptual mechanisms are disrupted such that the subject cannot even copy a picture of an object or tell a square from a rectangle. In *associative* visual agnosia, the subject can perform visual perception tasks, such as copying a figure reasonably well but cannot interpret the meaning of the form perceived. Riddoch and Humphreys (1987) postulated a third type they called *integrative* visual agnosia. In this type, perception is again intact at the early (e.g., copying) stage, but at a later perceptual stage the subject has difficulty integrating the different parts of the object into an integrated whole they can recognize. Thus, when given a picture of a toothbrush to recognize, the subject may be able to draw it in a fragmented way, bit by bit, but cannot put the bits together in his mind to form a concept or picture of a toothbrush. This is the type of agnosia that Michael has. All three types of visual object agnosia are usually associated with damage to both occipital lobes (*bilateral* damage).

The inability to recognize faces on sight (*prosopagnosia*) is also usually associated with bilateral occipital damage. It is therefore not surprising that it is often found in the same patients who demonstrate visual object agnosia. One possibility is that in some patients both prosopagnosia and visual object agnosia are consequences of damage to the system that represents complex parts. Mild damage to this system results in a problem in recognizing different faces, clearly a difficult task, as faces are complex and differ in subtle ways. More severe damage to this system not only results in prosopagnosia but also causes problems with recognizing complex objects. Because objects tend to be much less complex than faces and are easier to distinguish from other objects, more severe damage is necessary to cause visual object agnosia than to cause prosopagnosia. There are also cases of visual object agnosia associated with *alexia* (an impairment of reading) rather than prosopagnosia. In these cases the problem appears to be in the system that represents numerous parts, such as letters that make up a word and discrete parts that make up an object (Farah 1990, 1991). If this hypothesis is correct, it suggests that different systems or pathways in the occipital lobes are concerned with different types of visual representation. Thus, patients who appear to have damage in similar areas of the brain may in fact have damage to different pathways. The message for the neuropsychologist is clear: The site of a brain lesion at best provides a guide to the type of impairments the patient might have, but only a careful neuropsychological assessment can tease apart the subtle differences between many higher cognitive processes.

Michael also has a loss of color perception (*achromatopsia*) and a loss of color memory, both of which have been found in other patients with bilateral occipital lesions. He also experiences a loss of visual imagery. Although some reports exist of other patients with visual object agnosia experiencing such a loss, this is by no means always the case, and sometimes patients with damage in areas other than the occipital lobes have impairments of visual imagery. It may be that the individual differences in the ability to make visual images influence what happens after brain damage and that imagery may be mediated by more than one functional system in the brain.

Case Presentation

Background

In 1986 Michael was a healthy, 24-year-old Lance Corporal in the Army. He had been an average student at school and on leaving school had taken up a career in the armed forces, first as a seaman in the navy and then as a storeman in the army. His greatest joy in life was to ride motorcycles, and this recreation was to change his life forever. One day on leave, when he was riding alone, his motorcycle apparently swerved and hit a tree. Michael was admitted to the critical care unit of the main city hospital; he was in a deep coma and had multiple fractures where the left side of his body had been crushed. A CT brain scan revealed swelling of the right hemisphere of his brain, which was treated with a drug (mannitol) and hyperventilation, and his many ortho- pedic injuries were pinned and set. Within days of his admission, it became necessary to amputate his left arm. He had a rocky course over the next 2 weeks; his mother, who spent many hours at his bedside, was told it was "touch and go" at times. Five weeks after his accident, Michael regained consciousness and was able to open his eyes and obey requests. At this point, he was transferred to an orthopedic ward, where he remained for another 11 weeks.

Once Michael had left the critical care unit his head injury was virtually ignored while the surgeons grappled with his severe orthopedic injuries. In an acute hospital where wards and medical services are physically divided according to types of illness or damage, it is often difficult to decide where a patient with multiple types of damage should go. In Michael's case he clearly needed extensive orthopedic surgery and spe- cialist care; once in that service, he could talk normally and seemed cheerful and even "chirpy," which no doubt lulled the staff into thinking he had recovered from his head injury. In any case, there was clearly nothing further to be done for his brain either medically or surgically. The fractures in his left leg resulted in a twisted foot and a severe limp, which was partially corrected 7 years later by foot surgery.

My review of his hospital chart revealed minimal and conflicting information on his visual deficits. His mother said he was blind from the time he regained conscious- ness at 5 weeks, but at this time the only report ever made by a neurosurgeon during his 16 weeks as an inpatient stated that he had double vision (*diplopia*). A note made by the occupational therapist at 9 weeks stated that his sight was very bad but that at times he seemed able to look at an object and recognize it. A report by an ophthal- mologist at 10 weeks stated that he was *cortically blind* (i.e., blind as a result of damage to the visual cortex of the occipital lobes rather than as a result of damage to his eyes or the optic tracts). On discharge from the hospital at 16 weeks, he had mild spasticity of the right hand (his dominant, writing hand), and his speech and comprehension of language seemed normal. The New Zealand Foundation for the Blind assessed him as totally blind and enrolled him in their full-time, live-in reha- bilitation program.

Seventeen months after discharge from the hospital, Michael suddenly became aware of the moving lights of other cars when he was traveling as a passenger in a car at night. He also began to notice movement on the television. His rehabilitation therapists, excited by this, began an intensive program to improve his vision. Over the next 4 months, he progressed from being unable to read letters or words to being able to trace the outlines of letters and then recognize them. At this stage he was able to read short words, such as *it* and *the*, but he was completely unable to recognize any objects or people on sight. After another 3 months of intensive rehabilitation, he could recognize numbers, use a telephone, and locate his ashtray. He could read simple booklets and his digital watch. When shown a real object or a line drawing or photograph of an object, he could not recognize it, but he could describe the shape of the object and sometimes work out what the object was from his own description of its shape. His ability to recognize objects via touch, sound, or smell was completely normal. Even after many years of rehabilitation, which was at times quite intensive, Michael has remained unable to recognize most objects on sight and completely unable to recognize faces on sight.

Examinations by an optometrist 4 and 7 years after his head injury demonstrated that his sight had indeed recovered; his visual acuity was adequate and correctable to normal with glasses. More significantly, he had markedly reduced visual fields, leaving him with 5°–8°-degree central fields in both eyes. What this means for Michael is that he views the world down a tunnel. As long as the objects and pictures he is viewing are held at arms length and are small, he can scan them and see them in their entirety perfectly well, an important fact that allows his impaired vision to be ruled out as the cause of his higher cognitive visual disorders. Michael has no color vision in his right eye and moderately impaired color vision in his left eye.

A magnetic resonance imaging (MRI) brain scan carried out 6 years posttrauma (see Fig. 8-1) showed an altered signal, indicating dead brain matter (*infarction*) within the medial aspects of both occipital lobes, affecting grey matter and subcortical white matter. The area of damage was greater in the right occipital lobe, and the increased size (*dilatation*) of both occipital horns of the lateral ventricles suggested that this damage had been there, unchanged, for many years. The third ventricle, as well as the lateral ventricles, was mildly dilatated. The forward-traveling pathways to the temporal lobes were damaged on both sides, and on the right side the forward-traveling pathways to the parietal lobe were also damaged. No other areas of significant damage could be seen within the brain.

Neuropsychological Assessment

General intellectual and memory abilities   Assessments on the Verbal subtests of the revised Wechsler Adult Intelligence Scale (WAIS-R) 3 and 6 years posttrauma demonstrated that Michael's verbal abilities had stabilized; his Verbal IQ fell easily within the average range. He could repeat seven digits forward and five backward, demonstrating a normal attention span—an important consideration if a person is to be subjected to neuropsychological testing. He scored particularly well on tests of vo-

Figure 8-1 Michael's magnetic resonance imaging right hemisphere is on the left side of the scan. It shows altered signal within the medial aspects of both occipital lobes affecting grey matter and subcortical white matter, with the gliosis more prominent on the right. (Reprinted from Ogden 1993a, p. 575, with kind permission from Elsevier Science Ltd., Kidlington, UK.)

cabulary and comprehension, a good indication of his preaccident (or premorbid) verbal intelligence.

On tests involving the ability to think abstractly, he also performed well. For example, he had no difficulty giving the abstract meanings of proverbs. Along with consistent evidence that his performance on other frontal-lobe tests and his behaviors in a range of situations in daily life were generally appropriate, his performance suggested that his frontal-lobe functions fell within normal limits. This is an important finding in a person who has sustained a severe head injury, as frontal-lobe damage is very common in this group. Even a CT or MRI scan that shows apparently undamaged frontal lobes is no guarantee that extensive frontal-lobe damage has not occurred. The damage is often too diffuse to be visualized and involves shearing and tearing of the white matter tracts connecting the frontal cortex to the rest of the brain. Thus, neurobehavioral assessment of frontal-lobe dysfunction is essential given the subtle but significant influence of the executive deficits associated with damaged frontal lobes on a range of apparently unrelated abilities (see Chapter 10). Michael's general visuospatial abilities and Performance IQ could not be assessed because of his visual agnosia and tunnel vision.

On tests of verbal memory and new learning, Michael demonstrated moderately severe deficits, suggesting that he has some temporal lobe damage, at least in the left hemisphere. Indeed, his MRI scan showed that the forward-traveling pathways from the occipital to the temporal lobes were damaged on both sides. It is important to note that his verbal memory deficit was not severe, as in the case of H.M. (see Chapter 3). For example, in contrast to his impaired scores on formal tests of new verbal learning, Michael demonstrated good functional verbal memory for conversations that held significance for him. He can recall the gist of conversations he and I had up to 3 years earlier and has apparently normal or near-normal recall of the names and other semantic (factual) information about people currently in his life. When I telephoned Michael on my return from a year-long study leave overseas, on giving him my name, he immediately responded by asking me how my trip was and what new tests and rehabilitation ideas I had discovered that might be helpful to him. Many years later, when revising this book, I telephoned him "out of the blue" and he immediately recalled who I was. A long conversation about his life since I had last talked with him ensued, and he had no obvious difficulty with gross verbal recall. For example, within minutes of the beginning of our conversation he told me that Jill, his attendant carer, was there with him and that she was the same person who had been his attendant carer almost 10 years previously when we had been carrying out our research.

Michael probably also has some impairment of visual, nonverbal learning, but of course this cannot be tested because he cannot recognize visual patterns (other than simple shapes) or faces.

In apparent contrast to his reasonable verbal recall of life events since his accident, Michael has a striking loss of personal memories that extends back from his accident into his early childhood. The evidence for this loss is complex and extensive and suggests that the cause of his autobiographical retrograde amnesia lies predominantly in his inability to recall the dominant visual components and visual images associated with his personal memories. This explanation for his unusual and dramatic retrograde amnesia is supported by the observation that he can recall some aspects of his past if they are not visual and were thus stored, for example, as auditory memories. As an illustration of this, he remembers songs (melodies and words) from his past, and on regaining consciousness in the hospital after his accident he recognized all his friends when they came to visit him by their voices. Further details of Michael's autobiographical amnesia and my postulated explanation for it can be found in Ogden (1993a).

Language abilities and perception and recognition of letters and words Michael's speech is fluent and his comprehension normal. He can point accurately on command to lower- and uppercase letters displayed randomly on a page. He reads text slowly, apparently because of his tunnel vision, but accurately. Words in small print held at 1.5 m to compensate for his visual field constriction can be read fluently. His writing and printing of individual letters, words, and sentences spontaneously and to dictation are slow but generally accurate, and he can read his own printing. His reading of handwriting is slower and less accurate than his reading of print. His imagery of letters is intact. For example, when asked to imagine a letter and decide whether it has curved or straight sides, he is able to respond accurately.

Diagnostic tests of visual object agnosia   *Visual perception*: Michael's performance was 100% accurate on each of the following tasks:

a. Discrimination of line drawings of triangles with curved sides from those with straight sides
b. Pointing to the shortest and longest lines on pages of lines of different lengths
c. Pointing to and recognizing different shapes and sizes of the same shape (squares, rectangles, circles, hexagons, and so on) on pages of shapes and drawing shapes accurately on command.

In addition, Michael can copy line drawings of objects in a slow and disjointed fashion without recognizing what he is drawing (see Fig. 8-2). When asked what his copy of the turtle was, he said he did not know, but perhaps it could be a bird. He would not even guess the identity of the bird.

Visual recognition of objects: Michael's tactile and auditory recognition of objects, people, and animals is unimpaired, but he can recognize on sight only a few objects and animals that he has seen many times. On a formal test where he was shown 30 real objects, he could recognize only eight, all of which were objects he had been shown often as part of his rehabilitation program, such as an ashtray, eating utensils, and scissors.

When shown an object or a drawing of an object, his strategy is to describe its shape to himself and to guess what the object might be from his verbal description. A yellow feather he called a flower, a safety pin he called a clothes peg, and a vegetable peeler he called a razor. When shown a key, he described it thus: "a circle; there is a long, thin piece off one side; it is smooth on the top but seems to have a jagged edge on the bottom," but he could not recognize it. As soon as he picked it up, he recognized it instantly as a key.

His ability to recognize photographs, realistic three-dimensional paintings of objects, and line drawings of objects appears slightly more impaired than his ability to

Figure 8-2 Michael's copies of drawings. The models are in the left column and Michael's copies in the right column. (Reprinted from Ogden, 1993a, p. 578, with kind permission from Elsevier Science Ltd., Kidlington, UK.)

recognize real objects. For example, he recognized a real telephone in 4 seconds (he often uses a telephone in his own house), but he was still unable to recognize a line drawing of a similar telephone after 35 seconds of trying. I then said "ring, ring," and he said "Oh, is that what it is, a telephone!" One hour later, shown the same drawing, he was able to identify it correctly in 5 seconds.

He recognized two items, a house (8 seconds) and a spoon (6 seconds), in a series of 20 black and white photographs of common items. He was shown 30 realistic colored paintings of common objects and animals in context (e.g., sheep in a paddock, a baby eating from a bowl, apples on a tree, fruit in a bowl) taken from a series of books used for teaching 4-year-old children the names of objects and animals. He was asked to name specific objects in each painting and was able to name only two items correctly, a pen (3 seconds) and a "person" (4 seconds). He was unable to say whether the person was male or female, adult or child. He could identify some animals as animals after describing their form to himself, but he was not able to identify any specific animal correctly. In all the above experiments, he was given a minimum of 60 seconds before being permitted to give up, longer if he thought he might be able to recognize the item given more time.

Michael is also severely impaired in naming line drawings of single objects or living things. Of a series of 60 items, he named only three. This experiment, also used to assess category-specific visual recognition, is detailed in the next section.

Through the trials, Michael sometimes learns to recognize his descriptions of the objects he sees and becomes faster at identifying them with repeated exposures. When first shown a line drawing of an elephant, he attempted to describe its shape but was still unable to recognize it after 30 seconds. He was then told it was an animal, but this did not assist him. He was then given the names of five animals and asked which one it was. He correctly selected *elephant* and was able to point to the trunk. One hour later, he was shown the same drawing, and after 9 seconds he was able to identify it as an animal "because it has four legs," but he could not be more specific. When shown the same line drawing 2 years later, he was once again completely unable to identify it or even correctly categorize it as an animal.

Category-specific visual recognition: No broad category of object appeared easier or harder for Michael than any other one. He was shown a series of 60 line drawings falling randomly within each of the following categories: vegetables, fruits, plants, animals, insects, natural phenomenon, clothing, bathroom and household implements, tools, musical instruments, transportation, and body parts. In all but three categories, his recognition was nil. He recognized one object of the five in the categories of fruits (apple, 4 seconds), bathroom and household implements (toothbrush, 6 seconds), and clothing (trousers, 10 seconds), in each case after making a number of guesses based on its shape. He identified a line drawing of a butterfly as a plant, a cow as a dog, a truck as a house, and a spade as a hat stand. The toothbrush he described as "similar to a spoon or fork with bits coming up—a toothbrush!" When shown a drawing of a cat sitting upright facing the camera, he described it as follows: "Here is a face, and these look like legs; it must be a person!" His ability to recognize visually line drawings of living things was thus as severely impaired as his ability to visually recognize nonliving things.

When Michael was shown a page of 16 line drawings of objects and told that eight of them were different types of chairs and eight were different types of lampshades, his ability to discriminate between the two categories was well above chance. He made one error on the lampshades and two errors on the chairs. His strategy was to describe the form and see if his description was more similar to a chair or a lampshade.

Tactile and auditory recognition of objects: The same 30 real objects used in the visual recognition experiment were given to Michael to manipulate with his right hand, his left arm having been amputated. Large objects (e.g., telephone) were placed on the table in front of a blindfolded Michael, and his right hand was placed on the object. Small objects (e.g., a key) were placed in his right hand. He was free to manipulate the objects as he wished, and when necessary they were held steady while he explored them. All 30 objects were correctly named within 1–4 seconds.

While blindfolded, Michael was asked to name 20 sounds (given in the following order): water being poured from a jug into a cup, the rattle of a bunch of keys, brushing teeth with a toothbrush, the ring of a telephone, the sound of rain outside the building, footsteps, a noise of "baa-a-a" like a sheep, a door opening, a nose being blown, a match being struck on the side of a matchbox, the sound of a car starting up outside the window, a noise of "woof" like a dog, scissors cutting paper, a sniff, a noise of "moo" like a cow, a book page being turned, a door being closed, a noise of "quack" like a duck, the sound of a kiss, a cough. He named all sounds correctly within 1 second.

Semantic (factual) knowledge of objects: When given the name or other identifying information about an object or an animal (e.g., something that goes "miaow") and asked to describe it, his performance was normal with regard to function in almost all cases. When given the names, he was able to describe the function of the 30 objects used in the visual and tactile recognition experiments. He was also able to provide factual information and to describe the functions of living objects and natural phenomena (e.g., trees, specific animals, clouds, mountains). In contrast, he was frequently unable to describe accurately the shape of the object or living thing. For example, when asked what a cup was, he said it is made out of pottery or china and is for drinking. When asked about its shape, he said that it was hollow with a handle to hold it. When asked if he could visualize a cup, he said he could not but that he knows he picks it up by a handle to drink from, and it must be hollow to hold coffee. When asked what a canary was, he said it was a small bird that whistled, but he could not quite see its shape. He thought it had two legs. He did not know what the color was, but he thought it might be blue.

Visual imagery and the ability to draw objects from long-term memory   Michael can quickly and accurately draw from memory triangles, squares, rectangles, crosses, and circles. He can draw shapes of different sizes on command and lines of different lengths. For example, he responds accurately when asked to draw a line across the top of the page and underneath it a line of half the length of the first one. He can draw a large circle above a cross and a small circle below the cross. He can also draw on command some objects with simple shapes (e.g., a rugby ball, a basketball, a rugby field, an apple, a banana).

Michael can draw in a simplistic fashion some more complex common objects on command. He was able to draw a recognizable house and key (see Fig. 8-3), but his drawing of a flower looked more like a palm tree, and he drew a bed as a rectangle with four legs. He would not even attempt more complex or unfamiliar objects, such as a telephone or a broom, because he said he could not think how they might look. He was also unable to draw or visualize any specific objects, such as the house where he grew up.

When asked to visualize and describe a surf beach where he had spent a great deal of time before his accident (and has been to since), he said he could imagine the waves and the sand and hear the surf, but he did not describe the scenic surrounds of bush, cliffs, and rocky peninsulas. When asked the color of the sand, he said it was pale, when in fact the sands are distinctive black iron.

It appears, therefore, that Michael is unable to visualize (locate in long-term store or bring into awareness) objects and scenes from long-term memory store, or alternatively, he has lost the visual memory "templates" themselves. The drawings he is able to do and his verbal descriptions of visual forms from memory are impoverished and nonspecific and probably represent a stylized prototype of the object category. Michael also denies having dreams, perhaps suggesting a loss of the ability to generate visual images.

Figure 8-3 Michael's drawings of a key and a house from long-term memory. (Reprinted from Ogden 1993a, p. 580, with kind permission from Elsevier Science Ltd., Kidlington, UK.)

Prosopagnosia   Michael has a total inability to recognize any faces on sight, and this has not improved over the 17 years since his accident. Practice and familiarity do not help: He never recognizes his mother until she speaks although he sees her almost daily. He is unable to pick out any familiar face, including his own, in family photographs taken before and after his accident.

Michael was shown a collage of photographs of faces of people famous and well known to him before his accident and faces of people he would never have seen. When asked to point to any faces that seemed more familiar to him, he said that none seemed familiar. When asked to describe verbally from memory the very distinctive face of a famous NZ Prime Minister who had been in the public eye for many years before and after Michael's accident, Michael said (accurately) that he had a lopsided smile. When he was then asked to guess which of the faces on the collage was this man's face, he pointed to a face of an unknown man.

Michael's ability to discriminate gender, age, and expression of faces is also greatly impaired. He would sometimes guess gender correctly by the length of hair, but when this was controlled for, he performed at chance levels. When asked to say whether a face looked happy or sad, he would rely on the shape of the mouth and made numerous errors. When asked how old a baby in a photograph might be, he said it looked like an old man because it did not have much hair. Michael instantly recognized faces as soon as they spoke. When shown a photograph of a face and asked to match it to the identical face in a pair of faces, he performed correctly on all eight trials, but took a long time, generally matching the face by the hairline.

Michael could recognize face and body parts at a better than chance level if he knew that what he was looking at was a face part or a body part. He usually took a few seconds to make an identification and sometimes made errors, giving an incorrect but related body-part name; for example, a foot for a hand. With the instruction that he was looking at parts of the head, he was able to identify correctly an eye (2 seconds), a mouth (2 seconds), a nose (5 seconds), and an ear (16 seconds) when they were shown to him on separate cards. He was able to identify a face as a face, but he often made errors across species. For example, he identified pictures of the faces of a teddy bear, cat, and monkey as human faces.

When asked to point to face or body parts on himself, he had no difficulty. Given his tunnel vision, it was difficult for him to locate body parts on others while still being within arms reach, and he performed poorly at this task.

Color Perception and Color Memory   Michael could not identify any colors whether in isolation or in the context of an object. He commented that he saw everything as shades between white and black. When asked to name the color of tokens, he was correct only on white and black tokens. All other colors he named either white or pale, or black or dark. Yellow was white, and dark blue was black. When asked to group tokens according to their color, he made two piles; one he called dark, the other pale. This loss of color perception is termed *achromatopsia*, and it results from bilateral lesions in the area of the prestriate cortex extending to the temporal lobe, lesions that fit well with Michael's. When Michael was asked to give the colors of named (but not seen) objects, animals, or natural phenomena, he was usually correct with regard to natural phenomena that are frequently and stereotypically associated with their color name, such as blue sky, white clouds, blue sea, green grass, white snow. He made numerous errors on most nonliving and living things. For example, a banana was guessed to be either green or blue, and although he described a strawberry as a small, sweet berry that grows on low bushes and is eaten with sugar and cream, he could not visualize its shape or its color. Toast was dark and an apple was brown. He described a sparrow correctly as a small, common bird, but he was unable to visualize or remember its color. He guessed it to be blue, and when told it was brown, he said this did not enable him to visualize it. When asked what color his skin was, he first said it was blue; told that was wrong, he said pinkish white.

These difficulties with visualizing colors indicate a loss of color memory; whether this loss is a result of deficient color perception or an independent memory deficit is not clear. It has been postulated that impaired color perception may preclude the visualization, and thus the memory of colors, suggesting that other brain systems are incapable of supporting the recall of perceptually impaired color (Farah 1989). In contrast, a patient with bilateral occipital lobe damage and relatively intact color perception, but with a loss of long-term color memories, has been described (De Vreese 1991).

Personal and Social Consequences

Michael's inability to recognize objects or faces is, in a sense, almost more debilitating than being totally blind. He is always striving to recognize what he is sees, which can act as a barrier to learning how to cope without sight. Because he can read it is not necessary for him to learn braille, yet his tunnel vision makes reading extremely tiring. He sometimes comments on his inability to make mental pictures and his loss of dreams, but these impairments do not seem to worry him. The loss of one arm and his difficulty walking because of his old orthopedic injuries exacerbate his problems in moving about while trying to avoid objects that appear to loom up at the end of a tunnel and that he is not able to recognize.

His impaired ability to retain new information makes the task of rehabilitation difficult at times. For example, learning how to cook with one arm and an inability to recognize visually a saucepan, carrot, or tomato requires that everything in the kitchen be kept consistently in the same place. Michael forgets what goes where and has difficulty remembering to follow simple but important safety measures when cooking. He cannot go out alone because he cannot learn new routes like many blind people can and because his poor physical mobility makes this too dangerous.

His loss of preaccident autobiographical memories does not seem to upset him unduly, perhaps because his mother and friends have spent many hours telling him about his past so that he can gradually build up some sense of from where he comes. He remembers his old friends well (from their voices) but cannot recall anything they did together in the past. It is a credit to Michael's friendly and happy nature and great sense of fun that he has retained some good friends over the years since his accident. They still collect him and take him to their homes for a meal or party, where he enjoys drinking and socializing.

Given his many disabilities, it would be understandable if Michael often felt depressed and frustrated or became disenchanted with the ongoing grind of rehabilitation. Remarkably, this has not happened, and Michael consistently maintains his positive outlook. When asked how he does this, he replies that he is lucky to be alive and could be much worse off. As he says, he has regained his sight, and his ability to walk about is improving, especially with the latest operation on his foot. He does not appear to harbor any underlying feelings of bitterness or anger about his fate, although he does, of course, feel depressed at times about the future. If he were always happy, it would indicate that he had poor insight into his problems and suggest that he had sustained some frontal-lobe damage. Throughout his rehabilitation, Michael has generally sustained a high level of motivation, although with an increasing reluctance to proceed at the slow pace necessary to establish the sequential steps required to cope safely with activities of daily living.

After living in the Institute for the Blind, in his mother's home with a full-time caregiver and rehabilitation therapist, in a good friend's home, and in a home for young disabled people, 6 years after his accident Michael had achieved, at least in part, his dream of independence. He had moved into his own (rented) apartment, where he lived alone, with an attendant carer, Jill, coming in daily to help him and accompany him when he wanted to go outside the apartment. He had learned his way around the rooms and was skilled at using the telephone and microwave oven, washing dishes, and cleaning.

Ten Years On

When I first wrote this chapter in 1995, my conclusion about Michael's future was as follows: "It seems unlikely that he will ever be able to regain full independence, but given Michael's determination, this prediction may prove wrong." In 2004 when revising this chapter, I was living away from the city in which Michael lived, so decided to telephone him to check this prediction out. At that point I had not spoken to Michael for a number of years, but as soon as I introduced myself, he instantly recalled who I was and a long conversation ensued not only with Michael but also with Jill, his daily attendant carer. In this role, Jill has come to his house for a few hours a day on 5 days of the week for the past 12 or more years. She is now a grandmother, and clearly she and her family have become close friends of Michael's. As Michael joked, "Jill and I are like an old married couple, but without the sex!"

Michael, now 43 years old, is still the positive, effervescent person I remembered and continues to live life to the full. His response to my first question, asking him how he was getting on, was "Well I can see a little, but can conceive of all!" Some years previously he had received from the New Zealand Government Accident Compensation scheme some belated compensation, which, with the help of his carer, he invested wisely for his future, but that has also enabled him to follow some of his dreams. He purchased his own house, and in 1999, he flew to the United States with Lou, a friend he made following his accident. Lou worked for an organization called Bikers' Rights and assisted motor bikers injured in accidents. He and Michael became good friends, and Lou would often take Michael for trips in the sidecar of his Harley Davidson. Michael has always loved motorbikes, and the motorbike accident that almost took his life and certainly changed it forever has not in any way diminished his passion. The total amnesia for the accident itself and his very hazy memories of the many months of operations and pain that followed was probably a significant factor in allowing his love of riding bikes to remain untarnished.

Michael had a dream that he would love to ride Route 66 in the United States, and Lou said, "Why not?" Michael's mother was initially worried that he would end up in another accident, this time perhaps a fatal one, but she joined the dream believers after thinking about Jill's wise comment that Michael could sit in his big leather chair in his safe house for the rest of his life, or follow his dream, even if the risks were great. After much organization and planning, Michael and Lou flew to Los Angeles from New Zealand, and then to San Antonio where they picked up a Harley Davidson. They then proceeded to ride, with Michael in the sidecar, to New Orleans, Memphis (including Graceland), and Chicago, where they picked up Route 66 and rode to Los Angeles, Las Vegas, and back to San Antonio. In Chicago they came off their bike, and Michael suffered a bad gash to his left leg, which had been severely fractured in his original accident. The Chicago surgeon who sewed him up was a biker himself and stitched him in such a way that Michael could continue his journey across the States. On returning to New Zeland, his leg was a "mess" and further surgery was needed, but it was all worth it.

When they returned, Lou made up a photograph album of their travels but then realized that this wasn't much use to Michael. He then had the wonderful idea of putting together a series of musical CDs to remind Michael of their trip. For example, the first CD includes *Leaving on a Jet Plane, New Orleans, Memphis Tennessee, Carolina Blues, Miami Vice, The Painted Desert, Needles and Pins, Grand Canyon, Viva Las Vegas, Tombstone, Riders on the Storm, Waltz Across Texas,* and *Harley Davidson Blues.* Michael believes that he can remember parts of his trip, especially when cued by the songs on his CDs, which remind him of those locations or the music they enjoyed on their trip. Even if his memories of details of the trip are vague and nonspecific, the emotions of that trip—the feel and smell of the bike and his leather gear, the wind on his face, the different perfumes in the air, the music, often also linked to his past before he had the accident, and simply riding Route 66—are instantly and vividly brought to life for him by the music, and of course sharing stories with Lou, Jill, and his mother. With friends like Lou and Jill, who needs professional rehabilitation therapists! Michael's story is truly one of triumph over adversity, with a little help from friends.

Michael thinks he can possibly "see" a little better now, and he and Jill sometimes even go to movies (although he admits that it is the sound track rather than the visuals that allow him to follow the plot). He thinks that he can recall autobiographical memories laid down since his accident that involve sound, tactile sensations, and emotions. Certainly, his spontaneous recall of many of the tasks we did during the original assessments 10–13 years ago seem very clear. He had retained an excellent recall and understanding of the neuropsychological theories I had suggested might explain his visual agnosia and loss of visual autobiographical memories. Michael and I agreed to meet later in the year to reassess his visual agnosia and perhaps to carry out some experiments using functional MRI.

Discussion

Michael's case provides good examples of visual object agnosia and prosopagnosia. His visual agnosia could be classified as the integrative type because he can perceive simple shapes but not objects. Although he can copy drawings of objects, he does so line by line or element by element. Likewise, when verbally describing the shape of an object, he does so in a fragmented way. Michael's impairments of color perception and color memory and his inability to report dreams and use visual images make his case even more interesting to the researcher.

The main theoretical question raised by cases of visual agnosia and prosopagnosia relates to the fact that the disorders are modality specific. That is, the person continues to have access to knowledge about the object or face via the other senses, and it is only when the stimulus is seen that recognition and knowledge are blocked. What does this tell us about the way the mind is divided? Damasio, Damasio, and Van Hoesen (1982) provided one possible explanation in their study of prosopagnosia. In Figure 8-4, I have illustrated this in schematic form and extended it to include complex objects as well as faces. We can perceive information about an object or a face independently via all our senses. At this early stage, modality-specific perception presumably occurs in the appropriate sensory cortices (i.e., vision in the occipital sensory cortex, audition in the temporal sensory cortex, and tactile percepts in the parietal sensory cortex). Each percept is then matched to a modality-specific template (memory), and this process probably occurs in the adjoining modality-specific association cortices. When a match in one modality is made, it fires all the neural connections to other-modality associations with that stimulus. For example, when a visual match is made, it fires the neural systems that mediate the auditory, tactile, and olfactory knowledge about that object or face, and recognition occurs. The process of matching a percept to a memory template can be likened to unlocking a door leading to the room where full (multimodal) recognition occurs. The key can be in any sensory modality, which means that a patient with tactile agnosia could not recognize an object or face by feeling it but could gain access to the recognition system via vision.

This type of model can, of course, be developed and understood without any recourse to brain structures. A model is simply that, and this one provides only one of the possible explanations for the modality-specificity of the agnosias. It does, how-

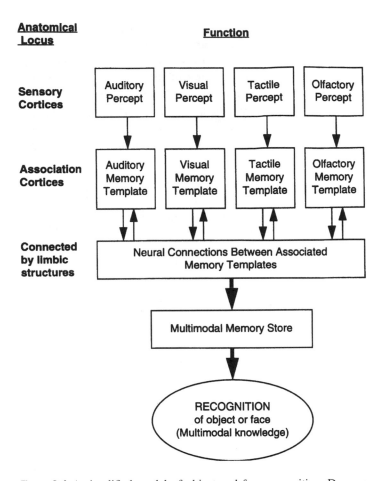

Figure 8-4 A simplified model of object and face recognition. Damage
to or dysfunction of the neural structures and pathways mediating visual
perception or the visual memory store for objects and faces could result
in visual object agnosia or prosopagnosia, but recall of mutimodal
knowledge leading to recognition of the object or face could nevertheless be activated via another modality (e.g., the sound, feel, smell, or
taste of the object or face).

ever, serve to illustrate the ways in which the careful study of patients with brain
damage and clearly defined neurobehavioral disorders can further our thinking about
how the normal brain might work. Ultimately, knowledge about brain–behavior relations will hopefully guide the development of logical rehabilitation strategies to help
these patients. In individual cases, a careful assessment following many of the same
principles and methods that underlie a formal research investigation can tell us what
rehabilitation strategies would be a waste of time and which ones are worth a try.
And of course, just observing what works for the individual, as Lou did for Michael

when he made up the music CDs to help him reexperience his dream ride across the States, is a "rehabilitation" strategy family and friends can often use effectively. The "Whatever It Takes" (WIT) model of rehabilitation (Willer and Corrigan 1994) (see also Chapter 10), would readily encompass Michael's long bike ride and the strategies used to enhance his memories of it later. In the WIT model, a range of commonsense principles, and rehabilitation strategies that follow from these principles, are utilized to assist the head-injured person to make the best of what skills he or she has in the easiest possible way and, most important, within the individual's own environment. Rehabilitation focuses on maximizing the ability to become involved in activities enjoyed by the individual rather than on concentrating on rehabilitating abilities that may be of little significance (e.g., remembering lists of meaningless words).

Another common line of theoretical inquiry touched on in the model above is the relation of mind to brain, which is often seen as a philosophical matter, though the neuropsychologist tends to take a more pragmatic approach. How do the neurobehavioral impairments that the patient demonstrates relate to the underlying brain damage? In Michael's case, we can feel reasonably confident that his various visual deficits are related to his bilateral occipital lobe lesions, as other cases in the literature have involved various combinations of these deficits in patients who also have lesions in the same area.

One possibility is that each of his impairments results from damage to different neural systems that lie physically close together within the visual cortex and the underlying white matter. It seems more likely, however, that some of his impairments result from the same basic visual cognitive deficit, and thus from the same damaged neural system. For example, as described earlier, the recognition of an object or a face probably requires forming a percept of it and then matching it to a stored visual representation (visual memory or template) in the mind. In visual agnosia and prosopagnosia, something goes wrong at this stage, and access into the knowledge system is blocked. It has been postulated that both the visual percepts and the stored visual representations or memories are displayed on a mental "visual buffer" or screen, where they can be mentally scanned or physically copied, or where the percept can be matched to a visual memory so that the recognition process can proceed (Kosslyn 1981, 1983; Farah 1984). In Michael's case there is a close match between his missing visual memories and the visual objects and other stimuli he cannot recognize, suggesting they both result in part from the same underlying cognitive deficit or deficits. His visual object agnosia and prosopagnosia could result from his inability at the late perceptual level to integrate the parts of an object or face that he sees into a spatially meaningful whole and also from his inability to integrate the elements of a visual memory of an object or face. Both deficits occur at the stage of inspecting the image (whether from a percept or a memory) in the visual buffer.

The explanation for Michael's belated recovery from cortical blindness 17 months after his accident is a mystery. Possibly some neurons in his visual cortex were disabled rather than permanently damaged at the time of his accident, and it took many months for the number of neurons necessary for useful sight to regain their function (perhaps via *remyelination*, or the formation of new neural connections). The recent overthrowing of the once "indisputable fact" that new neurons cannot form in the vertebrate brain provides another possible pathway for recovery. Recent animal studies have demonstrated that the number of new neurons generated in the dentate gyrus of rats doubled in response to associate-learning tasks that relied on the hippocampus, but not to associate-learning tasks shown to be independent of the hippocampus (Gould, Beylin, Tanapat, Reeves, and Shors 1999). Similarly, voluntary exercise in an enriched environment enhanced neurogenesis in the adult mouse dentate gyrus (Van Praag, Kempermann, and Gage 1999). Rats exposed to an enriched environment both before and after a cerebral insult demonstrated enhanced neurogenesis and decreased cell death in the hippocampus, coupled with improved cognitive performance, especially on spatial learning and memory tasks known to involve the hippocampus (Young, Lawlor, Leone, Dragunow, and During 1999). It also appears that the human hippocampal formation produces new neurons throughout adulthood (Eriksson et al. 1998). Although there is as yet no evidence that neurogenesis can occur in the occipital cortex of adult humans, the fact that neurogenesis in the adult human brain occurs at all surely raises the possibility that this might have occurred in Michael's case. In line with studies that demonstrate that specific activities appear to stimulate growth of specific neurons known to be related to that type of activity (Gould et al. 1999), perhaps some degree of neurogenesis was stimulated in Michael's occipital cortex by the intensive program to improve his vision instigated by his rehabilitation therapists when he first began seeing the moving lights of cars 17 months after his accident.

Observations by his attendant carer and by Michael himself suggest, however, that there is little evidence of any further increase in his visual fields over the past 12 years, suggesting that the recovery in sight that did occur was time-limited. Likewise, his visual agnosia, color agnosia, prosopagnosia, and loss of visual imagery appear to have remained substantially unchanged since I first assessed him. However, only a formal and detailed reassessment of his sight and visual fields, as well as of his cognitive impairments, could document accurately whether any further subtle changes have occurred.

For many clinical neuropsychologists, nurses, and rehabilitation therapists who work with patients like Michael, the theoretical insights provided by research studies are interesting but must take a backseat to the more urgent need to assist the patient to a state where he or she can regain a reasonable quality of life. To do so requires practical knowledge that often can be learned only by working with brain-damaged patients. Experienced rehabilitation therapists know, almost by intuition, when their patient can be pushed a little farther and when it is time for a rest or a change of activity. They learn how to predict and prevent the sudden outbreaks of aggression that can happen to any patient as a result of frustration and fatigue, and they know when a touch of humor will lighten the situation and help the patient to laugh at himself or herself. They know when a patient needs to cry and to express anger or helplessness, and they learn how to listen to what the patient needs to help him or her at these times.

The rehabilitation therapist must have an abundance of practical knowledge, patience, stamina, determination, compassion, and humor. The rewards come from working with a person like Michael, who in spite of massive disabilities, courageously continues to make small positive steps (and occasionally giant strides) while retaining his good humor and endearing himself to all who have the good fortune to come within his auditory or tactile orbit.

9

■

The Impaired Executive

A Case of Frontal-Lobe Dysfunction

The executive and personality impairments associated with frontal-lobe dysfunction are well known to all practicing neuropsychologists. In the 1930s and 1940s, frontal lobotomies in which the frontal lobes were completely removed or severed from the rest of the brain were a relatively common treatment for psychiatric disorders (Freeman and Watts 1942; Moniz 1954), although it soon became apparent that for many patients the results of the lobotomy were worse than the disorder it was meant to alleviate (Walsh 1994, p 176). *Psychosurgery* (brain surgery for the purpose of decreasing psychiatric symptoms) decreased substantially from the 1950s on, although centers in some countries still practice modified procedures called *leukotomies*. In these operations, the frontal lobes are partially disconnected from the rest of the cortex by sectioning the thalamofrontal fibers in the lower medial quadrant of the frontal lobe. These and similar greatly modified operations are reported to provide relief from the psychiatric symptoms with minimal frontal-lobe symptoms (McKenzie and Kaczanowski 1964).

Neuropsychologists do not, however, need to rely on the recipients of psychosurgery to become familiar with frontal-lobe impairments. Taken in all its forms, from mild to severe, it is probably the most common neuropsychological symptom cluster in the neurological population. It is common after closed-head injury and can also be a problem for alcoholics; sufferers of Korsakoff's syndrome; people with various forms of dementia, including Alzheimer's disease, Parkinson's disease, and Huntington's disease; patients with severe occupational organic solvent neurotoxicity; and, of course, in persons who have focal damage to the frontal lobes caused by a tumor, stroke, or penetrating object. Thus, assessment of frontal-lobe functioning is as integral a part of a basic neuropsychological assessment as is the assessment of verbal, visuospatial, and memory functions.

The now-outdated term "frontal-lobe syndrome" is still sometimes used as a shorthand way to characterize the wide range of impairments that can accompany frontal-lobe dysfunction. It has been labeled a *syndrome* because it comprises a range of cognitive and emotional deficits commonly associated with damage to the *prefrontal lobes* (the area of frontal cortex from the frontal poles extending back to, but not including, the motor association cortex, plus the basomedial portions of the frontal lobes). Such deficits may be mild to significant, and different combinations of deficits occur in different patients. The presence of a recognized pattern of frontal-lobe impairments, or the "frontal-lobe syndrome," is based on neuropsychological and behavioral evidence, not on neuropathology. Although brain imaging of patients who display a severe frontal-lobe syndrome may show a large area of infarction (dead brain tissue) in both frontal lobes, often no obvious or extensive damage to the frontal lobes is seen in people who display many frontal-lobe deficits.

The reasons that damage is not obvious are many, including imaging technologies that do not have the resolution to pick up small or diffuse lesions (e.g., in alcoholics or following closed head injury) or disconnection syndromes, in which the frontal lobes themselves are not damaged, but some of the fiber tracts that connect the frontal lobes to the other areas of the brain are not functioning. This nonfunctioning may be caused by physical damage to the pathways, as can occur in a closed head injury when the reticular formation that connects the brain stem to the prefrontal lobes is stretched and torn or because of a neurotransmitter imbalance. For example, in Parkinson's disease, which primarily targets the basal ganglia and not the frontal lobes, there is a decrease in the level of the neurotransmitter dopamine. Some of the numerous connections between the basal ganglia and the prefrontal lobes are mediated by dopamine; therefore, the frontal lobes of some people with Parkinson's disease may not function normally.

Because the functions mediated by the frontal lobes are so complex and diverse, it is tempting to call on disorders of the frontal lobes as an explanation for complex disorders that are otherwise difficult to explain. A good example is the frontal-lobe hypothesis of schizophrenia, which proposes that some of the symptoms of schizophrenia are related to frontal-lobe dysfunction, perhaps as a result of a neurotransmitter imbalance or as a side effect of the major tranquilizers taken by many people with schizophrenia.

The association between the frontal lobes and schizophrenia is controversial, but evidence for and against the frontal-lobe hypothesis of schizophrenia is being accumulated via increasingly elegant methods (Gershon and Rieder 1992). These methods include functional imaging techniques, such as positron emission tomography (PET), magnetoencephalography (MEG), and functional magnetic resonance imaging (fMRI), in which the activity of different areas of the brain can be visualized while the subject performs a particular motor or cognitive task (Crease 1993). Sophisticated cognitive tasks developed by cognitive neuroscientists to study normal subjects are also being used to test frontal-lobe hypotheses of schizophrenia. These tasks often use computers to produce experimental stimuli under highly controlled conditions and to analyze the complex results, which may include reaction times in milliseconds and eye-movement recordings. The cognitive experiments will not confirm or disconfirm neuropathology in schizophrenia but may demonstrate whether people with schizophrenia show subtle cognitive deficits similar to those displayed by people with confirmed frontal-lobe damage. The functional imaging techniques are more closely connected with neuro-pathology and may be able to demonstrate whether the frontal lobes of people with schizophrenia are abnormally active or inactive under conditions in which the subject is carrying out cognitive tasks thought to be mediated by the frontal lobes or, alter-natively, tasks not usually mediated by the frontal lobes (Gershon and Rieder 1992).

In summary, the range of deficits sometimes labeled the "frontal-lobe syndrome" is not a specific disorder with a specific cause but simply a shorthand way to describe a pattern of behaviors that occur when the prefrontal lobes are not working normally. It deserves a chapter of its own because of the association of frontal-lobe damage with many common disorders, from alcohol abuse to severe head injury. Phillipa, the woman whose case is described in this chapter, is at the severe end of the frontal-lobe dysfunction spectrum, with unambiguously bizarre and debilitating behaviors; yet it should be kept in mind that mild frontal-lobe dysfunction is often associated with subtle impairments, such as irritability, poor motivation, and a quickness to lose one's temper. All these impairments can disrupt the life of the sufferer and her family.

Theoretical Background

The Frontal Lobes as Executives

The frontal lobes, both in ontological and developmental terms, are the most recently developed areas of the brain. Because of their large size in man relative to other primates, they are often viewed as the seat of the highest and most complex cognitive activities. Rich connections between the medial and basal aspects of the prefrontal lobes and the upper part of the brain stem and thalamus mediate the state of alertness of the individual. The rich connections between the lateral prefrontal regions with all other cortical zones permit the frontal lobes to organize and perform purposeful and goal-directed behaviors based on the multimodal sensory information received from the posterior cortex.

Modern neuropsychologists have labeled the frontal lobes the *executive lobes* be-cause of their role in formulating, modifying, and executing plans of action (Luria 1973). If a person with frontal-lobe damage is involved in a well-learned, highly structured, concrete task, she will probably experience no difficulty. If the task is new, unstructured, and requires planning a strategy to initiate and complete the task, or if it involves thinking in terms of abstract concepts, then the person with frontal-lobe dysfunction may well show deficits.

How these executive functions can result in a poor performance on a neuropsy-chological test can be illustrated by the problems a frontally impaired person has when attempting to reproduce some of the Block Design items of the revised Wechsler Adult Intelligence Scales (WAIS-R) (Walsh 1985). In one item of this test, the subject is shown a picture of a square with a pattern of diagonal red and white stripes (see Fig. 9-1a). The subject must reproduce this pattern using nine blocks, each with two white

a b

Figure 9-1 The Block Design subtest of the revised Weschsler Adult Intelligence Scale Design (a) is one of the harder designs (the stripes are red and white) in the test. The patient is asked to copy the design using nine blocks, each of which has two white sides, two red sides, and two red and white sides. The poor performance of patients with frontal-lobe damage can often be improved if a grid is placed over the design as in (b). This divides the design into blocks and thus provides an external structure for the patient to follow.

faces, two red faces, and two faces with red on one side of the diagonal and white on the other. To carry out this task successfully, the subject must be able to conceptualize how to break the pictured pattern into block-sized units. This task is difficult or impossible for many people with brain damage, but people with parietal damage or frontal damage have the most difficulty. Frontally impaired subjects will improve their performance if a grid that divides the picture into block-sized squares is placed over the picture (see Fig. 9-1b). This grid provides an external structure to follow and relieves the person of the requirement of forming a mental concept to plan her strategy. Subjects with parietal damage cannot do the task because they have visuospatial perceptual and construction problems, and no amount of instruction or the provision of an external structure using a grid will help them.

Another difficult visuospatial task for some people with executive impairments is copying the Rey Complex Figure. When asked to copy this drawing, they often use a piecemeal approach, suggesting that their ability to plan a logical approach to this complex task is flawed. If, however, the figure is presented in sequential stages, their performance improves greatly. In contrast, presenting the figure in sequential stages to a person with parietal lobe damage may improve their copy to some extent, but they may still draw one section on top another and end up with a poor score. The disorganized copy of the Rey Figure illustrated in Chapter 10 (Fig. 10-1a) is that of a man who sustained a closed head injury and frontal-lobe contusions in an automobile accident. However, many people with focal prefrontal-lobe lesions perform normally when copying the Rey Figure, especially once they have recovered from the acute effects of their stroke or head injury (Damasio and Anderson 2003). For individuals with relatively small stable frontal lesions, the structure provided by the Rey Figure is probably sufficient to guide their drawing movements. This illustrates the range of performance ability, from normal to severe, that can be expected when assessing the test performances of patients with frontal lesions of various sizes and etiologies.

A common finding when assessing patients with executive deficits, which on the surface seems paradoxical, is that they often perform normally on traditional tests of intelligence, such as the subtests of the Wechsler Intelligence Scales. Usually their performance is enhanced because tests of intelligence are themselves highly structured and administered in a highly structured setting. With increasingly severe and bilateral prefrontal damage, some of these tests will be difficult for the patient if they require executive functions such as initiating plans without the help of an external structure (e.g., the more difficult Block Design tasks) and thinking abstractly (e.g., the Similarities subtest of the WIS batteries).

Executive impairments can result in problems in most areas of cognition, including memory. Working memory, or the ability to hold information in short-term store while it is manipulated or worked on in some way, is susceptible to frontal-lobe damage and may underlie other executive deficits, such as an inability to plan ahead. To plan ahead, one must hold in working memory current plans, tasks one must perform to work out the best future plans (e.g. check out various travel options), and possibly even past activities if their success or failure is helpful in planning future activities. All of this complex and interacting information must be manipulated in working memory; thus, if the efficiency of this system is impaired as the result of frontal-lobe damage, planning and organization will certainly suffer. The contribution of prefrontal systems to working memory may lie in the executive control of memory processes, rather than in the working memory processes themselves (Postle, Berger, and D'Esposito 1999).

Frontal amnesia is a term often applied to people who do not suffer from "true" memory impairments in the sense of experiencing difficulties with registering, encoding, or retrieving material, but who have apparent memory problems because of an inability to form plans that enable them to regulate the procedures and verify the outcomes of the various mental steps in the memory process (Luria 1971). For example, given a list of words to learn, the frontally impaired subject may be unable to organize the words to be learned in a logical way, such as building associations between words so that during recall one word cues another word. Providing external structure in the form of arranging the words in categories and pointing out how one category can lead, by association, to the next may help the subject. In contrast, providing these sorts of external structures and cues to a subject like H.M. (see Chapter 3), who has a true inability to memorize new material as a result of bilateral medial temporal lobe lesions, will not help him learn or recall word lists.

The everyday memory problems that are problematic for people with frontal-lobe dysfunction are often described as "forgetting to remember," or prospective memory. Thus, the individual who is asked by his partner to walk to the corner shop and buy the newspaper and a loaf of bread may arrive at the shop but forget what he came for. If he sees the newspaper on the counter his memory may be cued and he will purchase the paper, but forget the bread. Yet if he were given a list-learning test that required him to learn eight words, including newspaper and bread, he may well perform normally. H.M., of course, could neither learn the list of words nor remember to buy the newspaper or bread, even if he saw these items on the shop counter.

The ability to think abstractly is another important executive function frequently associated with the frontal lobes. Tasks that involve sorting cards into different categories dependent on feedback regarding errors (e.g., the Wisconsin Card Sorting Test) are viewed as tests of frontal-lobe integrity. These tests involve thinking abstractly. Certainly, frontally impaired subjects perform poorly on such a test (Milner 1963), but it is difficult to say with conviction that their failure is a result of their inability to think abstractly, to learn from their errors, to change from one mental set to another, or to plan and put into action a logical strategy to enable them to perform this complex task. Many recent studies using the WCST have shown that patients with nonfrontal brain lesions can also perform poorly on this test (Anderson, Damasio, Jones, and Tranel 1991; Grafman, Jonas, and Salazar 1990). The WCST and other similar tests nevertheless remain important assessment tools for executive dysfunction, but they must be interpreted in the context of a battery of other executive and nonexecutive tests, behavioral observations, and neuropathological information.

Other tasks considered to tap the ability to think abstractly include verbal tasks, such as asking the subject to explain the meanings of proverbs. A highly educated person with frontal-lobe damage may be unable to provide the abstract meaning for the proverb "A rolling stone gathers no moss"; instead, the patient may explain it literally. Although there is no doubt that frontally impaired subjects often experience great difficulty with tasks that include the ability to think abstractly, most tasks of this type involve so many abilities that it is often impossible to say with certainty why they failed. Indeed, different subjects may fail for different reasons (Messerli, Seron, and Tissot 1979). Caution must therefore be exercised when interpreting neuropsychological test results that suggest frontal-lobe dysfunction. Wherever possible, the specific reasons for failure on a test should be ascertained, and the subject should be assessed on different tests that rely to some extent on the same ability, to see whether these tests also end in failure.

The impact of impaired executive functions on everyday activities is often much more debilitating than the individual's formal test performance would indicate. Planning, preparing, and serving a relatively simple meal can become impossible. Shopping for groceries may be successful only if a list is constructed that groups different food types together in the order in which they appear along the aisles of the supermarket. Even then, if the individual does not cross off each item as he puts it in his cart, he might find that he has bought two of some items and missed others completely. Given that even relatively simple and immediate tasks are so difficult for the frontally impaired person, it is easy to understand that these people find their businesses collapsing around them and are unable to plan for a future family holiday.

The insensitivity of traditional neuropsychological tests to executive deficits lies in the tests' rigid structure. In recent years executive tests have been developed that attempt to mimic the more unstructured, dynamic environment of daily living. For example, the "Behavioural Assessment of The Dysexecutive Syndrome" (BADS; Wilson, Alderman, Burgess, Emslie, and Evans 1996) includes a number of tests that include requiring the examinee to plan ahead with little external structure to assist him, divide his time effectively among a number of tasks, and work out how to get a cork out of a tube given various tools (e.g., a beaker filled with water) and a number of rules about what cannot be done (e.g., lifting up the tube). Other assessment strategies require patients to perform tasks such as buying items in different shops and meeting someone at a specific time in a real-world environment such as a shopping mall, or mock-up of one. In this assessment situation, patients with frontal-lobe lesions are inefficient, break rules, and fail to complete tasks (Anderson, Hathaway-Nepple, Tranel, and Damasio 2000; Shallice and Burgess 1991). These tests go some way to overcoming the rigidity of traditional tests, and because the patients can see their similarity to the practical skills required in their day-to-day lives, they are more motivated to perform them.

The "Frontal Lobe" Patient

Phineas Gage, an efficient and capable foreman, was injured in 1848 when a tamping iron was blown through the frontal lobes of his brain. Although he physically recovered well from this horrific accident, he suffered a significant and permanent personality change as a result. His physician, J.M. Harlow (1868), described him as follows.

> He is fitful, irreverant, indulging at times in the grossest profanity (which was not previously his custom), manifesting but little deference to his fellows, impatient of restraint or advice when it conflicts with his desires, at times pertinaciously obstinate yet capricious and vacillating, devising many plans for future operation which no sooner are arranged than they are abandoned in turn for others appearing more feasible. His mind was radically changed so that his friends and acquaintances said he was no longer Gage.

One of the personality deficits that often accompany frontal-lobe impairments is the inability to inhibit inappropriate behaviors (called *disinhibition*). Phineas Gage demonstrated disinhibited behaviors when he was "irreverent, indulging at times in the grossest profanity (which was not previously his custom)." A lack of insight into one's problems and the effect one is having on others is another common and debilitating symptom of frontal-lobe dysfunction. Thus, Gage had "but little deference to his fellows," and almost certainly had no awareness of his problems. This lack of insight, coupled with another common frontal problem of being slow or unable to learn from one's mistakes and errors, makes successful rehabilitation extraordinarily difficult. The lack of insight is probably also related to another group of symptoms that includes a diminished sense of responsibility and concern for the future, impulsiveness, mild euphoria, a tendency to make inappropriate and childish jokes, and an impoverished ability to initiate activities or to act spontaneously.

Other difficulties include an impoverished ability to plan ahead and follow through a course of action and an inability to take into account the possible consequences of one's actions. Again, the case of Gage provides a good illustration in that he was often "devising many plans for future operation which no sooner are arranged than they are abandoned in turn for others appearing more feasible." The frontal amnesia that plagues subjects with frontal damage results not only in apparent memory impairments but, perhaps because of disinhibition, also encourages *confabulation* (the tendency to fill memory gaps with invented stories and facts with no apparent awareness that these stories are either incorrect or will be viewed as falsehoods by the listener). Another group of symptoms include the tendency to behave in an inflexible and rigid manner and to have difficulty changing one's opinion even in the face of clear evidence that one's behaviors or opinions are no longer correct or appropriate. *Perseveration* (the stereotypical repetition of sentences and behaviors) is also common. Finally, concrete thinking replaces the abstract attitude in some frontally impaired people. A number of texts provide more detailed descriptions of the frontal lobes, their rich connections with other brain areas, and the complex executive, personality, and psychosocial disturbances that typify dysfunction of them (Damasio and Anderson 2003; Stuss and Knight 2002; Walsh 1994, pp 133–195).

Case Presentation

Background

In the beginning stages of my doctorate, when I was searching the neurology and neurosurgery wards at Auckland Hospital for patients with unilateral lesions to assess for hemineglect, I came across my first unequivocal "frontal-lobe syndrome." Phillipa was referred to me 2 months after an operation in which most of her left prefrontal lobe had been surgically removed after she sustained a severe head injury. The frontal bone of her skull had been shattered, and the underlying brain was badly damaged on the left. Although she had some moderately severe damage to the right frontal lobe as well, I was interested in seeing whether she demonstrated right-sided neglect as a result of her left frontal lobotomy.

Phillipa was 35 years old; before her head injury (the result of an assault by a burglar) she had been an intelligent woman with a university degree in English literature who worked as a primary school teacher in a small town north of Auckland. She and her husband, Larry, had two children aged 8 and 10 years. Larry described Phillipa (as she was before her head injury) as follows: "She was a practical, positive person who did not suffer fools gladly. She could do three things at once and hardly ever seemed to get tired or uptight, even when the kids were acting up and she had another 2 hours' marking to do."

Psychological and Neuropsychological Outcome

Phillipa recovered amazingly quickly from the physical effects of her head injury and neurosurgery, but she was left with a mild weakness down her right side, restraining her from walking without assistance. Within a month of admission to the hospital, she was able to sit up in bed or in a wheelchair, and she rapidly became well known to all staff, patients, and patient's families connected with the ward. She would greet anyone who passed by her bed by calling out loudly, "Hullo you there. Come over here and talk to me." It did not seem to matter to Phillipa who she greeted in this manner: another patient's visitor, a doctor she did not know, or the woman who cleaned the floor. Most people looked embarrassed, replied with a brief "hullo," and moved rapidly away. Their exits would be punctuated by loud swearing from Phillipa, or comments such as, "You snaky bastard, run for your life!" Her inappropriate and disinhibited behaviors extended to a lack of appropriate modesty at times. She would, for example, undress in the ward (which she shared with five other women) without any attempt at modesty, regardless of who was in the room, including visitors. Her disinhibited comments and behaviors were totally at odds with the characteristics of the preaccident Phillipa and caused her husband and other family members' acute distress.

Phillipa was delighted when I sat down to talk with her and readily agreed to take part in the various tests I invited her to do. She was strongly left-handed and signed the consent form with flourish, roughly on the line where I pointed. She then proceeded to sign her name three more times up the left side of the page "just in case the first one isn't good enough." On the various paper and pencil tests of neglect (see Chapter 7), she demonstrated clear right-sided neglect; in addition, she was apt to embellish her drawings. For example, she drew only the left side of a daisy she was asked to copy but added a butterfly. Her copy of the Rey Complex Figure also demonstrated neglect and had various additional embellishments (see Fig. 9-2). When asked why she had added these lines, she replied, "Well, the whole purpose is to draw something interesting I have always believed!" Thirty minutes later, when asked to draw the Complex Figure from memory, she appeared to have no idea what I was talking about, but cheerfully drew some random squiggles and said, "There you are, that should be good enough even for you!"

Her rule-breaking behavior, typical of executive dysfunction, was dramatically displayed when I attempted to assess her on a tactile neglect task. The equipment for this test included a 15-inch-square wooden frame with a curtain hanging from it. Phillipa was asked to put one hand through the curtain to manipulate the magnetic shapes and letters distributed along a metal strip on the other side of the curtain and therefore hidden from her view. She was then asked to pick from a second group of shapes, using first touch and then sight, the shapes she had previously manipulated along the strip. Tactile neglect would be demonstrated if she did not identify the shapes that had been on the right end of the strip.

Unfortunately, I was unable to discover whether Phillipa had tactile neglect because she insisted on using her other hand to pick up the curtain so she could peek under it; telling her not to do it made absolutely no difference. She would verbally agree not to do it but then would go ahead and lift the curtain. I then tried holding her free hand to stop her, but her response was to lean forward and peer over the top of the curtain. By this time, I had abandoned the original aim of the test and was

Figure 9-2 The Rey Complex Figure model is in the top row, and Phillipa's copy, embellished with stars and flags, is in the bottom row.

more intrigued by her rule-breaking behavior. I offered her a chocolate biscuit if she did not try to peek behind the curtain (she had developed an insatiable appetite for chocolate and sweets since her head injury). She immediately agreed, but as soon as I placed her right hand through the curtain and guided her hand to a shape to feel, her left hand whipped out and lifted the curtain. Changing hands made no difference, and she managed to lift the curtain even with her weak right hand. I then tried yelling "stop" as soon as she began to lift the curtain, but this only had the effect of increasing her speed. She was unable to explain why she could not stop herself and found the whole thing very amusing.

Phillipa also perseverated at times, which was readily demonstrated when she was asked to copy me when I tapped out a simple rhythm on the table with my fingertips. She quickly picked up the first rhythm, but when I changed to a new rhythm and asked her to change as well, she replied, "Right you are, boss" and continued to tap in the original rhythm but added her voice, "ta ta ta taaa; ta ta ta taaa," in time with her tapping. Even when she managed to change the rhythm briefly, she would quickly revert to the first rhythm. On a test requiring her to learn pairs of words, she also perseverated, correctly pairing the word *cries* when given the word *baby*, but then going on to give *cries* as the response to *obey, school*, and *fruit*.

Phillipa's university degree in English literature provided strong grounds for an estimation of a superior premorbid ability to make verbal abstractions. This ability was severely impaired by her frontal lobe damage. She had trouble not only with providing abstract definitions for proverbs but also in thinking creatively or laterally in normal conversation. For example, asked about the support she was receiving from her family and friends, she replied that she did not see how they could support her when she was supported by the bed on which she was lying. When I gave her other definitions of support, such as caring, she replied, "Well, caring means looking after, and support means support and so they cannot be the same."

On formal tests of new verbal and nonverbal memory, Phillipa scored well below average. Her attention was hard to capture for more than a few minutes at a time, however, and her motivation to perform "boring" memory tests was poor; it was therefore impossible to assess her potential to store and retrieve information. She could certainly be viewed as having frontally mediated attention deficits that resulted in impaired new learning and memory. Her everyday memory for faces was good: She seemed to remember me without difficulty, but her memory for new names was variable, possibly the result of poor attention and motivation. Her memory for past events was hard to assess; however, her husband said she seemed to recognize different past occasions that he talked about, and she sometimes made comments to suggest she remembered them reasonably well. When her children came to visit, she often asked them questions about their activities and clearly remembered, for example, that her 10-year-old son played football and her daughter loved ballet.

In general, Phillipa had little insight into her condition. When asked why she was in the hospital, she was usually able to reply correctly that "I was bashed over the head, and then had a brain operation." When asked if she had any problems as a result, she would reply, "No, none that I can see and none that you can see." When asked about her family, she talked about them with little indication that she was concerned about her children or how they were managing without her. She would occasionally demand to go home and insist that she needed to return to her position as a school-teacher because the children would be getting lazy about their homework without her to push them, but she was easily distracted onto another subject. On other occasions she would confabulate when asked about her current situation and how she came to be hospitalized. She would spin a tale about coming down to Auckland for a visit and taking time off for a rest before she returned to her busy life up north.

During the 4 months she spent in the hospital, Phillipa rarely seemed depressed, although on a few occasions she was found sobbing uncontrollably. One of these times was precipitated by the nurse taking a bar of chocolate from her. She had developed a voracious appetite for sweets and was rapidly gaining weight. The dietitians had put her on a diet, and Phillipa seemed unconcerned by this as long as she was not able to see the chocolate or sweets denied her. On this occasion, she cried for 10 minutes or more, and no one could calm her. She finally seemed to run out of energy; when asked what had upset her, she had no idea.

Rehabilitation and Long-Term Outcome

Phillipa's primary rehabilitation while in the hospital was physical therapy, which proved to be a frustrating exercise for the therapists. She seemed incapable of carrying out even the simplest exercise on her own and required the continuous presence of the therapist to show her repeatedly what to do. Over the 4 months, the right-sided weakness resolved somewhat, but according to her therapist, this improvement resulted not from Phillipa's motivation but was the result of passive exercise and some spontaneous recovery of both her limb weakness and her right-sided body neglect.

With nursing support and home help, her husband elected to take her home 4 months after the accident. After struggling with a disinhibited, totally dependent person who bore little resemblance to the wife he once knew, however, he finally succumbed to the necessity of placing her in an institution. For him, the final straw was when he arrived home from work one day to find that his two children had run away (to the shed behind their scout den), leaving behind a note that read, "We are sorry to leave you Daddy, but Mummy doesn't want us any more, and she needs you more than us. Please look after Bluey (their pet parakeet) for us." The note was completed by stick drawings of two children holding hands with tears running down their faces and a bed with another stick person lying on it with a downturned mouth and one arm and fist raised. The home helper told Larry that she had come in from the garden on hearing shouting and swearing from Phillipa and had caught Phillipa in the act of throwing her full bed pan at her son and screaming at him to "get out." The home helper did her best to calm everyone down and did not realize until much later that the children had disappeared. They were found that evening, cold and frightened, and Phillipa was placed in a private psychiatric hospital 2 days later.

She has remained in psychiatric nursing homes ever since, and her husband and children (now adults) visit her about once every 3 months. It took many months of psychotherapy before any of them could put their guilt behind them and get on with their lives. Larry said to me when by chance I bumped into him years later:

> Phillipa is exactly the same as she was when she left the hospital. She seems to enjoy our visits and never seems to realize how long it has been since we last saw her. She seems to have no concept of time. If we stay too long, she starts yelling and swearing, and within minutes of us leaving the nurses say she has completely forgotten we were ever there.

Discussion

Frontal-lobe damage and the impairments it causes can range across the entire spectrum, from behaviors that are so subtle that it is difficult to tell if they are even abnormal to the extreme behaviors exhibited by Phineas Gage back in 1848 and Phillipa today. Many of the functions mediated by the frontal lobes are important for social interaction, so the consequences of all degrees of frontal-lobe dysfunction can be considerably disruptive. For example, even relatively minor frontal-lobe damage, such as that following serious alcohol abuse or moderate closed-head injury, can result in some behavior disinhibition. In turn, this disinhibition can render aggressive behaviors more likely and less predictable in some individuals, especially if they had a tendency toward violence before their brain damage occurred. Because alcohol acutely affects the optimal functioning of the frontal lobes in people who are not alcoholics and have no frontal damage, it comes as no surprise that the consumption of alcohol by alcoholics or head-injured people can, for a short time, increase to dangerous levels the disinhibition, lack of insight, and aggressive tendencies of the drinker. The fear and apprehension that many families suffer as they wait for the man of the house to return home after a regular drinking session are only too common.

Frontal-lobe damage must never be used as an excuse for violent behavior; rather, in cases where violent behaviors increase following frontal-lobe damage, rehabilitation strategies that include clear, concrete, frequently repeated rules of behavior, unambiguous boundaries of acceptable behavior, and immediate repercussions for unacceptable behaviors must be put in place.

It is important to be aware that frontal-lobe damage per se is not invariably accompanied by an increase in aggressive behaviors. In many cases, the frontally impaired person may become more passive than previously; indeed, passivity was one of the primary types of behavior change sought by psychiatrists when they referred their patients for frontal lobotomies.

After extensive bilateral frontal-lobe damage such as that sustained by Phillipa, rehabilitation may prove impossible and institutionalization inevitable. In such tragic cases, family members probably suffer much more than the patient, given the latter's lack of insight into her changed personality. Perhaps the best a therapist can offer is counseling to support the patient's family through their grief for their loss and to assist them to overcome feelings of guilt so they can move on with their lives.

10

■

BEATING THE ODDS

SEVERE TRAUMATIC BRAIN INJURY AND THE IMPORTANCE OF ONGOING REHABILITATION

The following speech,[1] given to a traumatic brain injury (TBI) support group by Neil, a 22-year-old former university student who had sustained a severe TBI (also called severe head injury) 3 years previously, provides a moving prologue to this chapter:

> This time three years ago, I was an *A* student at university studying third-year engineering. I was a good sportsman and enjoyed a great social life. One afternoon while riding my motorbike home from university, I hit the center lane of the motorway for some reason. I broke my neck, badly damaged my right arm, and I suffered severe head injuries. For the nonmedical of you, that means I bashed shit out of my head.
>
> I don't know much about the rest of that year, but I'm told that I spent 3 months in hospital, which included 1 month in the hospital's critical care ward, at $4000 a day. I came out of hospital in a wheelchair to live with my parents, and my mother was given leave from her job to look after her 25-year-old baby. I say baby, because that was about the level I was at. I needed help with everything. I needed constant attention. I needed to be retaught everything.
>
> Mum was given a break on the weekends when she returned to her job and Dad relieved her of nursing duties. On two mornings a week, I went to the hospital for occupational and physiotherapy. I made good progress, but then even this minimal rehabilitation was stopped once I had got to the stage that I could beat my therapist at chess. They said that there wasn't much more they could do for me. As I said before, I don't know much about the rest of that year; I spent my time popping in and out of reality, but I do know that I hated being so dependent on my parents, and I hated what this must have been doing to them.
>
> Everyone was amazed at the progress I was making. By the end of the year, I could walk without the walking stick, and apart from the arm, there didn't seem anything wrong with me except that I couldn't say a whole sentence before I had forgotten what I was going to say, forgotten what we were talking about, forgotten who I was talking to. I had no short-term memory at all.
>
> Over the following year, I continued to make good progress. I went to Australia with my brother and cousins for the World Cup rugby matches. That trip gave me a

1. The speech that begins this chapter is printed with the generous permission of the writer, Neil G., and Jude Hay, who first printed the speech in her master's thesis.

great deal more confidence, and by the end of it I was walking quite confidently amongst big crowds of people. However, on my return to my parents' home, I sank further and further into depression. Where was I heading? What will I be doing in 10 years' time? What will I do today?

I was given a computer so that I could finish my degree, a $4000 machine that took me 6 months to learn to operate even the simplest programs. I tried hard and I remained very determined, but there wasn't one day I didn't think about suicide. A friend took me up to the YMCA, and he got me to join the gym there, which was probably the best thing I could have done. I was embarrassed about my appearance, but I went there every day and I improved each time, until I had got to the stage where I felt quite proud of what I could do. My arm was amputated at the end of that year, and what a relief that was. It had just been an albatross to me and I now felt a lot better.

At the beginning of the following year I tried to get back into university by redoing my last full year. However, it soon became obvious that it was still far too early even for that and I stopped going. The neurosurgeon suggested that I should start going to the Concussion Clinic at the hospital, where I went for three mornings a week. I'd never heard of a head injury before my accident, so going to this place certainly opened my eyes to it. Sure I'd played rugby for nearly 20 years and had been knocked out quite often, but only for seconds at a time. With this accident I was out for more than three months. Being able to talk with people who knew what I was going through helped me a lot.

I still had a lot of time that I wanted help filling. I was finally referred to the Rehabilitation League to learn how to do simple jobs all over again, so that one day someone might want to employ me. Since starting there I have been a lot happier. Everyone has got to have a reason to get out of bed each day, and I feel that I am making progress again. Being able to stand here and give this speech to you is a big achievement for me now. I am sure that you would all appreciate that the old nut is a pretty complicated system, and that every head-injured person is affected differently by it, but like any injury it requires stimulation for it to heal. Before the Rehabilitation League took me in hand, I wasn't going anywhere; just sitting at home each day. The point I am wanting to make to you with this speech is that if the system is going to spend this huge amount of money just to keep us alive, then they have got to spend that extra bit to give us some proper rehabilitation, or if money is the main concern here, then they should just let us die with some pride.

Neil's words highlight the despair and frustration experienced by many victims of TBI whose lives are saved as a result of the sophisticated neurosurgical techniques and advanced critical care facilities now available in most major hospitals throughout the Western world. Yet the rehabilitation of these patients is largely "hit and miss" because of a lack of resources committed to the development and maintenance of expensive rehabilitation units. The availability of good rehabilitation services for the severely head-injured does, of course, vary across and within countries, but even those regions fortunate enough to be well endowed with such facilities often find it impossible to provide for the increasing number of TBI victims who survive because of improved acute care.

Why are rehabilitation units so difficult to establish and maintain? One reason is probably political: the head-injured population is often viewed as a burden on society, and many victims, because of their brain injury, lose the ability to protest effectively their plight. Many severely head-injured people (and often their families as well) rapidly fall to the bottom of the socioeconomic ladder because of the treatment costs and their inability to work. Many victims of TBI are young males who are already unemployed and in a low socioeconomic group even before their TBI. Fighting the system to provide better rehabilitation facilities therefore falls to families, friends, and the professionals who care for the head-injured. These are the very people who have to struggle day after day looking after the needs of the head-injured, a role designed to produce burnout if good support systems are not in place. It is hardly surprising, therefore, that they find the task of persistently campaigning for better facilities almost impossible.

The rehabilitation of head-injured people is far from straightforward, another fact that acts against the establishment of successful programs. Head-injured people have organically based problems with memory, planning, and organization; impaired judgment; a poor ability to learn from their mistakes; poor motivation; and emotional mood swings as a result of diffuse shearing injuries, brain stem injuries, and focal damage to the frontal and temporal poles. They also suffer from lowered self-esteem, a loss of confidence, and psychosocial problems that impinge on every aspect of their own and their family's lives. In addition, many victims of TBI have to adapt to permanent physical disabilities, such as *hemiplegia* (a paralysis or weakness of one side of the body). Progress is often slow and unrewarding, and prediction of the ultimate attainable level of recovery is almost impossible. This uncertainty, along with fluctuations in the individual patient's progress, can lead to feelings of depression, anger, frustration, and hopelessness in both the victim and the family. It is no easy task for rehabilitation therapists to encourage a balance between motivation to strive for improvement and grieving for losses, acceptance of disabilities and development of a new self-identity for the brain-injured person.

Despite these difficulties, the complex art and science of head-injury rehabilitation is developing rapidly, with new techniques being assessed in the many excellent rehabilitation units springing up in the United States and, to a lesser extent, in the United Kingdom, Australia, and New Zealand. There is no single "right" way to carry out successful rehabilitation, although there are many "wrong" ways. What does seem fairly certain is that the problems of the head-injured need to be addressed in a number of different ways, preferably by a team of people working collaboratively, but in which individual therapists each practice their own specialty. It is common for a head-injured person to require physical therapy, speech therapy, occupational therapy, cognitive rehabilitation, and individual and family-centered psychotherapy and psychoeducation. The need for input from each of these specialties can continue for many years.

I could have chosen many case studies to illustrate the all-too-common problems and frustrations suffered by severely head-injured people. Many, like Neil, have suffered when the therapists who worked with them for a while reach a point when they said they could no longer help, leaving the patient in limbo. Even in rural areas and small towns where resources are few, however, much can be done to help these people to regain a fulfilling life, and I have chosen such a case to present here in the hope it will motivate others to persevere even when support and hope for success are scarce.

Theoretical Background

The literature on the neuropathology, assessment, and rehabilitation of TBI is extensive, and rarely a month goes by without the publication of a new book on some aspect of the subject. The area of rehabilitation in particular is constantly updated, and it would be foolhardy to attempt to summarize this area here. Rather, I provide some basic information about the neuropathology of severe TBI and it's common cognitive, behavioral, emotional, and psychosocial consequences, as these aspects are generally well established and agreed on by most professionals in the field. I will also reference and comment briefly on some of the rehabilitation methods that have been used in an attempt to assist recovery within each of these areas of impairment.

Neuropathology

Head injuries can be of three types: penetrating, crushing, and closed. In a *penetrating* TBI the skull is pierced or broken and the brain beneath damaged (e.g., from a bullet wound or when the skull is broken by a sharp object in a car accident). The consequences may be less severe than in a severe closed TBI if the damage is restricted to a small part of the brain. The deficits will be related to the functions mediated by that area of the brain. A *crushing* TBI, in which the head is caught between two objects (e.g., under the wheel of a car) is the rarest type of TBI; often the most serious damage is to the base of the skull and the nerves that run through it rather than to the brain itself.

Closed head injuries (CHI) are by far the most common. They occur when the head suddenly accelerates (e.g., when a car runs into your car from behind), decelerates (e.g., when your car hits a telegraph pole), or rotates (e.g., when you receive a punch to the head that is hard enough to knock you out). There is no penetrating wound, and the damage is caused by the movement of the soft brain mass inside the bony skull. Diffuse damage to nerve fibers (diffuse axonal injury) occurs because of the stretching and shearing of the fibers as the brain vibrates and rotates on its axis. This type of damage is widespread but is often most severe at the level of the brain stem, and the reticular formation (RF) is especially vulnerable at this point. Damage to the RF results in lowered arousal of the cortex, particularly the prefrontal areas, which contributes to many of the frontal-lobe symptoms of CHI. Arteries and veins may also be torn, leaking blood into brain tissue and causing diffuse disruption, or sometimes resulting in a significant area of focal damage where there is a substantial hemorrhage.

Further areas of focal damage can be caused by the brain surface rubbing on the sharp ridges and edges inside the skull as the brain continues to rotate when the skull stops. The sites most commonly damaged are the inferior (orbital) frontal lobes and the inferior anterior temporal lobes. Focal injuries also occur as the brain hits the skull on impact, and these include *coup* injuries, in which the damage is at the site of the impact, and *contre-coup* injuries, in which the impact causes the brain to accelerate inside the skull, resulting in it hitting the skull opposite the point of impact and damaging the brain region directly opposite the site of impact. Thus, when a car is hit from behind, frontal lesions may result from a contre-coup injury as the brain accelerates inside the skull and hits the bony skull around the orbits; from a deceleration injury when the head hits the windscreen; from the brain moving inside the skull after impact; and from RF shearing and tearing when the brain vibrates and rotates at the level of the brain stem. It is therefore little wonder that frontal-lobe deficits are so common following CHI. Damage to the temporal lobes, also very common, results in the memory deficits that underlie many of the most difficult rehabilitation problems.

The damage that occurs in the first few seconds of an accident is sometimes called the *first injury* (Gronwall, Wrightson, and Waddell 1998). Unfortunately, in severe CHI, the neurological damage often does not stop there. A *second injury* can occur if the victim is trapped in a way that blocks breathing (perhaps because of vomit that blocks the airways or from an injury to the nose or face), which reduces the oxygen supply to the brain. Other injuries may result in the loss of a significant amount of blood, lowering blood pressure and reducing the supply of blood and oxygen to the brain. Rapid acute care at the site of the accident thus involves clearing the airway, stopping bleeding, and replacing lost blood with a transfusion to protect the brain from second injury while the patient is transported to hospital.

Many people who sustain a severe CHI do not die on impact but die days or even weeks later. These deaths or a worsening of the patient's condition are often the result of the *third injury*. These complications include swelling of the brain as the escaping fluids from damaged cells and blood from torn vessels cause a rise in intracranial pressure, and the brain swells and fills more of the skull. If the brain becomes too tight, the blood has difficulty circulating through it, which can result in ischemia (loss of oxygen), causing areas of the brain to die. If the intracranial pressure rises too much, the blood circulation can be cut off entirely, and the brain dies. Many of the technologies used in critical care units are designed minimize the brain swelling, keep blood pressure at the correct level, ensure an adequate intake of air and oxygen and the removal of waste products like carbon monoxide, and restrict the levels of water and salt in the body to limit the flow of tissue fluid into the brain.

Blood clots can also accumulate in the days immediately following the accident; not controlled or evacuated, they too can elevate intracranial pressure, with the same devastating results. Some blood clots form quickly outside the coverings of the brain (an *acute extradural hematoma*), and these need to be evacuated immediately by a neurosurgeon, or they will quickly result in the brain being pushed down through the cerebral aqueduct (called *coning*), resulting in death. In some cases *chronic subdural hematomas* form slowly over a period of days; these are particularly common in elderly people and can follow even a quite minor injury. Posttraumatic *hydrocephalus* can also occur days or even weeks after the accident, when the cerebrospinal fluid (CSF) circulation is blocked by blood or scarring following the brain injury, also causing a rise in intracranial pressure. Sometimes hydrocephalus resolves without intervention, or sometimes the neurosurgeon removes the blockage or inserts a shunt into the ventricle to drain the CSF into the pleural or abdominal cavity. The vastly improved technologies now used in critical care units to control the complications that constitute the third injury have significantly increased the numbers of severely head-injured people who survive. The quest now is to find ways to improve the long-term outcome for these survivors, and this is a mammoth and difficult task for the rehabilitation specialists and the families of victims.

Assessment of Severity and Outcome of TBI

In the acute stages, a commonly used measure of severity is the Glasgow Coma Scale (GCS) (Teasdale and Jennett 1974, 1976), a 15-point scale that assesses motor responses, verbal responses, and the stimulus necessary to provoke eye-opening. The patient is usually first assessed at least 6 hours after the accident to avoid the confounding effects of alcohol and other noncranial contributors to a confused or comatose state. A score of 8 or lower means the patient cannot open her eyes, obey commands, or utter words and is viewed as an indicator of severe TBI. A score of 9–12 is usually considered a moderate TBI, and a score of 13–15, along with an initial loss of consciousness of 20 minutes or less, is usually considered a mild TBI (Rimel, Giordani, Barth, Boll, and Jane 1981). In some cases the GCS must be carried out immediately, as later assessment is impossible if paralytic drugs are used in the critical care unit for controlled ventilation.

The assessment measure used most often by neurologists and neurosurgeons to assess global outcome is the Glasgow Outcome Scale (GOS) (Jennett and Bond 1975). It includes five levels of outcome: good recovery, moderate disability, severe disability, a persistent vegetative state, and death. Jennett, Teasdale, Braakman, Minderhoud, and Knill-Jones (1976) found that the GOS at 6 months was a reliable predictor of ultimate outcome because patients' GOS category did not change after that period. The GOS is obviously a global measure and is not useful for assessing specific problem areas. Therefore, it has limited value for individualized rehabilitation planning.

Detailed assessments by neuropsychologists, speech pathologists, physical therapists, occupational therapists, and vocational rehabilitation specialists using both formal assessment tools and behavioral observations of the individual interacting and coping in the real world (in home, social, and work settings) form the basis of a rehabilitation program. These assessments need to be repeated as the individual changes over time. Thus, a patient who was classified as having a moderate disability by the neurosurgeon at both 6 months and 2 years may have recovered significantly during those times in areas of efficiency of information processing, ways of coping with memory problems, improvement in insight, and reduction in the frequency of inappropriate comments when interacting socially. These improvements may have resulted in a change from being unable to cope with social interactions or concentrate on a task for more than a few minutes, to a return to work, albeit part-time and at a lower level than before the accident.

Another often-used measure of the severity of TBI is that of posttraumatic amnesia (PTA) (Russell 1971), which refers to the state of disorientation and confusion that often follows a return to consciousness, when the patient seems unable to attend to and acquire new information. Its duration is thought to be related to the severity of the TBI and to give an indication of prognosis. Assessment is often difficult, especially as the patient may have islands of memory within the period of PTA. Although tests have been developed to assess memory and orientation aspects of PTA, including the Galveston Orientation and Amnesia Test (GOAT) (Levin, O'Donnell, and Grossman 1979) and the Westmead PTA Scale (Shores, Marosszeky, Sandanam, and Batchelor 1986), other consequences of PTA such as slowness, impaired verbal fluency, and slowed reaction time are not included (Snow and Ponsford 1995). Thus, the common measures of PTA should therefore be used only as an approximate measure of outcome.

Neuropsychological, Psychiatric, and Psychosocial Outcome of Severe TBI

Because CHI causes widespread diffuse damage, and focal areas of damage can also occur, wide-ranging cognitive deficits can result (Lezak 1995). In addition, motor, sensory, and emotional deficits are common. As damage to the RF, frontal, and temporal areas occurs to a lesser or greater degree in most severe closed head injuries, some combination of attention, information processing, executive, and memory problems will be found in most cases.

Common *executive* (frontal-lobe) deficits (Stuss 1987; Stuss and Knight 2002) include a lack of motivation, a poor ability to initiate actions, poor planning and organizational skills, a decreased ability to change a mindset or a behavior from an established one to a new one, a poor ability to think abstractly, and an increased dependence on external structure to guide behaviors and cognitions. Patients with frontal-lobe problems demonstrate a decreased awareness of their own deficits, an inability to learn from the feedback of others and their own mistakes, inappropriate behaviors, slowed thinking and response, poor ability to learn new information because of difficulty in attending to it and organizing the material they wish to remember in a logical way, and difficulty in focusing attention on the task at hand, especially when other noises and distractions are present.

Memory deficits for new verbal and nonverbal material are common as a result of temporal lobe damage, and in some cases there is a period of retrograde amnesia that extends back in time before the TBI. Patients with left hemispheric damage often have word-finding problems, and if they have sustained areas of focal left hemispheric damage in language areas, they may have difficulties with producing or comprehending speech (see Chapter 5). Patients with parietal lobe damage may have difficulties finding their way around. With right parietal damage in particular, they may demonstrate neglect or inattention for the left side of space (see Chapter 7). On occasion patients sustain damage to their occipital lobes, which can result in visual-field defects and, in cases where the damage is bilateral, may result in *visual agnosia* (the inability to recognize objects on sight) or *prosopagnosia* (the inability to recognize familiar faces on sight) (see Chapter 8).

Some deficits, such as attention span, lack of awareness, and word-finding problems, may spontaneously resolve with time (perhaps as stretched nerve fibers in the RF recover and bruising of brain tissue subsides). Other deficits, such as finding one's way around, may recover to some extent as the brain finds new pathways to mediate the tasks required of it. Some functions, such as severe memory deficits following temporal lobe damage, may never recover, but the patient may learn ways to compensate for the lost ability (e.g., by using a diary to compensate for memory loss). Some patients never recover a sufficient range of functions to be able to live even semi-independently, usually the result of severe frontal and temporal lobe damage. Useful rehabilitation cannot be achieved because such individuals are so lacking in insight and awareness that they cannot learn from their mistakes or learn to accept and cope with their new lowered ability levels or even learn to use a diary consistently to compensate for memory problems.

The psychiatric and psychosocial disorders that not uncommonly follow severe closed TBI include personality changes (often as a result of frontal-lobe damage), emotional lability, irritability, an inability to inhibit aggressive and violent reactions, and poor control of the expression of (often inappropriate) emotions. Depression and suicidal thoughts may occur years after the TBI, when progress has plateaued and the patient has regained the ability to be aware of his changed cognitive and psychosocial status. Fatigue; loss of confidence, self-esteem, and independence; changes in sexuality; and family disruption or breakup are all common, long-lasting consequences of TBI (Grant and Alves 1987). Many of these problems result from a combination of the neurological damage and the psychological reactions of the head-injured person to his changed status. The wider psychosocial consequences of family disruption, loss of employment, and decreased social and sexual activities are an understandable but tragic nonneurological consequence of the TBI (Bond 1975; Brooks 1984; Brooks and McKinlay 1983; McLean, Dikmen, Temkin, Wyler, and Gale 1984; Oddy, Humphrey, and Uttley 1978; Ponsford, Sloan, and Snow 1995).

Rehabilitation

Rehabilitation programs for the severely head-injured range from minimal or no rehabilitation following discharge from the acute hospital; to weekly outpatient treatment sessions with physical therapists, occupational therapists, and speech therapists— sometimes with little overall collaboration and planning between the therapists; to intensive long-term, live-in or day rehabilitation programs in which different types of therapy are integrated into a holistic program planned and constantly updated to meet the individual needs and goals. Some programs include cognitive retraining, often using computerized tests (Sohlberg and Mateer 1989; Gianutsos 1992), although the aspects of this approach that, for example, involve repetitive memory exercises have been criticized for lack of effectiveness in improving memory skills (Ponsford 1995; Robertson 1990).

A holistic approach is based on the premise that the cognitive, psychiatric, and functional aspects of TBI cannot and should not be separated. Proponents of this approach utilize intensive live-in or day programs in which individual and group therapy sessions aim to assist TBI victims to become more aware of their strengths and weaknesses in all areas including cognitive, social, and emotional; develop compensatory skills in all areas; and participate in vocational counseling (Diller 1976; Ben-Yishay 1978; Prigatano 1991). These programs are expensive to run, and because they are so complex, their effectiveness is difficult to evaluate accurately. However, for those fortunate few who have access to such programs, they do appear to increase self-esteem and productivity and result in less emotional distress than do less complex and holistic programs (Prigitano 1994). Cognitive behavior therapy has been used successfully for anxiety and obsessive-compulsive disorders (Williams, Evans, and Fleminger 2003) and depression (Khan-Bourne and Brown 2003) in TBI patients.

Combined approaches can also be very effective and usually combine theories and methods from neuropsychology, cognitive psychology, and behavioral psychology in an intensive day program (Wilson 1997). For example, in this model, cognitive theory might inform the design of a rehabilitation strategy. Errorless learning (Baddeley and Wilson 1994) is an illustration of this; for people with significant memory problems, learning using a trial-and-error approach can result in confusion, as the person cannot remember their mistakes and thus cannot learn to avoid them. The errorless learning strategy uses a graduated learning procedure that does not require the individual to guess the answer. For example when learning the name of their therapist they may first be told the name and be shown it written down, and then be shown the name with the last letter deleted and asked what the name is, and so on with letters removed one at a time until they can remember the name after being cued with only the first letter. If they cannot remember the name they are told not to guess, and the therapist provides the correct answer and asks them to repeat it.

A combined approach commonly also includes psychoeducation seminars and group and individual exercises designed to increase insight, enhance strengths, and find ways to compensate for memory and other problems. The social milieu of the program is important, as it is for the holistic approach, as the peer group who advance through the program together learn from and support each other.

In any effective program, it is important to include social activities and individual and family counseling along with retraining daily living skills (Ponsford et al. 1995). Group psychotherapy with other head-injured people can assist clients with reality testing and help them become aware of their deficits, allow them to practice social skills and rebuild confidence in a safe environment, and serve as a support group. Some programs emphasize the importance of rehabilitating the individual within his or her own home and community using a range of approaches and therapy models and concentrating on practical applications of theory and outcomes important to the individual. The "What-ever-it-takes" (WIT) model of Willer and Corrigan (1994) is the best known example of this approach.

Vocational retraining is essential where there is a possibility that the TBI victim might be able to return to some sort of work. Programs that include one-to-one on-the-job vocational training with a "job coach" appear to have the greatest success rate in terms of returning the individual to paid employment. Usually, employment is at a much lower level than before the injury and may be part-time. It would be costly to employ a job coach for each brain-damaged client, which often leads to using the job coach for a limited period only. There is a hidden cost in this strategy, however, as severely head-injured persons may be unable to maintain consistent work attendance without regular "booster" visits from the job coach, often for the duration of the client's working life. Once the client is well established in a set routine in the job, these visits may be as infrequent as once every 2 months.

Rehabilitation programs are of little use if they do not result in further improvement of the head-injured client's productivity and quality of life than would occur spontaneously over time. Improvement is often difficult to measure, especially given the dubious ethics involved in providing no rehabilitation to some head-injured people to obtain an appropriate control group for comparison. Group measures may not be particularly valid, in any case, because no two head-injured individuals are alike in their premorbid characteristics, degree of brain damage, level of family support, and goals for successful rehabilitation. Nevertheless, it is important to measure improvement in individuals and within programs not only to satisfy the insurance companies but also to encourage the clients, their families, and the staff, who put so much emotional energy into the programs they run.

Many attempts to develop scales to measure improvement of different aspects of rehabilitation have been made (Diller and Ben-Yishay 1987). The Ranchos Los Amigos Scale (Hagen 1982) is an 8-point rating scale commonly used to assess improvement in inpatient medical rehabilitation programs. Staff members rate the patient's spontaneous responses to stimuli in the environment, from no response to purposeful and appropriate responses. Numerous functional rating scales have been developed for use in long-term rehabilitation programs (Diller and Ben Yishay 1987). These scales assess various behaviors: basic activities of daily living, the ability to problem-solve, and the appropriateness of social interactions. Of economic importance is the assessment of work productivity, which has been assessed as return to paid work and the number of months and years the individual remains in work. Although many head-injured people are able to return to employment after participating in a rehabilitation program, the number of head-injured people who remain in work years later is much smaller.

Rehabilitation of the multiple and complex problems associated with severe TBI is challenging, but there have been many advances made in this area over the last decade. That there are many models of TBI rehabilitation is probably a good thing, as often a program that works well for one person fails miserably for another. The work is expensive, tiring, and tedious, and improvement is often both minimal and slow to occur. Many clients, even when they are able to return to paid employment, are unhappy and dissatisfied with their jobs and their lives, often because of their ongoing lack of awareness about the severity of their deficits; they often continue to believe they can return to work and life at their premorbid levels. This type of un-awareness is neurologically based (Prigatano 1991) and is often impossible or extremely difficult to change. Without awareness, acceptance of disability and the establishment of a new self-identity are not possible. Despite all the problems with rehabilitation, the alternative of condemning the severely head-injured to a life of total dependence with little opportunity to find even small pleasures in life is even more expensive, in terms of both economics and human misery.

Although organized rehabilitation programs are becoming increasingly common as public and private health authorities realize the importance of a high standard of rehabilitation, not only for the individual's future well-being but for economic reasons, there are, of course, many TBI victims who live in an area where such programs are not available. In such cases, a program can be organized on an individual basis, utilizing a range of different therapists and approaches, and perhaps following as closely as possible the "Whatever-it-takes" model. Sam, the case that follows, illustrates this approach. For a number of excellent case studies that utilize a more formalized combined neurorehabilitation approach, the reader is referred to Barbara Wilson's (1999) book of case studies.

Case Presentation

Background

At the time of his TBI, Sam was a 21-year-old university student in his final year of a 3-year undergraduate degree in geography. He had left his childhood home a year earlier for an apartment he shared with three other students. He maintained regular contact with his family and generally went home to mum "for a decent feed" each Wednesday night. His parents had been divorced for 11 years, and his mother lived with his two teenage siblings and worked full-time as a school teacher. His father, an accountant, had remarried, and he and his second wife had two children aged 6 and 9 years.

The accident occurred at 6:00 PM on a Saturday night when Sam was driving home after a football game. His best friend, Andrew, was in the front passenger seat, and later their team mates reported that they had all been having "a few beers" after winning their match that afternoon. Sam, they said, had not had very much to drink, and in fact he was generally known to be careful about not driving when he had been drinking. The driver of the other car in the crash was later found to be responsible for it. He had jumped the red light at an intersection, impacting with the left (passenger side) of Sam's car, which then smashed into a lamp-post on the other side of the intersection. The other driver and Sam's friend Andrew were killed on impact.

Sam was admitted to the department of critical care at the city hospital in deep coma (GCS of 6). Apart from a number of broken ribs, Sam's main injury was to his brain. He had no skull fractures, but a computed tomography (CT) brain scan initially showed some hemorrhage in the posterior parts of the lateral ventricles and in the fourth ventricle and some hemorrhage around the brain stem. There was evidence of *contusion* (bruising) in the left cerebellar hemisphere and in the frontal region on both sides but mainly on the left side. Sam's vital functions were taken over for him (i.e., he was ventilated and had a tracheostomy), and he remained in this state for 4 weeks, at which point he was weaned from the ventilator. He remained virtually unresponsive for another month before his level of consciousness began to improve slowly. By this stage he could understand some speech but could not speak, and he was able to perform some purposeful movements with his left hand in response to command. He had a right-sided hemiparesis and a weak left arm. He was transferred to the neuro-surgical ward, where he underwent intensive physical and occupational therapy for 6 months. When he was discharged from the hospital to his mother's house 8 months after his TBI, he was fully orientated to time and place and could move himself in his wheelchair, feed himself, understand speech quite well, and speak fluently, al-though in a rather flat monotone.

Seven years after his TBI, Sam lived independently; he was employed and enjoyed life most of the time. By that stage he appeared to have reached a fairly stable state in his recovery, and in the 6 years that had elapsed since his discharge from hospital, he and his family worked continuously and courageously to enable Sam to reach this state. Their's is a success story that provides examples of many of the positive out-comes that can occur for all family members, even after such a tragedy.

Neuropsychological Assessment

Verbal abilities   Seven years after his TBI, Sam was assessed on a simple test of verbal comprehension, the Short Token Test (De Renzi and Faglioni 1978), on which he earned a perfect score, demonstrating that his comprehension and ability to respond to instructions were good. He was then given the revised Wechsler Adult Intelligence Scale (WAIS-R). Although his Verbal IQ fell in the middle of the average range, there were some marked differences between the subtest scores. On the Vocabulary subtest, he scored at the top of the high average range, indicating that his premorbid ability would have been at least at this level, probably higher. At the other extreme were his Arithmetic and Digit Span scores, which fell at the bottom end of the low-average range. Sam was only able to reverse two digits backward, and he had great difficulty with all but the easiest of the Arithmetic problems. He improved a little when he was given the problems to read rather than having to hold them in working memory and also when he was permitted to use paper and pencil to work them out rather than having to manipulate the numbers mentally. After a TBI, the ability to process complex or multiple pieces of information is compromised, and mental arithmetic exposes this deficit. Sam's Comprehension, Similarities, and Information scores were average and therefore somewhat low for someone of Sam's estimated premorbid ability and level of formal education. These results suggest some impairment of the ability to retrieve some well-learned factual information and problems with making verbal abstractions.

Sam could read slowly but fluently, and although he was unable to write with his dominant right hand because of a weakness, he was able to form clumsy letters correctly with his left hand. His speech was slow but understandable, and he occasionally had word-finding problems. These problems became apparent when he was given a test of oral word fluency, which requires producing as many words as possible in one minute, beginning with a specified letter. His score on this test showed mild impairment.

Visuospatial abilities   Sam's WAIS-R Performance IQ fell at the top of the low average range, pointing to a significant drop from his estimated premorbid ability on visuospatial tasks, especially under time pressure. One of the major problems following TBI is a slowing of response speed; as the Performance subtests are all timed, scores are generally lowered after severe TBI. Sam's weak right hand also made it difficult for him to manipulate the test materials. Sam was allowed to take as long as he needed to complete each test to determine whether he had true visuospatial problems in addition to his slowness. He was able to complete most of the problems, but he demonstrated a marked difficulty on Object Assembly, a jigsaw puzzle test in which no clues are provided as to what the finished object might be. This lack of guiding external structure was probably the cause of Sam's poor performance on this test, as on three items he was unable not only to complete them but was also unable to work out what the finished items might be. To test this theory, on another occasion he was provided a picture of the finished objects, showing how each piece fitted to make the whole. With this guide he was able to complete all items correctly. Patients with severe visuospatial problems, often resulting of parietal lesions, are less likely to be assisted by external guidelines. Sam's damage was diffuse, but he also had bilateral frontal-lobe contusions, and his frontal-lobe damage probably impaired his ability to perform abstract tasks, to organize and plan a logical approach to tasks, and to learn from his mistakes. Therefore, attempting to do a jigsaw puzzle without knowing what the object is will be a rather hit-and-miss affair for these people.

Frontal-lobe problems   Sam demonstrated mild to moderate frontal-lobe problems on a number of tasks. In addition to his mild word initiation problem, his difficulty processing complex information efficiently, and his inability to complete Object Assembly without a clear external structure or pattern to guide him, Sam also demonstrated a poor ability to plan and organize his actions ahead of time, even when he had an external structure to follow. This difficulty was apparent when he tried to copy the Rey Complex Figure (Osterreith 1944; Taylor 1969) (see Fig. 10-1a). He seemed

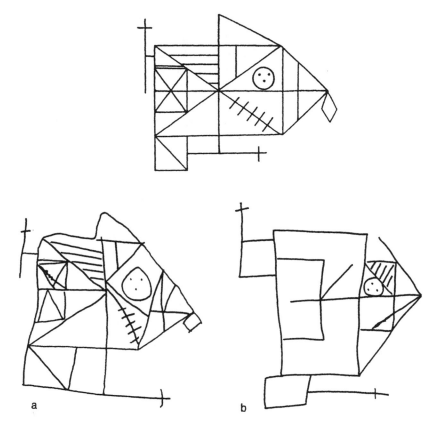

Figure 10-1 The Rey Complex Figure Model is in the top row; (a) is
Sam's copy of it, and (b) is his recall of it 30 minutes later.

unable to follow any logical sequence, and his resulting score fell more than three
standard deviations (SD) below the mean score for men of his age (Spreen and Strauss
1991). Another problem usually associated with frontal-lobe dysfunction is difficulty
making verbal abstractions. An example of this problem was provided by Sam's concrete responses when asked to explain proverbs on the Comprehension subtest of the
WAIS-R. Asked to explain "strike while the iron is hot," Sam replied, "It is no use
trying to iron your shirt when you have just turned the iron on. You have to wait until
the iron heats up." He was also given the Wisconsin Card Sorting Test (Grant and
Berg 1981), a test that requires sorting cards into categories depending on verbal
feedback from the examiner as to the correctness of the previous responses. This test
assesses the ability to follow rules, to change one's mindset from one category to
another, and to learn from errors. All these abilities appear to be mediated primarily
by the prefrontal lobes; thus, sorting tests are excellent tests of the integrity of the
frontal lobes. Sam's performance was poor on this test. Although he managed to sort

to the first category, he was unable to change and keep to the next category, returning to the first category even after being told that it was incorrect.

Sam also demonstrated evidence of frontal-lobe impairment in his everyday behaviors. One year after his head injury, he had only minimal insight into his deficits and as a result was usually cheerful, and at times quite euphoric. Asked what he thought the future held for him, he usually replied that he supposed he would have to return to the university to finish his degree the following year, and then he would travel for a while. His family and friends said his personality had changed significantly. Before the accident, he had been a quick-witted young man with a tendency to sarcasm and a quick temper. The new Sam was easygoing, slow-witted, and rather childlike in his conversation. His childlike conversation was a result of his concrete responses and comments and his poor ability to think abstractly. Although his social behaviors were not particularly inappropriate, his lack of social insight occasionally caused some annoyance. For example, one night his brother brought his new girlfriend home after a date and was sitting in the lounge with her. As his brother explained, "Just as we were getting into it, in comes Sam, plonks himself down on the couch beside us, and starts talking. No hint would get rid of him, and I finally had to get up and push him out. My girlfriend thought I was being really unkind to my poor dolt of a brother, and nothing was ever quite the same between us after that!"

Seven years after his accident, Sam's insight into his difficulties had improved markedly, undoubtedly a major factor in his successful rehabilitation. Head-injured people whose insight is permanently impaired are extremely difficult to rehabilitate because they cannot learn from their mistakes and often tend to behave in socially inappropriate ways. This behavior can embarrass friends and family until the head-injured person is increasingly left out of social events. Although Sam did not lack insight, he did suffer from other frontal-type deficits. When asked what he saw as his main difficulty, he replied:

> I feel a sort of void in myself. I can't seem to find the motivation to do things I know I should do, even if I know I will enjoy them if I can only get started. I know I should exercise, but it is such a struggle to start, and I know I should make the effort to go to parties, but unless someone pushes me, and comes and gets me, I find myself sitting in front of the television instead. Sometimes I get really frustrated with myself. I guess I am just lazy.

Sam may, of course, be "lazy" but more likely his lack of motivation and difficulty initiating activities are results of his frontal-lobe damage. The best way to assist people with these problems is to provide structure and to organize their activities for them, including telephoning them to remind them that it is time to get dressed for a social occasion and picking them up and going with them to the venue. Friends and family members of a head-injured person can help by sharing these tasks because it can be a tedious and time-consuming role if left to one family member. Sam was assisted with his poor motivation to improve his physical fitness by Lance, a head-injured ex-university student who had discovered that a daily workout in the gymnasium helped him overcome severe depression. He decided he wanted to help others in the same situation and began by taking on Sam as his "buddy." At first, Lance sometimes had to pull Sam from bed and push him into the car to get him to the gymnasium; but after 6 months of taking him to the gymnasium three times a week, he was able to arrange to meet Sam there, and Sam would usually arrive on time.

This type of "buddy" system can sometimes work quite well, especially if the "buddies" share some premorbid characteristics. Lance and Sam were the same age, came from similar socioeconomic and cultural backgrounds, and shared a similar sense of humor. Despite the cognitive impairments that made their return to university impossible, they nevertheless had some intellectual interests in common. This relationship highlights the point that even severe head injury does not change every aspect of the personality and intellect. It is important to discover and emphasize the characteristics that are not changed by the head injury because these characteristics can form the basis for the individual's gradual reconstruction of his self-identity. Once they had established a firm relationship, Sam and Lance were also able to support each other in grieving for their losses; at times, they were even able to laugh at themselves and their mistakes, as both suffered in similar ways.

Memory Impairments

Sam's immediate memory span for repeating digits forward was six digits, which is in the normal range. He did not have an extensive retrograde memory loss (i.e., loss of memories of events or facts that occurred before his accident), and although he could not remember the accident itself or the 2 weeks before it, his memories before then were largely intact. An extensive period of retrograde amnesia is uncommon following head injury, and most people lose only those memories that are laid down immediately before the head injury occurs. Sam did, however, suffer a permanent and significant impairment in learning new verbal and visual information. This difficulty is termed *anterograde memory impairment* because it refers to difficulty in remembering information and events that occur after the head injury.

Anterograde memory problems are arguably the most common and debilitating of the cognitive deficits resulting from severe head injury. Like many other head-injured victims, Sam found he had difficulty remembering the names and faces of new acquaintances, and he would forget what he meant to do that day or what food items he had walked to the shop to buy. Two years after his accident, he enrolled in one class at the university but found he could no longer remember the lecture material, and any information he managed to glean from his textbook quickly faded. On formal memory testing, his difficulties were confirmed. On a test where he had to learn a list of 12 unrelated words over 12 trials, he had considerable difficulty, and by the twelfth trial had learned only seven of the words. One hour later, he was able to recall only four of the words. His recall of the Rey Complex Figure, 30 minutes after copying it, was extremely impoverished, falling more than 3 SD below the mean score for men of his age (see Fig 10-1b).

The memory problems suffered by head-injury victims are often the result of damage to the temporal lobes, but before reaching this conclusion, the possibility that frontal-lobe damage may be contributing to the deficits should be explored. Frontal-lobe dysfunction causes apparent memory difficulties because new information is not structured or encoded in long-term memory in a meaningful way as it is learned. As a result, it is difficult to recall the material later because it has been stored in a haphazard manner.

People with frontally mediated memory impairments can often be assisted if the material they are trying to learn is carefully and logically structured for them. For example, if a person is trying to learn a list of words, the words would be grouped first according to some meaningful principle. A shopping list might be grouped as breakfast items, lunch items, bathroom items, and so on. The later recall of the information might then be facilitated by providing the appropriate cues. In Sam's case, he was given a second list of 12 words, but this time he was assisted in grouping them by forming associations between some of the words. Using this strategy, he increased the number of words he learned by the 12th trial to nine, and more important, he was able to recall eight of the words an hour later. His visual memory was also aided by structuring the stimulus carefully when learning it. He was given a parallel version of the Rey Complex Figure to copy (the Taylor Figure; Taylor 1969), but this time he was guided so that he copied it in a logical manner. His copy improved to near-normal levels, and his later recall also improved, although not to the same degree as his copy.

Although structure certainly helped Sam's new learning ability, he still demonstrated a marked deficit on a range of verbal and visual memory tests. This deficit remained even on recognition tasks, which are usually much easier than tasks that require spontaneous recall. An example of such a task is the Recognition Memory Test (Warrington 1984), in which the individual reads 50 words or views 50 photographs of unknown faces and then must choose the words or faces he has just seen from pairs of words or faces. Each pair contains one item that was just seen and one item that was not seen. This test is unlikely to be difficult for people with frontal-lobe damage, but people with significant memory problems as a result of temporal-lobe damage are likely to show impairments on the task. Sam's scores on this Recognition Test fell at the 10th percentile for words and at the 25th percentile for faces. Thus, whereas Sam's frontal-lobe dysfunction may contribute to his memory problems, it is likely that his poor ability to learn new information resulted primarily from bilateral temporal-lobe damage, probably of greater severity on the left side, which would be consistent with his greater verbal than visuospatial, nonverbal memory problems and with the right-sided limb weakness he sustained.

Memory problems resulting from temporal-lobe damage are less likely to be helped by the provision of external structure, and memory retraining programs have so far not been successful. People with these types of memory problems are best helped by training them to use a diary in a consistent and logical manner to substitute for their memory loss. Sam and his family agree that the diary Sam carries everywhere is the most important rehabilitation aid he has. Sam has dubbed his diary the "Book of Independence," and he says he views it as an extension of his brain. It took many long and tedious months to train Sam to use his diary in a consistent manner (Solhberg and Mateer 1989), and on many occasions he contemplated "giving it away, and relying on Mum to tell me what to do and when to do it." During the first 2 years of Sam's rehabilitation, even his mother sometimes despaired of his ever learning to use his diary so that it would remove some of the stress from her. As she remarked, "When he was told about a future appointment, he would not have the initiative to get out his diary immediately and write the appointment in, and within 5 minutes he would have forgotten the details. Even when we made him write in his diary, he would forget to look in it regularly, or he would put it down somewhere and forget where it was." Seven years after his head injury, Sam always wears a money belt in which he keeps not only his money but, more important, his diary. In addition, he carries a simple electronic diary that he programs first thing each morning to bleep at the times when he must remember important activities. When he hears a bleep, he looks in his diary to see what activity he is meant to remember. Sam also regularly looks in his diary at breakfast, lunch, dinner, and before going to bed. After years of struggling, the diary has become a habit that he no more has to think about than to change into his pajamas before retiring for the night.

To people with intact memories, all these regulated procedures seem incredibly tedious and hardly worth the trouble. To Sam and his family, the regulated use of his diary spells independence, and the ultimate outcome has been well worth the years of struggle necessary to form this habit.

Personal and Social Consequences

Obviously, a severe head injury changes the victim's life permanently. For some, happiness and fulfillment is lost forever, but for others who are more fortunate in terms of family and other support systems and rehabilitation facilities, a new life can be forged from the remnants of the old one. Sam was one of the fortunate ones, but his good fortune owed much to his own courage and determination and to the love and perseverance of family and friends.

Three years after his head injury, Sam began attending the Rehabilitation League on a daily basis; there he was given experience working in different occupations, including activities such as packing parts, gardening, assisting a builder, and filing papers in the office. His ability to cope successfully with each of these activities was assessed. After 18 months, he was given a trial in the office of a computer firm helping the other office workers as needed. He was able to cope with this situation in the mornings only, and even 7 years later finds he is too tired to work more than 4 hours each weekday. He become rather bored and frustrated with this work and was given training in copying computer programs onto disks to fill client orders. He still performs this job and now has the additional responsibility of recording client orders and sending the disks and invoices to the clients. Sam still finds his work frustrating at times but he has come to terms with the fact that he may never be able to cope with a more difficult job.

Sam's failed attempt to return to one class at university just 2 years after his head injury resulted in his becoming seriously depressed for some weeks—at times contemplating suicide. At this time he found individual psychotherapy helpful. Over a period of 6 months, Sam expressed feelings of anger that this happened to him, grief for the many things he had lost, and guilt about the stress and sadness he had caused his family. Not until this time did he begin to talk about his friend, Andrew, who had been killed in the accident. He gradually came to terms with many of his losses and began to entertain the possibility that he could find some fulfillment in life, even if he had to give up many of his old plans and dreams and lower his sights before he could achieve any happiness. A turning point came for Sam when he decided it was up to him to live for Andrew as well as for himself and that from that time on he would look forward, not backward. Although he certainly continues to experience bad days when he feels frustrated and "low," he has never felt seriously depressed since that time.

Head injury is a family affair, and the stress on family members can be even greater than that on the head-injured victim. Often the family's stress takes its toll many months and years after the head injury. In the early stages, relief that their child or partner has survived and seems to be recovering in leaps and bounds compensates and perhaps masks the enormity of the changes that have occurred in their loved one. As time passes, however, the everyday stresses of coping with the head-injured person's physical, emotional, and cognitive problems take precedence. Perhaps most difficult is the "change in personality" that often becomes increasingly apparent. Such a change is probably a combination of frontal-lobe dysfunction causing inappropriate behaviors and a lack of insight; memory problems resulting in dependence on other family members; and feelings of apathy, depression, anger, irritability, and frustration that the head-injured person displays. These emotions may be a result of the brain damage but are exacerbated by the victim's psychological reactions to his tragic circumstances.

Family-centered practice (Perlesz, Furlong, and McLachlan 1992) is one therapeutic model that can be helpful to all family members in the early stages after head injury if information about the consequences of head injury, how to cope, and how to assist in rehabilitation is given at the right time in a sensitive way. It can also help later in the rehabilitation process when the therapist can facilitate the process of adaptation for the family by easing the pain for family members as they come to terms with what the head injury has meant for them. In the year immediately after his head injury, Sam's family members seemed receptive to the information they were given. With the help of the psychologist, they worked out a support system so that the entire burden of caring for Sam would not fall on Margaret, his mother. As the years passed, however, and Sam's rate of recovery seemed to plateau, the family's hope that Sam would ultimately regain his old identity and full independence faded, and helping him with his rehabilitation became a chore.

Three years after his head injury, Sam's family reached a crisis: His mother was exhausted, and Sam's siblings, tired of dealing with his problems, were spending less and less time at home. Donald, Sam's father, had agreed that Sam could spend every second week with him and his family, but this arrangement had quickly run into difficulties because Sam often became irritated with his two half-siblings, leading to arguments with Donald that sometimes nearly reached the point of a physical fight. Donald also felt that Sam was lazy and should be able to cope with full days at work. Both families agreed to try family-centered therapy when Donald's wife, Julie, reached the end of her tether and said that if Sam stayed with them again, she would leave home.

As Sam's family members expressed their feelings within the family group, they learned to recognize when and in what areas their family system was struggling to cope. They were thus able to devise creative and supportive strategies that allowed the system to change in such a way to minimize the stresses on each family member. An important corner was turned when the family viewed a video taken of Sam once a month during the 6 months he was undergoing physical, occupational, and speech therapy as an inpatient in the hospital. This video was moving in that they had forgotten how far Sam had come. In particular, Donald was able to release deep feelings of grief and to revive feelings of respect and love for his son.

Sam also made progress during these family-centered sessions. It seemed that hearing his family's stories and focusing on the changes in their lives rather than in his allowed him to reclaim some responsibility for the healthy functioning of the family. He agreed to cooperate in a cognitive-behavioral program that involved a family member holding up large warning signs when Sam began to show signs of becoming irritable. For example, if Julie noticed Sam becoming irritated with the children, she would hold up a sign saying "1st Warning: You are becoming irritable." If this did not result in Sam's calming down or leaving the room, she would hold up a second sign saying "Warning 2: Calm down or leave the room." If this did not have the desired effect, a third sign would be displayed saying "Final warning: Leave the room immediately." This intervention was highly successful and often resulted in the children, followed by Sam, breaking into giggles. It was effective because of the external cueing it provided for Sam and also because Julie was not in the position of having to argue with Sam, which invariably upset both of them even further. Within a month the signs were no longer necessary because Sam and the children had learned for themselves what caused Sam to become irritable and voluntarily stopped the chain of events before a problem arose. To assist Margaret, the family support system was reestablished, and Sam's friends were approached about taking Sam out on weekends. At this stage in Sam's rehabilitation, the importance of each family member taking up his or her own life again was stressed.

Finally, Sam was ready to build a new self-identity. Before he could begin this process, he grieved for the old Sam and said goodbye to those parts of him that were lost. Many therapeutic techniques were used to assist the new Sam to emerge. Throughout therapy emphasis was on new skills, and mistakes, problems, and difficulties were played down. New skills, including positive thoughts, were written in a special section in Sam's diary by Sam and other family members and friends. These new skills were reviewed regularly, and new instances that strengthened those skills were sought. Sam was also given practical training to help him with communication, sometimes with other family members joining him in role playing. Lance's entry into Sam's life and their regular sessions at the gymnasium gave him back a pleasurable feeling of physical control and a new friend who was able to empathize with Sam because he, too, had survived and overcome a severe head injury.

Gradually Sam's level of confidence and self-esteem increased. Four years after his head injury, he moved into an apartment with two other people his age, neither of whom were "disabled." This move was successful, and he remained in that apartment for 18 months. He finally found the confidence to invite a woman out, and after 2 years they married and in time had two children. Sam's wife says she cannot imagine the old Sam his brother sometimes talks about and loves him just as he is. Sam and his partner go to his mother's house "for a decent feed" most Wednesday nights, although he telephones first to make sure Margaret has no other plans. Margaret recently remarried and no longer organizes her life around Sam's needs. Sam's relationship with his father, Donald, and his family is generally peaceful; Donald confided in me that whenever he finds himself becoming annoyed or frustrated with Sam's easygoing attitude and lack of initiative, he watches Sam's rehabilitation video. As he said, "It never fails to make me cry, but I always feel better afterwards, and I find myself spending more time with my other children."

Discussion

Severe head injury occurs primarily among young men, and modern critical care technologies and medical knowledge have ensured that many more victims now survive than in the recent past. The diffuse axonal and cortical damage and, in many cases, focal damage that are the hallmarks of severe closed head injury ensure that cognitive impairments are usually wide ranging and long lasting. Unfortunately, rehabilitation research and practice techniques have not kept pace with acute-care technology, and many who survive face a life of dependence and misery.

It is far from established that any specific model of rehabilitation works in terms of increased productivity (e.g., return to paid employment or school), a decrease in the number and severity of cognitive and emotional problems, and an increase in the quality of life (e.g., happiness). In general, however, it appears that intensive, long-term rehabilitation programs are best, especially if they include cognitive retraining, activities of daily living training, psychoeducation (for both client and family), establishment of community support networks, individual and group psychotherapy, and retraining in social skills. In addition, it seems important to include vocational retraining on the job, ideally with a system in place for infrequent but regular maintenance checks of the client's work performance throughout the client's working life.

Families and friends of the head-injured are also victims and need support, assistance, and sometimes even "permission" to live their own lives without guilt once the critical stages of the head injury are passed. Families who are supportive in the early stages after the head injury may become discouraged and "burned out" as the years pass and the head-injured person's progress plateaus, especially as psychosocial problems are often significant for 1 or more years after the CHI. Inappropriate behaviors continue, the head-injured person still suffers periods of depression or has displays of uncontrolled violence and aggression, and his motivation to work or participate in hobbies may remain low. It is hardly surprising in such cases that families break up.

Many stories of TBI victims and their families do not have particularly happy endings, unlike Sam's case. With support and determination, a willingness to give up dreams and ambitions that can no longer be realized, and determination to work toward new, attainable goals, it is possible for some head-injured victims to achieve a fulfilling life and leave the tragedy that halted the old one in the past.

11
■

THE UNSEEN INJURY
MILD TRAUMATIC BRAIN INJURY

My first impression of Rachel was of a tall, attractive young woman who conducted herself in a composed, mature manner. If I had been asked to estimate her age, I would have said she was at least 16, possibly older. Even after discovering she was only 14, I often found it difficult to think of her as a "young" teenager, primarily because of her mature and thoughtful outlook rather than because of her appearance. At times it would come as a surprise to find that many of her life experiences (e.g., relationships with boys) were those of an "average" 14-year-old girl and that she was not as emotionally mature as she first appeared.

Rachel was referred because of difficulties she had been experiencing following a mild closed traumatic brain injury (TBI) 2 months earlier. Rachel's doctor and mother were concerned because her problems were emotional as well as cognitive and had been "dragging on" for many weeks. As Rachel commented, "No one really believes my problems are because of my head injury anymore, because I seem so normal and healthy on the outside. Sometimes even I think the head injury was a red herring, and I am going crazy." The skepticism of friends, family, and even the medical profession about an organic cause for Rachel's problems typifies the attitude of many to the postconcussional syndrome and its treatment and is the reason why many sufferers and rehabilitation specialists call it "the unseen injury."

Rachel's story falls at the severe end of the spectrum of outcomes that can follow mild TBI. Many people appear to suffer no or minimal problems after such an injury; others have some problems that resolve after a few weeks. Nevertheless, from 5% to 25% of people who lose consciousness for only a few seconds or minutes following a blow to the head, or who do not lose consciousness at all but "see stars" and feel dazed for a brief period, suffer from a consistent array of postconcussional symptoms for a considerable length of time (Bohnen, Twijnstra, and Jolles 1993; Gronwall, Wrightson, and Waddell 1998). Some people seem more susceptible to these symptoms than others, which seems to be in part a function of how quickly they return to work or school and the demands their work places on their concentration, memory, and problem-solving abilities. As a high achiever at school, Rachel fell into this category of people at risk for a significant postconcussional syndrome (PCS). Her premorbid personality characteristics and developmental stage may have been additional factors in how some of her symptoms were expressed and their long duration.

Theoretical Background

Definition and Neuropathology

No universal standard exists for defining mild closed TBI except that it is caused by a blow to the head. *Closed* TBI refers to a head injury in which the skull is not penetrated (although it may be fractured) and the brain exposed. Only about 10% of TBIs are *open*, referring to the skull being broken so that the brain is exposed (Grafman and Salazar 1987). In this chapter TBI will refer to a closed head injury. The most commonly used definitions of mild TBI include a combination of the following: a period of unconsciousness of 20 minutes or less, a Glasgow Coma Score (GCS) of 13–15 on regaining consciousness (usually corresponding to spontaneous eye opening, an ability to obey commands, and a verbal response that may be incoherent or confused), hospitalization not greater than 48 hours, and a period of posttraumatic amnesia (PTA) of less than 24 hours (Rimel, Giordani, Barth, Boll, and Jane, 1981). Many people who sustain a mild TBI may lose consciousness for only a few minutes, or not at all, and have a PTA of a few seconds only, but even these people can suffer from postconcussional symptoms (Bohnen et al. 1993).

A computed tomography (CT) study of 500 patients with mild TBI found that 7.2% had small brain lesions (contusions and subcortical hemorrhages) typically located in the inferior anterior frontal and temporal lobes. In a subgroup of 171 patients who had a loss of consciousness of 10 minutes or less, 7.6% had CT abnormalities (Sekino et al. 1981). With the greater imaging powers of magnetic resonance imaging (MRI), lesions not revealed by CT are being exposed (Voller et al. 1999; Wilson 1990). Levin et al. (1987a) reported that 14 of 16 consecutive patients admitted with mild or moderate TBI had lesions imaged by MRI, especially in parenchymal tissue, that were not seen on CT. Diffuse axonal injuries caused by stretching and tearing of nerve axons are also a possible consequence of mild TBI, although these injuries obviously would be minimal compared with severe head injury. This type of damage could nevertheless result in transient disruption of the reticular formation system (RF), causing lowered cortical arousal and the consequent common problems of fatigue, hypersensitivity to noise, and emotional lability.

Gronwall and Wrightson (1975) have shown that the effects of mild TBI are cumulative and that young adults who sustained two mild head injuries had poorer scores on a test of information processing rate. These patients also took longer to recover than a comparison group who had sustained only one head injury.

Neurobehavioral and Psychosocial Deficits after Mild TBI

In the hours and days immediately following a mild TBI, the victim may suffer headaches and feel nauseated, extremely tired, and possibly confused and disoriented. The best treatment at this stage is to sleep and rest. Most people feel fully recovered 2 weeks later, and many are able to return to work without difficulty, especially if the work is not too taxing mentally or physically (Ponsford 1995). Some people, however, suffer some symptoms that constitute the PCS for varying lengths of time and in varying degrees of severity (Wrightson and Gronwall 1999), with Levin's (1995) review of six major studies concluding that at 3 months after a mild TBI, two-thirds of the patients were still suffering from neurobehavioral deficits. The most common of the cognitive symptoms are deficits in concentration; decreased ability to focus on the task at hand, especially in a noisy or distracting environment; an impairment in processing complex information; and problems with recent memory. These deficits are usually assessed by performance on standard neuropsychological tests of attention, information processing, and new learning and recall. In day-to-day life, sufferers notice that they have to put much greater effort into learning and recalling names of new friends and facts in school; they become irritable in noisy environments; and if their work requires concentration, memorizing information, or processing new information, they tire very quickly, develop headaches, and soon find themselves falling behind in their work or schooling.

The physical and psychosocial effects of mild TBI have a neuropathological basis (lowered cortical arousal from frontal-lobe dysfunction) and follow from the victim's and others' reactions to the victim's cognitive problems. Common symptoms include fatigue, nausea, changes in sleep and eating patterns, periods of dizziness, hypersensitivity to noise, lessened tolerance to alcohol, irritability, anxiety, and depression. Some sufferers have a lack of insight into their problems, although this occurs less commonly than after severe head injury. If the PCS continues for many weeks or months, sufferers may gradually lose confidence in their ability to work and maintain relationships, resulting in frustration and irritability and a lowering of self-esteem. Family disruption often occurs as family members struggle to cope with the problems of the head-injured person. Some sufferers may even come to believe they are going crazy or become so depressed that they feel suicidal, especially if they have not obtained information about PCS and do not relate their problems to the mild TBI they sustained weeks ago.

Cross-Cultural Issues in Assessment

The proportion of people who suffer from PCS varies widely across studies. Levin et al. (1987b) compared etiology and outcome in three trauma centers and found marked sociocultural differences among victims of mild TBI as well as significant disparities in the neurobehavioral outcomes at each center. Further study of memory performance at baseline and at 1 month after head injury demonstrated that the baseline performance of patients at two of the centers (in Galveston, Texas, and in San Diego, California) was better than that of patients at the third center (in the Bronx, New York). In fact, the memory scores of controls in the Bronx group were similar to the baseline scores of the head-injured groups at the two other centers (Mattis and Kovner 1978). The three control groups (one for each center) did not differ with respect to age, years of education, or socioeconomic background; therefore, it seems likely that cultural differences and cultural inappropriateness for some ethnic groups of the standard memory tests used to assess outcome caused the variations in memory outcome. If each center had not used its own control group or had relied on published test norms for comparison with scores of the head-injured groups, the conclusion that more individuals in the Bronx group were suffering from the PCS might have been incorrectly made.

Studies carried out in New Zealand (Ogden and McFarlane-Nathan 1997; Ogden, Cooper, and Dudley 2003) add support for the importance of not assuming that nonwhite ethnic groups growing up alongside their white peers in an apparently similar environment will necessarily perform at the same level as their compatriots on all tests. This may be the case even for tests that do not appear to be culturally biased (Ogden 2001a). The argument that the nonwhite ethnic groups are less accomplished at cognitive tasks generally was also found to be spurious in the New Zealand studies. In one study, 20 non-head-injured Maori men from a poorly educated, low socioeconomic group aged 16–25 years (the group most affected by head injury) performed at above-average levels (compared with western norms) on the revised Wechsler Adult Intelligence Scale (WAIS-R) Block Design subtest (a test of pattern perception and construction), but below average on the WAIS-R Vocabulary subtest. Their performance on the Oral Selective Reminding Test, a memory test involving learning a list of 12 unrelated high-frequency words over 12 trials, was above the "normative" score of a group of pakeha (white) New Zealand men of a similar age, education, and socioeconomic group, but the Maori men's scores on the memory passages of the Wechsler Memory Scale (WMS) were below the average of similar American and New Zealand age and education groups. In this test the subject is read two short stories and then asked to recall them (Ogden and McFarlane-Nathan 1997). These findings have been supported by further studies comparing healthy young Maori men and women with healthy pakeha controls (Ogden et al. 2003).

One possible explanation for these variations in performance is that Maori culture and art emphasize complex visuospatial patterns not unlike those that constitute the Block Design Test, but Maori children do poorly in school subjects such as English, which are based on Western culture and vernacular. Although they share a considerable vocabulary with pakeha New Zealanders, many common English words have taken on a different meaning for this group of young Maori men. These factors might explain their poor performance on Vocabulary. Their excellent memory performance on the Selective Reminding Test might be explained by the considerable oratory skills for which Maori people are greatly respected and their amazing (to the pakeha) ability to recall and recite their genealogy for many generations back. This genealogy is passed down orally to the children from their elders. Perhaps as a result they have developed particular skills in learning word lists. Their poor performance on the WMS memory passages seems a clear example of an understandably lowered performance on a culturally inappropriate test, as these stories are very "Americanized." Given that Maori children are generally less suited to Western-style schooling and educational material than their pakeha peers, American-based stories are likely to be even more foreign and uninteresting for Maori than for pakeha. Indeed, the young Maori men, after being read stories of the same length about common Maori experiences, performed at a higher level when asked to recall them. Young pakeha men from the same socioeconomic group gained lower scores on the stories about Maori experiences than on the WMS stories (Ogden et al. 2003).

These examples provide some important lessons. First, when assessing the neurobehavioral outcome of a group or individual who is culturally different from the sample on which the assessment instruments were standardized, it is important to assess a control group or subject who is matched not only on the usual variables of age, education, and socioeconomic group but also matched as to cultural background and ethnic identity. Second, we should be aware of the cultural inappropriateness of many of the neuropsychological and psychiatric assessment instruments used to assess the effects of brain damage. If we could use different assessment instruments developed according to the interests and skills of Afro-Americans or the New Zealand Maori and standardized on these groups, we would likely find that these cultural groups, appropriately assessed, perform at a higher level than groups of age, education, and socioeconomically matched white Americans or pakeha New Zealanders on the same tests. Third, given that mild TBI affects people across all ethnic groups, especially young men in urban areas (as the result motor vehicle accidents, football injuries, and assaults), the importance of skepticism when assessing studies of PCS that do not have a carefully matched control group cannot be stressed enough.

Rehabilitation

In the first instance, victims of a mild TBI should rest and sleep until PCS symptoms resolve. When they no longer have significant headaches, can cope with conversations under noisy conditions, and no longer need afternoon naps and need to retire to bed early, they should return to normal activities for shortened hours, gradually increasing their hours until they are working normally again. University and school students and people employed in jobs that require concentration, problem solving, or fast reaction times are more at risk for developing PCS than those who work in routine, nonpressure jobs. These at-risk persons should take additional care to return to work gradually, guided by their symptoms. Some people, even after following such a program, continue to experience PCS for months or years. For these people, it may be that a vicious neurological-psychological cycle is set in motion. The fatigue, irritability, and memory problems cause disruptions in the lives of family members; consequently, negative interactional patterns are established, resulting in further stress on the head-injured person, who becomes even more irritable and unreasonable. Such family dynamics are common after mild TBI, especially if the head-injured person and the family have not been given sufficient information about TBI and have not had any rehabilitation. Family therapy may assist the family in seeking ways to change unhelpful patterns and to enhance interactions that lower the stress on the head-injured person and encourage recovery. Often information about PCS, even when received many months later, can relieve the victim of thoughts that he is going crazy and can provide the family with an explanation for their difficulties.

Case Presentation

Background

Before her accident, Rachel was the top student in her class at school; she enjoyed music, art, swimming, aerobics, and skiing. Rachel planned to attend the university to study fine art when she completed school at the age of 17 years. Her mother, younger sister, and friends perceived her to be an extrovert. As her best friend, Louise, commented, "Rachel was always involved in something exciting." She was popular at school and had a good relationship with her mother, who was only 35 years old and led an active working and social life. Her younger sister, Jody, was also considered exceptionally talented, and at the age of 12 she was already an accomplished violinist. The girls' parents were divorced, and their Maori father, who lived in a rural part of New Zealand, was seen as something of a "misfit" by the girls' pakeha mother but "a laid-back dude" by his daughters. Rachel and Jody usually spent a few carefree weeks in the summer with him before returning to their very different city lifestyle when school began again.

In the August of her fourteenth year, Rachel was on a skiing holiday with Louise and Louise's parents. On the last day of the holiday, she hit a stone while skiing and fell, hitting her head hard on the bottom of a pylon supporting a chair lift. When Louise reached her a minute later, she seemed dazed and a little confused, but after resting for 10 minutes she was able to stand up and ski the short distance to the base facilities. She was checked by the ski patrol staff, who said she may have had a brief concussion and should rest and not ski again for a few days. Louise and her parents noted that Rachel seemed confused and was unable to remember much for about 4 hours after the accident. After a night's sleep, Rachel felt somewhat better and was no longer confused, although she did complain of a continuous headache. They drove back to Auckland the next day. After a checkup by her family doctor, Rachel rested for the week of school holiday left before returning to school at the beginning of the final term of the year.

Three days after starting school, she returned home in the early afternoon, distressed because she could not concentrate and could not rid herself of a dull headache. From this time on her school performance deteriorated, and art was the only subject with which she could cope. The art room was quiet, and the students worked at their own pace. On her doctor's suggestion, she reduced her school hours to 3 a day and slept in the afternoon. She still could not keep up with mathematics and soon dropped that subject, retiring to the art room earlier each morning. At home she was irritable, morose, lacked energy, and spent her evenings in her room listening to music. Her mother and friends tried to entice her to socialize, but with little success. Home became either a morgue or a battleground, depending on whether Rachel was in "her morose mood or biting our heads off at the slightest thing."

Neuropsychological and Psychosocial Consequences

Two months after her head injury, Rachel was referred by her doctor for a neuropsychological assessment and counseling. At the initial interview, it was apparent that her mood was extremely depressed and that Rachel believed she had suffered brain damage that had been underdiagnosed by her doctor. She was in tears as she said:

> I can't remember anything and I can't think clearly any more, and that has to mean brain damage. I'll never be able to finish school now, let alone go to university. I don't see the point in living like this. I have no energy to do anything, and my friends are soon going to stop asking me out. I don't blame them. Who wants a brain-damaged friend?

Her mother and sister, who were both at the interview, were shattered by these revelations and quickly tried to reassure her that she was not brain-damaged and that head injury took up to 2 years to recover from.

The next stage of the interview comprised an assessment of Rachel's emotional state and the possibility that she might be suicidal. Rachel said she had thought it would be better for everyone if she died; but said she had not planned any way to do it and did not think she had the courage or energy anyway. Rachel agreed to talk to her mother if she again had feelings that life was not worth living. More realistic information was given to the family about mild TBI and PCS. Rachel's fears of having suffered significant, permanent brain damage were counteracted, and they discussed the possibility that she might need a few months but was not likely to need as long as 2 years to regain her previous level of functioning completely.

Rachel returned for three further individual psychotherapy sessions to help her gain control over depression. During this time she was encouraged to pursue recovery more actively by pacing herself carefully at school, by attending only those classes she felt she could cope with comfortably, and by spending as much time as her body (and brain) demanded resting and sleeping. She and her mother explained PCS to her teachers and friends, who were supportive.

Rachel's mood lifted, and she was given a neuropsychological assessment. Rachel's ethnicity was both pakeha and Maori, but she had been socialized and educated in a pakeha system. Her academic success at her largely pakeha school and her strong relationships with her pakeha peers indicated that it was appropriate to assess her using tests normed on a white population. Most of her scores on the Verbal subtests of the Wechsler Intelligence Scale for Children-Revised (WISC-R) (Wechsler 1974) fell in the "superior" range, demonstrating that her vocabulary, general knowledge, and verbal comprehension and abstraction abilities were probably unimpaired. Her only significantly lowered score (and this fell in the "average" range) was the mental Arithmetic score. She was unable to hold long problems in memory while she worked them out. This difficulty improved when she was able to have the written problems in front of her and to use a paper and pencil to work them out. On the Performance subtests of the WISC-R, she lost points for slowness, although when given unlimited time she was able to do most of the items of each subtest. Because of her slowness, most of her scores fell in the "average" range.

Rachel was then given the Paced Auditory Serial Addition Task (PASAT) (Gronwall 1977), a test that puts demands on sustained attention and concentration, working memory, and performing multiple mental tasks under time pressure. It is thought to measure information-processing capacity, which is often considerably reduced after mild TBI. Performance on this test correlates highly with the symptoms of PCS, and repeated assessments on the PASAT over time provide a good indication of recovery from the head injury. When performance nears normal levels, the client is usually ready to return in a graduated way to work or school. Rachel became distressed during the second trial of the PASAT and refused to continue.

Rachel's scores on tests of new learning and memory fell in the "average" range, a considerable drop for her. In addition, she found these tests very tiring. Her copy of the Complex Figure was above average, and her later recall of it fell in the "average" range. Both scores were considered low for her, especially given her superior artistic ability.

On tests of frontal-lobe ability, Rachel did not demonstrate any difficulty. Her ability to initiate words beginning with a specific letter in one minute (Oral Word Fluency) was within normal limits, and she had no difficulty changing set on the Wisconsin Card Sorting Test. Her copy of the Complex Figure was well organized and structured.

Following this assessment, we decided she should not return to school for the few remaining weeks. Her friends' end-of-year examinations were coming up, and they were working hard preparing for them. Rachel found it stressful not to be sitting the exams, and she felt she was "getting on her friends' nerves." At this stage Rachel was having difficulty sleeping at night; typically, she would nap in the afternoon, feel wide awake at night, and finally fall asleep at about 4:00 AM. Various interventions were attempted to reestablish a normal sleep pattern, but success was minimal. Unable to sleep, Rachel often awakened her mother to talk, so her mother was clearly suffering from sleep deprivation as well and was understandably worried about Rachel's apparent lack of improvement. By this time, some 12 weeks after her TBI, Rachel was doubting that such a small bump on the head could cause so many problems and thought that she must have a psychiatric condition. I helped Rachel to explore this possibility, and she decided that the PCS might still be having an influence but that her loss of energy and emotional reactions to losing her ability to do well at school had resulted in her feeling depressed and losing her self-confidence. She decided she wanted to give her mother and sister a rest from worry and to give herself "some fresh air." As she commented, "I feel stagnant and useless and dead." She arranged to stay with her father and his extended family in a rural seaside town for 10 weeks until the start of school in the new year.

Rachel returned as planned the following January; physically she looked much healthier and happier. Her holiday had been a great success, and she said she had slept well, raced around swimming and boating with her cousins, and thought not at all about schoolwork. Her headaches had disappeared, and she found she could concentrate throughout the reading of an entire book. She had also become fascinated by her Maori heritage and had spent many happy hours listening to her great-grandmother tell of her own childhood and the myths and legends of her tribe and ancestors.

It was decided to repeat some of the neuropsychological tests before Rachel started school again. Her approach to the tests was more energetic, and she managed a 3-hour session without tiring. On the Performance subtests of the WISC-R, she was much faster, improving her scores markedly, even considering the "practice" effects of her previous assessment. Her results on both the verbal and nonverbal memory tests also improved significantly to "superior" levels, and on the PASAT she achieved scores within one standard deviation (SD) below her age norm. Clearly, there was still room for improvement on this test, but it was decided that she could return to school, mornings only at first, and with individual tuition in some classes (math and French) to help her make up for the classes she had missed.

A careful social schedule was also arranged so that she would not become overtired and return to poor sleep patterns. She was permitted a nap in the afternoon if she needed one but was instructed to set her alarm so that she did not sleep for more than 1 hour. A "good sleep habit" program was instigated immediately to train her to relax before she went to bed and to use her bedroom for sleep only. She was prepared in advance for the possibility that her recovery pattern would not always be smooth and that at times she would feel herself slipping back. This was normal and did not mean she was not recovering. She was given self-help strategies to get her past these possible difficult "patches." Rachel found that she could cope with school, and her sleep patterns stabilized. She gradually built up her sporting and social activities. Within 6 weeks she was back in her regular class and, as she said, "going on nearly all six cylinders."

Discussion

Rachel's case illustrates many of the organic, psychological, and social factors that complicate the assessment and rehabilitation of people who have ongoing problems after a mild TBI. Her age was a further complicating factor. Adolescence is a time of rapid physical, hormonal, and emotional change; when these changes are added to the stresses of performing at a high academic level, it is perhaps not surprising that the sudden onset of typical postconcussional symptoms caused such an extreme disruption in Rachel's life. Older groups also seem to be more susceptible to PCS (Rutherford 1989), possibly because of the brain's decreasing capacity for recovery following insult.

Why PCS is so idiosyncratic is not fully understood, but it is likely that the interaction of a range of organic and psychological factors is responsible for the variable susceptibility of people to what appear to be only mild blows to the head (Dikmen, Temkin, and Armsden 1989). Previous head injuries, a premorbid history of serious emotional or psychiatric problems, alcohol or solvent abuse, the developmental stage, and a demanding job are all likely to be factors that increase the potential for a significant PCS. In some cases, malingering can be a factor, especially where there is monetary compensation for problems related to the head injury. In many such cases, PCS can be viewed as a psychological construct without an organic basis. In true cases of PCS, where there is an underlying organic cause, there is very often some psychological overlay; it is as important to prevent these psychological symptoms from developing as it is to manage the rehabilitation of the organically mediated symptoms. Whereas some cases of extended PCS may be primarily the result of neurological damage (as supported by MRI findings of diffuse lesions following mild TBI), it is possible that many cases of PCS that continue for months or years have become almost purely "psychological." These people should not, however, be viewed as malingerers but as suffering from a poorly managed PCS.

Research studies have shown that good management for mild TBI incorporates the following steps:

a. Following the head injury, the victim should be advised to rest for 1–2 weeks before attempting to return to work. Clear oral and written information should be given to the head-injured person and the family about the various problems that sometimes occur after a mild TBI and when and where to seek further help and advice on how to overcome these problems.
b. People at risk for the PCS should be checked 2 weeks after the head injury to ensure that they are embarking on a gradual return to work. People who still report significant cognitive problems at that time should be neuropsychologically assessed and referred to a rehabilitation service that can design a program suited to their specific needs.

Rachel had her own insightful analysis of her painful struggle with the PCS and her ultimate success in overcoming it:

> After my head injury slowed my brain down, I couldn't cope with not being the best in class. I think having such a bright sister made it worse; I could see she would catch up and overtake me soon. I really thought I must have brain damage and although the doctor said I would be myself again in a few weeks, and then a few months, and then 2 years, it seemed to me no one really knew what was happening to me, or they were too afraid to tell me. That was when I even thought I might be going crazy—I know the first signs of craziness often start about my age—and the

head injury had nothing to do with it. I think I just gave up then. Even if I did get better, imagine still being in the same class when I was 16 with a lot of 14-year-olds, including my sister. Once I gave up, it was better in some ways, except Mum wouldn't let me just stay in my room all day, and I could never sleep at night.

After I came to see you, I felt better for a while and that it really was the head injury, and Mum and the school took the pressure off a bit. I hated doing those tests before I went away, especially that one where I had to add the numbers. I was sure I had brain damage after that. It was such a relief when we decided I should get right away from Auckland, and you told me to leave all my school books behind and just have a good time doing whatever I felt like. I think once I got up north, and Dad and my cousins didn't really care about my head injury or that I had failed at school and treated me the same as always, I began to feel like the old Rachel again. It was great really getting to know all my *whanau* (family) up there, and finding out about my Maori side, and learning about my *tipuna* (ancestors). I found I was quite quick at picking up Maori words and remembering long Maori names, so perhaps my ancestors were working on my brain and fixing it! Mainly, I think, my energy came back, and even when I did feel tired I was no different from any of the others, falling asleep lying in the sun on the beach. I was pretty tired by nighttime, and mostly I had no trouble sleeping all night.

I must say I was a bit scared when I came back and not looking forward to going back to school. Once I got there it was okay, though, and it was quite amazing to be able to think again and to remember stuff I'd had in class the day before. I suppose I do think now that I did have a postconcussional syndrome; it certainly sounds like the articles you've given me to read. I guess I just never gave my brain space to recover. It had lots of time, but I was so stressed it couldn't use the time efficiently. I have learnt something from it all. I'm not going to get so tied up in my work and having to be top of the class again. I really think if I had not cared so much about my work, I would have not got so depressed and given up so quickly, and I would not have had such a problem with dropping behind for a while. It was all or nothing for me I think, and that was the problem. I couldn't cope with doing it all, and doing nothing made me think I had lost it.

When asked what "take-home message" she might have for other teenagers who have problems following a mild TBI, Rachel replied:

> I would tell them to read the story of the tortoise and the hare and to give up on being a hare for a bit and try out the slow but sure tortoise walk. I figure it is best to risk being a bit boring like a tortoise but move steadily forward than to go like a hare and collapse before the end!

Eight years after Rachel's TBI, a telephone call to her mother revealed that Rachel had quite quickly regained her preinjury, extrovert personality and within 2 years was once more back at the top of her class in most subjects. She had continued to explore her Maori heritage and had enrolled in the Maori language class and the *kapa haka* group (Maori cultural group) at school. After leaving school she went on to university where she completed, in the minimum time possible, a degree in fine arts, with her artwork often incorporating Maori design and symbolism. Now aged 22 years she was traveling and working in Europe with friends before deciding whether to return to university to complete a higher degree or take up a career.

12

∎

Explosions in the Mind

A Case of Subarachnoid Hemorrhage

It was a hot midsummer day with not a cloud in the sky, and Danielle, her husband Adam, and their two children, 12-year-old twins Emma and Andrew, were on their last day of their summer holiday before the twins had to return to school and Danielle and Adam to work. They were staying in Danielle's parents' holiday home at Piha, a ruggedly beautiful black sand surf beach west of Auckland. As it was a Sunday, the crowds were out, and between the lifeguards' flags, the surf was alive with screaming, happy children on body boards, and parents trying to keep track of them. Adam was surfing on the big waves out the back, and Danielle and the twins were competing on their body boards to see who could catch the longest wave. Suddenly, without warning, Danielle's head exploded (as she recalled later). Fortunately she was in waist-deep water and she managed to stagger out of the sea, collapsing on the sand. The twins, realizing she was not behaving normally, grabbed her board and rushed out of the surf to her side. She managed to tell them that she had been hit on the head by a surfboard, and was feeling very sick.

By this time people had begun to crowd around and the lifeguard on duty came over to see what was wrong. Danielle managed to walk into the lifeguard station with the guard's help and lay down on the couch while he checked her skull. "Can't feel any bump, and there is no blood," he reported, "so I think you must be just concussed." By the time the children managed to attract Adam's attention and he caught a wave to the beach, Danielle still had a thumping headache, and as the light made it worse (*photophobia*), was lying with a wet cloth over her eyes. Adam and the children helped her back to their cottage, and when she still hadn't improved 2 hours later, they decided to go home to Auckland and take Danielle to the Accident and Emergency Department at Auckland Hospital. After having a number of tests, including a computed tomography (CT) brain scan, they were told that Danielle had suffered a subarachnoid hemorrhage (SAH) and had not been hit by a flying surfboard at all. The doctor explained that the sensation of being hit on the head and an exploding headache was common when an aneurysm on an artery feeding the brain burst, expelling blood at high pressure into the subarachnoid space around the brain. Danielle was admitted to the neurosurgery ward for further tests and treatment.

This scenario of a healthy adult being struck down by a sudden, terrible head pain is almost diagnostic for a SAH. Some die immediately from the hemorrhage, whereas others lose consciousness or perhaps die over the next few days. Many, like Danielle, remain awake but become confused and drowsy. Most people who survive the initial hemorrhage undergo neurosurgery to clip off the source of the bleeding, usually an aneurysm, or endovascular coiling of the aneurysm to occlude it. Recovery is variable, with long-term outcomes ranging from severe generalized brain damage resulting in a global cognitive deterioration and paralyzed limbs to a return almost to pre-SAH cognitive abilities with no physical impairments.

Even those who suffer a mild SAH, have an uncomplicated medical course, and return to their job and social life within 3–6 months of their hemorrhage more often than not experience some persistent neuropsychological or psychosocial difficulties. Research into outcome following SAH carries some important messages for health professionals who are in a position to provide helpful and accurate information about SAH to the victim and family or who are involved in the patient's neuropsychological assessment and rehabilitation (Hackett and Anderson 2000; Hop, Rinkel, Algra, and van Gijn 1998; Ogden, Levin, and Mee 1990; Ogden, Mee, and Henning 1993a, 1994; Ogden, Utley, and Mee 1997).

In recent years there has been an increase in the identification of incidental un-ruptured intracranial aneurysms (UIAs). These are sometimes identified during brain imaging and angiography following a SAH resulting the rupture of another aneurysm but are also occasionally found in nonsymptomatic adults who have undergone a magnetic resonance image (MRI) of the brain to screen for some unrelated problem. The issue of whether or not to treat UIAs is a controversial issue and will be discussed in the next section (Towgood, Ogden, and Mee 2004).

Theoretical Background

Definition and Causes

Spontaneous subarachnoid hemorrhage is a rare form of stroke that usually occurs in previously healthy people. Most victims fall in the 45- to 60-year age group, although SAH can occur at any age. Indeed, when a young person is reported to have collapsed unconscious while playing an energetic sport, the cause is often a SAH. Both sexes can suffer a SAH, but studies show that more women than men are affected.

In most cases SAH is the result of the spontaneous rupture of a cerebral aneurysm, a balloon-like weakening on the wall of a cerebral artery (Af Bjorksen and Halonen 1965), although in from 7% to 25% of cases, *cerebral angiography* (a radiograph of the arteries) fails to reveal an aneurysm. These latter cases are categorized as *non-aneurysmal* SAH (West, Maru, Eisenberg, Tuerk, and Stuker 1977). Head trauma, tumors, and infections, as well as a hemorrhage from an arteriovenous malformation (a congenital and abnormal tangle of blood vessels), can also result in a SAH.

Why cerebral aneurysms occur in some people but not others is not known. The percentage of autopsied cases revealing aneurysms is about 2% (Jellinger 1979), and estimates of aneurysmal rupture as the cause of death in whole populations are less than 1%. The international yearly incidence of SAH is about 10:100,000 (Bonita and Thomson 1985; Parkarinen 1967). About 40%–50% of people who suffer a SAH die at the time of the initial bleed or within a month (Bonita and Thomson 1985). Those who survive may be left with a range of deficits from very mild to severe, and recovery varies. Some studies have shown that most patients have not fully regained their premorbid levels of higher cognitive and psychosocial functioning 1–7 years after the SAH (Ogden, Levin, and Mee 1990; Ogden et al. 1993a, 1994, 1997; Vilkki, Holst, Ohman, Servo, and Heiskanen 1989, 1990).

It is important to identify risk factors for the rupture of cerebral aneurysms with the ultimate aim of reducing these risks and the sometimes devastating consequences of SAH. A number of studies have identified cigarette smoking as a risk factor (Bell and Symon 1979; Bonita 1986; Fogelholm and Murros 1987; Ogden, Mee, and Henning 1993b; Taha, Ball, and Illingworth 1982), and Bonita (1986) found that a history of treatment for hypertension in addition to smoking increased this risk significantly. Other studies, however, failed to find an association between hypertension and aneurysmal SAH (Keller 1970; McCormick and Schmalstieg 1977). Clinical impression suggests that a sudden rise in intracranial pressure (such as that caused by sneezing, coitus, or defecation), a transient rise in blood pressure associated with physical strain, or a sudden emotional shock might precipitate an aneurysmal SAH in some cases.

In one large study, almost all the victims of SAH (or their next of kin) in a defined geographic area over a 3-year period (257 patients) were given a questionnaire about the occurrence of stressful events in their lives in the year preceding their SAH. Their responses were compared with a control group of 100 hospital patients. The results demonstrated at a high level of statistical significance ($P = .00001$) that SAH is preceded by many more moderately stressful events or one or more extremely stressful events (such as a family death, divorce, or bankruptcy) much more frequently than they precede hospitalization for illnesses such as orthopedic or skin problems (Ogden et al. 1993b).

Diagnosis and Treatment

Subarachnoid hemorrhage   When an aneurysm ruptures during a SAH, blood is expelled under high pressure, and it disperses around the brain in the space between the *pia mater*, the fine covering that clings to the surface of the brain, and the next covering, the *arachnoid mater*, so called because the blood vessels within it give it a spidery appearance. This space is thus called the *subarachnoid space*, and it communicates with the subarachnoid space around the spinal cord. Cerebrospinal fluid (CSF) produced by the choroid plexus lying in the ventricles flows out into the subarachnoid space. Therefore, when an aneurysm ruptures into the subarachnoid space, red blood cells are usually found in the CSF when a lumbar puncture is performed. This is one of the diagnostic signs of SAH, along with the sudden and severe headache experienced by the victims, a stiff neck caused by an inflammatory response to the blood around the base of the brain and spinal cord, and most important, the confirmation of an aneurysm on one of the arteries.

The aneurysm can be visualized using *MRI angiography* (where magnetic resonance imaging is used to visualize the arteries) or by a more invasive technique called angiography. This involves injecting a radioactive dye into the vessels of the brain and taking radiographs as the dye moves through the vessels, showing up their outlines. The neurosurgeon and neuroradiologist can then decide whether the aneurysm is treatable by either surgical clipping or by endovascular coiling (International Subarachnoid Aneurysm Trial Collaborative Group, 2002). If surgical treatment is decided on, a 3–4-hour operation is performed under a general anesthetic. The skull and *dura* (tough covering on the outside of the brain beneath the skull) are opened and the brain gently retracted to allow the surgeon to trace the artery back to the aneurysm, so that a small metal clip can be placed over the neck of the aneurysm. Once this is done, there is almost no chance that the aneurysm will bleed again, and the patient is therefore "cured."

Increasingly, the much newer technique of coiling is utilized to occlude the aneurysm and prevent it from rupturing again. In this procedure, a microcatheter is introduced into the arterial system leading to the aneurysm and the tip of the catheter positioned in the neck of the aneurysm. A stainless steel delivery guidewire is then pushed up the catheter, and when it is positioned at the neck of the aneurysm, a positive electric current is applied to the guidewire, which results in the detachment of a tiny soft platinum coil that is released into the aneurysm sac. Many coils are thus inserted until a dense packing of the aneurysm is achieved. The coils attract blood cells, platelets and fibrinogen, which results in clot formation. Coiling can be carried out under a local anesthetic but is usually done under a general anesthetic for the comfort of the patient. Coiling usually takes 2.5–3 hours.

Each procedure has good and bad aspects, and in many cases one type of procedure will be more suitable for the shape, size, and position of the aneurysm than the other. Clipping is much more invasive, requiring opening the skull and major neurosurgery, with all the complications that that might entail. However, clipping has a high success rate in permanently occluding the aneurysm. Coiling does not require neurosurgery but often the aneurysm is not fully occluded, and when this happens, further procedures are required to prevent the risk of further bleeding. Aneurysms without clearly defined necks are not easily able to be coiled. However, coiling techniques are improving rapidly, and this method holds the best promise for the future.

In a small number of cases the decision is made not to treat the aneurysm, perhaps because the patient is too sick or very old, or because the aneurysm is in a position that would be impossible to reach. Some aneurysms are much more risky to treat than others; for example, giant aneurysms over 25 mm in diameter located on the tip of the basilar artery have a significant risk of rupturing during surgery or coiling, almost certainly causing death, as the basilar artery lies along the brain stem. It is much less risky to treat a 10-mm aneurysm in the anterior circulation (e.g., on the middle or anterior cerebral arteries or the anterior communicating artery—all very common aneurysm locations). In cases in which the risk of treating the aneurysm is too high, the patient is treated with good medical care and advised to give up smoking and reduce hypertension.

Damage may have been caused at the time of the SAH by the blood around and sometimes within the brain tissue if the blood was expelled under pressure into the brain, resulting in a hematoma. Damage may also be caused by the surgery (or less often by the coiling) and by the various complications that sometimes follow SAH. The most serious of these complications is *vasospasm,* in which the arteries react to the blood around them by going into spasm, which can result in a loss of blood and oxygen (*ischemia*) to the area of brain supplied by that artery, causing an ischemic *stroke* (an area of dead or damaged neural tissue). At present, a great deal of research is being conducted on drugs to prevent and treat vasospasm.

Other complications include *hydrocephalus*, in which the exit to the lateral ventricles is blocked by blood, causing the ventricles to dilate, thus increasing the pressure inside the head. This condition usually corrects spontaneously over time, but when it does not, the neurosurgeon places a valve and tube called a shunt into the ventricle, which allows the excess CSF to drain safely into the abdominal or heart cavity.

Throughout the patient's hospital stay, her condition is graded according to a scale that takes into account how alert and oriented the patient is and whether she has any neurological deficits, such as a hemiplegia or language difficulty. On admission, this grade is assumed to reflect the severity of the hemorrhage and assists the neurosurgeon in decisions regarding surgery and other medical treatments. The patient's grade continues to be monitored because it indicates complications such as vasospasm that may occur days after the SAH or surgery. In addition to this SAH scale, the Glasgow Coma Scale, developed to assess the severity of head trauma, is also often used.

Unruptured intracranial aneurysms   As mentioned in the introduction, sometimes one or more UIAs are identified following a SAH, and incidental UIAs can also be identified during an MRI brain scan carried out for some other purpose. When this occurs the crucial question is whether the patient will be better off if the aneurysm is left untreated or is treated electively. If the patient is untreated, she will be followed up at regular intervals to ensure the aneurysm is not growing too large and will be advised to decrease risk factors for rupture such as smoking and hypertension. Although treating the aneurysm with either clipping or coiling will generally be much less risky than treating an aneurysm that has ruptured, both clipping and coiling UIAs can result in damage to the brain, and even death in rare cases. For some patients, long-term (usually mild) cognitive deficits result from this brain damage.

Very often, if the UIA is harbored by a patient who has suffered a SAH from another aneurysm, the UIA is treated once the patient has recovered from their SAH.

This is because of studies indicating that these people are at a higher risk for aneurysm rupture. However, when an incidental aneurysm, especially a very small one, is discovered in a healthy person, the natural history of aneurysms rupturing over a lifetime must be weighed up against the risks of treating the aneurysm. The research on spontaneous rupture rates of aneurysms is controversial, but a reasonably well accepted figure is that their rate of rupture is 1%–2% a year (Inagawa and Hirano 1990; Juvela, Porras, and Poussa, 2000). Thus, for most people who harbor an incidental UIA, it will never rupture and they will die of other causes, hopefully in old age. Many factors such as the age of the individual, and the location and size of the aneurysm will influence the risk of rupture, and these factors need to be taken into consideration. In addition, the individual's own feelings about harboring a UIA are very important; for some it is like living with a time bomb in their heads and affects their quality of life, whereas for others, it quickly becomes forgotten and they carry on regardless (but hopefully having given up smoking). Thus, even if the neurosurgeon thinks it is feasible and not too risky to treat the aneurysm, the ultimate decision lies with the individual.

Neuropsychological and Psychosocial Deficits after SAH

There are numerous difficulties in the neuropsychological assessment of a group as diverse as SAH patients. By its very nature, SAH involves the likelihood of diffuse disruption to brain cortices, at least in the period immediately subsequent to the hemorrhage (Grote and Hassler 1988; Smith 1963). In addition, there may be more localized areas of disruption as a consequence of vasospasm and ischemia that can occur over a period of days after SAH (Crompton 1964). It is therefore hardly surprising that cognitive and psychosocial impairments can differ dramatically from patient to patient.

Clearly, the overall picture of cognitive outcome following SAH is dismal: More than half the victims of SAH die or become demented (Bonita, Beaglehole, and North 1983). Even given that results of cognitive studies can apply only to patients who have a reasonably "good" neurological outcome (i.e., are not left with any obvious neurological disability such as weak limbs or difficulties with verbal communication), cross-study comparisons are often difficult because of differing selection criteria, methodologies, follow-up periods, and test batteries. Nevertheless, recent large, prospective, longitudinal follow-up studies (i.e., studies that enroll subjects at the time of their SAH rather than retrospectively and assess them over time) have demonstrated a pattern of impairment in patients with a good neurological recovery that is generally consistent with mild diffuse cortical damage (Ogden et al. 1993a, 1997; Stabell 1991). Although the cause of the diffuse damage is different from that occurring after moderate to severe head injury, the long-term cognitive and psychosocial symptoms are remarkably similar.

Memory deficits following SAH have attracted particular attention, perhaps because of the importance of memory as a factor in the patient's rehabilitation and return to a normal lifestyle and because of the many studies reporting memory impairments after SAH (Ljunggren et al. 1985; Ogden, Levin, and Mee 1990; Ogden et al. 1993a; Stenhouse, Knight, Longmore, and Bishara 1991). A few studies have reported that the rupture of anterior communicating artery aneurysms is more likely to result in memory deficits and, in some cases, global amnesia, than is rupture of aneurysms at other sites (Bornstein, Weir, Petruk, and Disney 1987; Stenhouse et al. 1991; Vilkki 1985). Other studies have not, however, supported this finding (De Santis et al. 1989; Ljunggren et al. 1985; Ogden, Levin, and Mee 1990; Ogden et al. 1993a; Vilkki et al. 1989), and in general, the site of the ruptured aneurysm has not been found to correlate with the type of cognitive impairment (memory or other impairment) or the severity of impairment (Ogden et al. 1993a).

Other impairments that commonly occur after SAH, even in patients who have a good neurological recovery, include deficits in perceptual speed and accuracy, difficulties with concept formation, abstraction and cognitive flexibility, and impairment of form perception and visuospatial constructive ability (Bornstein et al. 1987; Ljunggren et al. 1985; Ogden et al. 1993a; Sonesson, Ljunggren, Saveland, and Brandt 1987). Memory problems are most likely to be noticed because they affect all areas of everyday life; for some people, however, other deficits may be just as debilitating although less obvious. For example, a person whose work involved a high degree of visuospatial ability (e.g., architect, artist, carpenter, taxi driver) could be disadvantaged by a subtle impairment of visuospatial function so that much greater effort was required to carry out tasks that would have been relatively easy before the SAH.

Psychosocial symptoms commonly reported by SAH patients and their families include excessive sleepiness, fatigue, a lack of initiative, withdrawal of interest in former activities, decreased self-confidence, anxiety, depression, irritability, headache, lowered libido, heightened sensitivity to noise levels, and attention and concentration problems (Ljunggren et al. 1985; Ogden et al. 1994, 1997; Ogden, Mee, and Utley 1998; Sonesson et al. 1987). The most frequent and pervasive symptom is fatigue. In one large follow-up study of 89 "good recovery" SAH patients, 86% still suffered from excessive fatigue 12 months after SAH (Ogden et al. 1994), and 4–7 years following SAH, out of a group of 123 ex-patients, 35% suffered from daytime sleepiness (Ogden et al. 1997).

Many "good recovery" patients are unable to return to the occupation they had at the time of their SAH, especially if it involves concentration, long hours, or complex decision-making. Others may return to their occupation but at a lower level or with reduced hours (Ljunggren et al. 1985; McKenna, Willison, Lowe, and Neil-Dwyer 1989; Ogden, Levin, and Mee 1990; Ogden et al. 1994, 1997; Ropper and Zervas 1984; Vilkki et al. 1990). Primarily healthy middle-aged people are affected by SAH, and their ability to return to employment at the same earning capacity is clearly important both financially and for retaining healthy self-esteem. Most people in this age group find it difficult to retrain for other work, and with the high rates of unemployment currently found in many countries, securing a job often requires good psychosocial skills as well as intact cognitive functions.

The overall poor psychosocial outcome for some individuals may be explained in part by the fatigue and irritability the individual experiences when struggling with subtle and unrecognized cognitive impairments. The negative effect of such emotions on family members and work colleagues can be considerable, and a vicious cycle resulting in a general decline in well-being can soon be established. Therefore, recognition of and information about a range of cognitive and psychosocial impairments contribute to the overall rehabilitation of SAH victims. If cognitive deficits are permanent, individuals can be assisted in adapting their lifestyle and career accordingly.

Case Presentation

Background

At the time of her SAH, Danielle was a 36-year-old mother of twins, who worked as an assistant from 8:30 AM until 3:00 PM 5 days a week in a daycare center for preschool children. Although her health was generally good, she did have some of the risk factors associated with an aneurysmal SAH. She had been a heavy smoker for 20 years, although over the last few years she had reduced the number of cigarettes she smoked each day to 10. A retrospective questionnaire given to Danielle and her husband 2 weeks after her SAH demonstrated that she had been stressed by a number of events over the last year. Her father had been diagnosed with lung cancer, and Danielle spent a lot of time assisting her mother with his care and supporting her emotionally. Her husband Adam had been laid off from his clerical job and had had difficulty obtaining another, resulting in significant financial stress on the family.

Following her SAH on admission to the neurosurgical ward, Danielle was noted to be drowsy and confused with a severe headache, but no other neurological signs. A computed tomography (CT) scan demonstrated a moderate amount of blood around the brain, and an angiogram showed a 10-mm aneurysm on the bifurcation of her right middle cerebral artery (MCA). The aneurysm was successfully clipped 24 hours after her admission to hospital, but 2 days after the surgery Danielle's condition deteriorated. Her left arm and left side of her face became weak and numb, and she had difficulty speaking clearly as a result of dysarthria. Blood-flow studies indicated probable narrowing of the right MCA (*vasospasm*), causing lowered blood flow and the development of an ischemic deficit or stroke in the right hemisphere. She was treated by artificially raising her blood pressure with drugs and by giving her increased volumes of intravenous fluids. She was also given the drug nimodipine, a calcium channel blocker that appears to protect the cells in the brain suffering from early ischemia, thus preventing them from dying. Over the next few days, Danielle's arm and face weakness and numbness resolved along with her dysarthria, and her level of alertness also improved to normal levels. However, an MRI brain scan showed an area of infarction (*stroke*) approximately 2 cm in diameter in her right parietal cortex. Danielle was discharged from hospital 3 weeks after her SAH with instructions to rest at home for 3 months before returning to work.

Danielle felt her recovery was quite good over the first 3 months when she remained at home. She managed to get plenty of rest, including a break each afternoon before the twins came home from school. As she was not permitted to drive for 6 months, this made life somewhat difficult, but she thought that being forced to walk more was probably good for her. She had not been able to smoke while in the hospital and found that she was able to give up smoking completely when she returned home. Whenever she felt the urge to smoke she thought about the trauma she had just been through, and that was enough to maintain her resolve to remain smoke-free.

On returning to work, she found that her fatigue levels were so great by early afternoon that she had to have a rest when the children in the daycare center were having their sleep. She also felt that she was often "not quite with it" during meetings of the staff when they planned new activities. Her memory for the names of parents and new children at the center was also problematical at times, and she found that she needed to keep a diary with lists of all the children's names in the back of it, as well as notes of daily meetings and activities. Danielle also found that by the end of the day she was easily irritated by her own children's demands or even by the noise of the television when they were sitting quietly in front of it. On more than one occasion, she had dissolved into tears when Adam came home from work and asked her how her day had been. These changes in her behavior were worrying to her, as before her SAH she had looked forward to the quality time she spent with her children when they came home from school, and she was not the kind to "get emotional easily."

Before her SAH Danielle had particularly enjoyed the activity at the daycare center they called "Making Things." This involved drawing, cutting out, and making models with the children. Danielle now found that she had some difficulty with this and that her drawings and models were now more like those of the 4-year-old children she taught. At home, she also found that she could no longer sew her children's clothes; first she found that cutting out the fabric resulted in some very weird shapes, and second, she found that maneuvering the fabric under the needle of the sewing machine was impossible for her.

She told her neurosurgeon about these difficulties at a follow-up appointment 4 months after her discharge and a month after returning to work, but his examination did not reveal any weakness or numbness of her left arm or hand which might explain her difficulties. He did, however, find that she had a left-sided visual field deficit or *hemianopia*, which meant that she had a loss of vision in the lower left quarter of her visual field. He explained that this was caused by the small stroke she had sustained in her right parietal lobe, and that it should not cause her any difficulties as she would compensate for it quite spontaneously simply by moving her eyes or head. This made sense as Danielle had not been aware of it before, and had not noticed any difficulty with, for example, reading. Danielle also expressed anxiety about the possibility of a further SAH, and although the neurosurgeon tried to allay these fears she remained concerned. He suggested that he refer her for a neuropsychological assessment and counseling to help her cope better with work and give her an opportunity to talk about her fears of another SAH.

To provide an example of how a neuropsychological assessment is written up, Danielle's report (with identifying details changed) is reproduced here. It is couched in straightforward language, as it was intended for Danielle and her husband as well as her neurosurgeon and general practitioner.

Neuropsychological Assessment Report

Client: Danielle Mackey; d.o.b. 23rd February 1966
Address: 16 Charles St., Auckland
Date of assessment: July 2002
Age at assessment: 36 years
Referral: Follow-up neuropsychological assessment 5 months post-SAH

Tests given
> Beck Depression Inventory (BDI-II; Beck, Steer, and Brown 1996)
> Stait-Trait Anxiety Inventory (Spielberger 1983)
> National Adult Reading Test, 2nd Edition (NART)
> Wechsler Adult Intelligence Test, 3rd Edition (WAIS-III)
> Wechsler Memory Scale, 3rd Edition (WMS-III)
> Rey Complex Figure: copy and delayed recall
> Oral Word Fluency
> Wisconsin Card Sorting Test
> Trail-making Test
> Hemineglect Tests (Ogden Scene Test and Albert Line Cancellation Test)

History   Mrs. Mackey (Danielle) sustained a subarachnoid hemorrhage (SAH) in February 2002. An aneurysm at the bifurcation of the right middle cerebral artery was successfully clipped, ensuring that Danielle is extremely unlikely to experience another SAH. Danielle unfortunately had rather a "stormy" course following the surgery, including vasospasm that resulted in a small stroke in her right parietal lobe. She recovered well from this and was discharged from hospital 3 weeks later. After 3 months at home, she returned to her occupation as a child care assistant in a daycare center, 5 days a week from 8:30 AM until 3:00 PM. She was referred by her neurosurgeon for an assessment and counseling by her neurosurgeon as she was experiencing some difficulties both at work and at home.

Danielle described problems with fatigue and irritability, and she has discovered that she can no longer sew or help the children at the day-center where she works with their model-making activities. She also has ongoing concerns about the possibility of having another SAH, in spite of knowing that her aneurysm has been safely clipped off.

Client presentation   The assessment was conducted over two 3-hour morning sessions 3 days apart. Adam attended the first hour of the first session with Danielle—an hour-long interview to assess Danielle's coping abilities and ongoing problems. Danielle was given a number of tests designed to evaluate her current thinking and memory abilities. On a questionnaire designed to assess depression, she scored within the normal range, but on a test designed to assess anxiety, she demonstrated mild levels of general anxiety as well as some anxiety about the current situation. Her anxiety about having to do the neuropsychological tests was not unusual or surprising, as she said she had never been a particularly good student at school and had preferred sports and home economics. However, she relaxed when it was explained that the tests were not to see how clever she was but just to get an idea of her strengths and any weaknesses that might have resulted from her SAH and the small stroke she had.

Danielle was cooperative and concentrated well throughout the assessment and was clearly doing her best on the tests, although she was visibly tired at the end of the 2-hour assessment on the second day.

Psychological assessment   Danielle is a pleasant woman who is understandably anxious about the ongoing difficulties she is experiencing in a number of areas. Adam has been supportive since the SAH, and without his help, Danielle's recovery would have undoubtedly been much slower than it has been. The Mackeys are in agreement about Danielle's major problems, which include excessive fatigue and sleepiness. Danielle finds she needs 12 hours of sleep each night and often has a nap after lunch. She is sensitive to noise levels and finds it hard to concentrate when there are a lot of things going on at once. Given that they have twins aged 12, high noise levels and a lot of activity are often unavoidable.

Danielle's recent memory is poor; for example, she often forgets what she is about to do, especially if it is not routine or she has not written it down. She also has a lot of difficulty remembering the names of new children and parents at the daycare center. She will be permitted to drive again in 2 months, but Adam doesn't think she should drive for quite some time, as he feels she would be unsafe; he commented that when she was a passenger and he was driving, at times she seemed to be unaware of traffic and people, especially on their left. For example one day when they had stopped at a pedestrian crossing she told him he could drive across it without realizing that two children were just stepping off the sidewalk. She also becomes irritable very quickly, and has a "short" temper. This is particularly upsetting for Danielle, as she was a very calm person before her SAH.

Her hobby of sewing is no longer possible, as she cannot seem to cut out patterns any more or use the sewing machine. Although she still likes to read, she finds it too tiring to concentrate for too long. On the positive side, she has given up smoking and walks to work every day. Danielle commented that they had not yet reestablished their previously good sexual relationship, as she was always exhausted by the time they went to bed.

Neuropsychological assessment   *Overall cognitive abilities*: Danielle's pre-SAH IQ is estimated to be in the "average" range, based on her educational history (passed the national exam aged 16 years and left school at 17 years), her occupation as an assistant child-care worker, a test of premorbid ability (the NART), and her highest WAIS-III subtest score on Vocabulary. Tests of reading and writing demonstrated that her fluency was in the average range. Her WAIS-III Verbal IQ fell in the average range, but her Performance IQ was low average. The reason for this difference becomes clearer when the Index Scores are examined, along with her other test results.

Verbal abilities: Danielle has an average Verbal Comprehension Index Score, and on a test of oral word fluency she scored within the average range.

Visuospatial abilities: Danielle's Perceptual Organization Index Score fell in the Low Average range. She had particular difficulty with two tests involving visuospatial construction and reasoning, Block Design and Matrix Reasoning. These results were supported by her copy of the Rey Complex Figure, which was drawn in a very piece-meal manner, with two details missing from the left side of the figure, indicating unilateral visual hemineglect (an unawareness of stimuli in the left side of space). Mild hemineglect was also apparent on the Ogden Scene test where she missed the tree on the left side of the drawing, although she was able to copy it when it was pointed out to her. Her drawing of the scene was generally somewhat disorganized. She missed only two lines on the very far lower left corner of the Albert line can-cellation test, which may have been a result of mild hemineglect exacerbated by the visual field loss she has in the lower left of her visual field.

Attention, concentration, processing speed, and working memory: Danielle's im-mediate attention span was average, and her ability to sustain concentration throughout the test sessions was quite good, although she did require a brief break every 30 minutes. She scored in the low average range on the Processing Speed Index. This was because of a slower than average time on both the subtests that make up this index, Digit-Symbol Coding and Symbol Search, as well as her tendency to skip some of the symbols on the left of the page on Digit-Symbol Coding. This latter problem is another indication of her left hemineglect. She also had slower than average scores on both Trails A and B, although on these tests, which involve connecting sequential letters and numbers scattered across an A4 page, her hemineglect was signaled only by the much longer time she took to find symbols on the left of the page.

Danielle's Working Memory Index Score fell at the lower end of the average range, primarily because of her score on the difficult Letter-Number Sequencing task, which fell 1 SD (standard deviation) below the mean. As her ability to repeat strings of digits backwards was also a little low, it is likely that Danielle's ability to concentrate is mildly impaired. This finding is not unexpected only 5 months following a SAH, and her concentration is likely to continue to improve with time. She also had difficulties with one of the working memory subtests of the WMS-III, Spatial Span, but this appeared to be the result of a more general visuospatial confusion rather than con-centration or working memory per se.

Executive abilities: On tests of organization, forward planning and changing mental set, Danielle's results were mixed. Her poor copy of the complex figure certainly suggested disorganization and poor forward planning, but this is more likely to be a result of impaired visuospatial perceptual and constructional abilities as a result of her right parietal lesion. In support of this, on more specific tests of executive functions Danielle did not show impairment. Although her performance was slow on the Trails B task where she was required to change mental set between numbers and letters, she was also slow on Trails A, where changing mental set was not required. This suggests that her below-average performance on this was more likely to be a result of a slowing of information processing and her hemineglect. She obtained an average score on Oral Word Fluency and on the Wisconsin Card Sorting Test, with both tests involving changing mental set and mental flexibility. She also scored in the average range on tests of verbal abstraction (WAIS-III Similarities and the Proverbs in the WAIS-III Comprehension subtest). In summary, Danielle appears to have intact executive abilities, which will assist her in making use of strategies to overcome her visuospatial problems, as well enhancing her ability to find solutions to psychosocial and occupational challenges.

Memory abilities: On the WMS-111, Danielle performed within the low average to average range across all subtests. On all the verbal memory tests she scored in the average range, although on the Word List memory test she took more trials than average to commit the words to long-term store. This reflects her difficulties with remembering names, but indicates that if she takes the time to go over new names a number of times, she will be able to remember them. On the visual memory tests she scored in the average range on the Face Recognition test, suggesting that she can remember faces; thus, she might want to try and actively visualize the face that goes with each name in her strategy to improve her recall of names. Her lowest scores were on Family Pictures and Visual Reproduction, but her performance suggested that this may have been a consequence of her visual hemineglect rather than a visual memory deficit per se.

Summary   Danielle's neuropsychological test results support the problems she reports in day-to-day life and are entirely consistent with her stage of recovery only 5 months after a SAH, as well as her small right-hemispheric stroke. She has a mildly impaired ability to concentrate and becomes confused and irritated when she is tired or is bombarded with too many things going on at once. She also has difficulty remembering new names and keeping track of appointments. These problems are likely to resolve with time, and Danielle can help herself by ensuring that she gets enough rest and continues to use a diary to assist her memory. She would be wise to reduce her working hours to mornings only for a few months and then gradually increase them until she is back to her pre-SAH hours without feeling excessively fatigued.

Danielle's main impairments are those related to her small stroke, and these may not recover fully. She has mild left visual hemineglect that may resolve over the next few months, but in the meantime she should not drive and should be extremely careful when crossing roads or when in other situations where full attention to the left is important. For example, she should avoid situations in which she is in sole charge of children playing on outdoor equipment or near water, and she should not oversee children near traffic. She might feel more useful at the daycare center if she took on other activities such as story time and general inside play and child-care rather than activities that involve construction of models. Painting with young children may be therapeutic, however, as her paintings may be as interesting as those of her young charges! Danielle seems to have retained her sense of humor, and this is a most valuable characteristic that will surely assist her rehabilitation. Danielle's executive abilities are not impaired, and this is the most important finding of all, as this signals that she will almost certainly be able to rebuild her life so that it is once again full and satisfying.

Conclusions   Danielle's problems of sleepiness, hypersensitivity to noise, difficulty in concentrating, slowed response times, irritability, emotionality, and poor verbal memory are all problems commonly found after SAH. Her hemineglect and decreased visuospatial abilities are a consequence of her right parietal stroke. It is not surprising that Danielle is having difficulty coping with caring for noisy and demanding pre-school children, especially given that she also has to cope with two children at home. As only 5 months have elapsed since Danielle's SAH, further improvement is very likely, especially of those symptoms related to her SAH. Following are some ideas that may assist Danielle during her recovery.

Recommendations   *Occupation*: If possible, Danielle should reduce her working hours to mornings only so that she can rest in the afternoons before her own children return from school. Danielle's language skills remain excellent, and she should perhaps concentrate on these activities at the daycare center rather than on construction activities. She should not take on responsibilities for overseeing children while they are involved in potentially dangerous outside activities or near water.

Visuospatial abilities: Danielle has sustained some damage to an area of the brain that mediates some visuospatial abilities, including those important for sewing and driving. She also has mild hemineglect, which is an unawareness of stimuli to the left of her body. She therefore must not drive or participate in activities that might be dangerous until a further assessment demonstrates that she has fully recovered (which is not a certainty).

Memory: Because her verbal memory remains somewhat impaired, allowances must be made. Danielle can assist herself by keeping a regular diary of names, appointments, and tasks she wishes to accomplish and reading it at regular intervals throughout the day. A further aid would be to take time each evening to write in her diary a careful plan for the following day.

Family: Danielle's family members have also had some difficult times since Danielle's SAH, and they have agreed to come to some family therapy sessions to explore constructive ways they can work together to reclaim their happy family spirit again.

Rehabilitation

The Mackey children attended two therapy sessions with their parents, and together they planned ways they could make life easier for their mother. The children came up with the following ideas: help Dad cook two meals a week when Mum is especially tired; take Mum breakfast in bed every Sunday; keep the noise levels down by playing our tapes and the television in our bedroom with the door shut and invite friends home in the weekends only, after first checking to see if Mum feels okay; do not upset Mum by arguing with her, even if she is wrong; take turns at vacuum-cleaning the house; keep our room tidy even if it means hiding everything in the cupboard until we have time to clean up properly; and do our homework without Mum having to hassle us.

Adam agreed to help them with these plans and said he would pay them to help around the house. The twins then agreed to keep a record of what they did, including when they "mucked up" by arguing with Mum or not doing their homework without being hassled, and said their Dad could give them less pay unless they did something extra to help Mum. Danielle appeared to be rather amused by this discussion but agreed that her children's plans would help her greatly. She commented that they might get tired of doing all those housework tasks pretty soon, but her daughter assured her that "It will be worth it if you get properly better and we can have fun again." The twins' plans did work most of the time, although their parents later decided that in 1 week out of every 3 they could have a break from meal preparation and vacuuming.

Danielle discussed the findings of her neuropsychological report with the director of the daycare center, who was very understanding and supportive. For the next 3 months she worked in the mornings only, and she enjoyed this immensely. She regained her confidence, and sometimes she stayed to have lunch with the other childcare workers before going home to rest. Within a year she was once more working until 3 PM every day, although she still found that a 45-minute rest after lunch when the children were resting made a difference to her ability to cope positively with the rest of the day and evening. She continued to use a diary and spent time practicing the names of new children and parents while visualizing their faces. Her anxiety over her memory problems dissolved as a result of knowing that these were a common consequence of SAH and would probably improve over the next 6 months.

A reassessment of Danielle's memory and visuospatial abilities 6 months later showed a considerable improvement in her memory and a complete resolution of her hemineglect, but only minimal improvement of her visuospatial problems. Thus, although she no longer missed items on the left of her copy of the complex figure, her copy was still rather messy, and she still found it too difficult to sew or make models with the children. However, she said her painting skills had improved to about a 5-year-old level, which made her the expert in her class of 3- and 4-year-old children.

A month after the neuropsychological assessment I saw Danielle with Adam for a few therapy sessions to look at ways Danielle might overcome her fear of having another SAH. Danielle admitted that this concern was preventing her from resuming sexual relations, and that this was becoming a barrier between them, as she avoided intimacy in case it led to an expectation of intercourse. Asked how she thought she had come to have this fear, she explained that she had read an article about SAH which had listed sexual intercourse as an activity that could precipitate a SAH. Adam was clearly relieved by Danielle's explanation of her reluctance to make love and her coolness toward him, and they were then able to talk about it at home.

Danielle already knew that she did not have a higher-than-normal risk of having another SAH because an angiogram of all the blood vessels in her head had demonstrated that she had no more aneurysms. Also, the surgeon had assured her that the chances of the clipped aneurysm rebleeding were extremely small. Most aneurysms have probably been present for many years before they rupture, and the chance that a new one would develop is unlikely. Just to be on the safe side, Danielle stopped smoking after her SAH, and she planned to learn to cope better with stress via therapy and yoga.

In an attempt to reinforce her intellectual knowledge that SAH was in fact quite rare and that she was unlikely to have another one, I gave her several articles on SAH. Like many people, Danielle suspected that health professionals sometimes tell patients "little white lies" if they think it will make them feel better. I thought that reading for herself that a wide range of researchers and clinicians share the view that she is probably safe from a further SAH might allay her fears at the emotional level. She read many of the articles and became quite intrigued by the medical aspects of SAH and its treatment. As a consequence, she said she was now convinced that she was safe, and although she might never entirely overcome her fear, it was now at a level she could live with comfortably. Reading the articles made her realize how lucky she had been to survive at all, let alone to recover so well. A month later Danielle reported with a laugh that they had successfully made love on three occasions over the last month, without even a mild headache resulting, and they now felt ready to increase the frequency of this very pleasurable rehabilitation activity to three times a week!

Discussion

Indeed, SAH is an "explosion in the mind," and the consequences can be devastating. In population terms, averaged across all age groups, SAH is a relatively rare form of stroke. Within the middle-aged population, however, it is not particularly uncommon, and for middle-aged hypertensive smokers and people under stress the risk increases significantly. The finding of an incidental UIA is becoming more common as costs for imaging the brain using MRI decrease, allowing screening for a wide range of suspected brain pathologies. For a healthy person with no symptoms from their UIA, the decision to have elective treatment is obviously not an easy one. Neurosurgery or endovascular coiling are both serious procedures that carry a small risk of hemorrhage during the treatment as well as posttreatment complications (International Study of Unruptured Intracranial Aneurysm Investigators 1998; Raaymakers 2000; Raaymakers, Rinkel, Limburg, and Algra 1998; Towgood et al. 2004). For some patients, a UIA feels like a "time bomb" in the head, and living with the anxiety this causes may be worse than the relatively low risks (when compared with the outcome of a SAH) of elective treatment to occlude the UIA.

Although we do not know the pathology that underlies the common problems that follow SAH in patients who make a good physical recovery, one possibility is that blood breakdown products are deposited in the meninges, resulting in an encephalopathy (Ropper and Zervas 1984; Sonesson et al. 1987). It has also been postulated that as a result of extreme increases in intracranial pressure and the brief period during which intracranial circulation may be arrested immediately after SAH, a transient ischemia may occur (Grote and Hassler 1988; Smith 1963). Either of these hypotheses is congruent with diffuse cortical damage, the brain pathology that best explains the pattern of symptoms that occur.

In addition, patients who suffer localized cortical damage as the result of vaso-spasm and ischemia may well show additional cognitive impairments known to be associated with that brain area, as in Danielle's case. In patients with an uncomplicated course and a good neurological recovery, most cognitive impairments, including the verbal memory problems sometimes apparent in the early weeks, have usually recovered to pre-SAH levels within 12 months after the hemorrhage (Ogden et al.1993a).

For people who survive a SAH, a number of interventions can assist their return to a fulfilling, productive life. First, the importance of clear and factual information cannot be overstressed. In most cases, as with closed head injury, such information allays more fears than it produces. For example, when a patient is discharged from the hospital having made a good physical recovery, written information about the possible short- and longer-term effects of the SAH and how to cope with them will help to avoid a vicious cycle developing. If it is not understood that excessive sleepiness, hypersensitivity to noise, and irritability are common symptoms, the person may misinterpret his feelings and behaviors, his family will react inappropriately, and sensible precautions such as having frequent rests, returning to work gradually, and avoiding noisy environments will not be taken.

As all medical specialists know, some patients can be given important information clearly and sensitively and yet not "hear" it or take it in. This is hardly surprising given that the patient and his family are often in a stressful situation at the time. For this reason, it is helpful to provide written information as well as discussions of the issues as often as seems necessary. It is often at the follow-up appointment that the neurosurgeon or psychologist realizes that the patient has not fully understood information they were given previously, and it is a useful strategy to explain everything of importance again, even if the patient does not request any specific information.

As in Danielle's case, for people who experience ongoing subtle but nevertheless debilitating problems, counseling or therapy that can address the psychological aspects of recovery is often helpful. Information can be easily misinterpreted, especially given in isolation. For example, although some people suffer a SAH while having sexual intercourse, they are probably equally likely to suffer one while engaged in some other strenuous activity, such as jogging. In all cases the aneurysm is probably at the point of rupturing anyway, and the sudden increase in blood pressure or intracranial pressure simply precipitates it then rather than later. Exploring misconceptions early and preventing fears from growing are much better than trying to allay them once they have taken hold.

This discussion about the importance of giving and continuing to give clear information provides me with an excuse for relating one of my favorite anecdotes. I was carrying out a follow-up neuropsychological assessment on a woman, whom I will call Ruth, who had suffered a SAH 3 months earlier. She had just come from her follow-up assessment with her neurosurgeon, who had been pleased with her progress. This particular neurosurgeon is exceptionally good at explaining complex operations and risks to his patients in a straightforward way. As a result I had found that most of his patients, even when stressed by the fact that they were about to have a serious operation, had an excellent grasp of what was wrong with them, the operation procedures, and their other treatments. Ruth, an intelligent woman who had an uncomplicated recovery from her hemorrhage and neurosurgery, was praising her neurosurgeon's skills to me and remarked that her operation had been quite long and in fact had taken about 4 hours. She said she was amazed that the surgeon could concentrate for that long. I replied that it was indeed amazing and obviously required special skills, and I commented that brain surgery like hers in particular often took even longer than 4 hours. At this Ruth exclaimed, "You mean I had brain surgery? Well I'll be blowed!" Despite the fact that her neurosurgeon had explained the operation to her in detail, two or three times, complete with drawings of the arteries, the aneurysm, and how the aneurysm was clipped, and despite the fact that she had had the hair shaven from one side of her head and had a large piece of skull removed and replaced with very visible sutures, she was unaware that the operation had actually involved her brain! Presumably the surgeon and other hospital staff (including me) never mentioned the word *brain*, assuming that she realized that when you operate on arteries inside the head, it must involve the brain. Ruth had absorbed other complex information, however, and was able to explain that her surgeon had clipped a weak spot on one of her arteries in her head.

This anecdote provides a good lesson in not assuming that what is common knowledge and language to the health professional may not be to the patient. When I told the neurosurgeon this story, it was his turn to be amazed. He now makes it very explicit to his patients that he is going to perform *brain* surgery!

13

■

Twenty Years Too Late

Organic Solvent Neurotoxicity

The focus of this chapter is a 38-year-old man named Peter. When he was 32, Peter would probably have been described by his friends as a typical New Zealand family man. He worked hard as a spray painter so that he could pay off the house mortgage and provide his children with a higher quality of life than he had growing up. He and his wife enjoyed each other's company and socialized on weekends with other couples and families with similar interests. Peter's three sons were his pride and joy, and he spent quality time with them playing sports and taking them fishing and swimming.

Today Peter is unemployed, and his life revolves around visits to the psychiatrist to help him overcome depression. His marriage is under severe stress, and he and his wife no longer see their friends. His children fear him, and they and their mother visit the family therapist weekly for help with school and behavioral problems and to learn ways of coping with Peter's changed personality and irrational, sometimes violent, behavior toward them.

What has happened over a few years to turn this once-happy family inside out? This family is a victim of a potentially common and preventable neurological disorder called occupational organic solvent neurotoxicity (OSN). Because of a lack of effective education about methods of protecting himself in his occupation as a spray painter, Peter has been exposed to high levels of neurotoxins over many years and has sustained irreversible brain damage as a result. Sadly, the story of Peter and his family is not uncommon, and the points I hope this chapter will make could equally well have been made by telling the similar stories of many other clients I have assessed, mostly tradesmen between the ages of 35 and 55 years.

Vast numbers of workers are potentially exposed to organic solvents that are widely used in industry in paints, glues, adhesives, and degreasing or cleaning agents and in the production of plastics, textiles, printing inks, polymers, dyes, agricultural products, and pharmaceuticals (NIOSH 1987). Long or intense exposure to many of the solvents used in these industries can result in chronic OSN. The symptoms tend to have a slow and insidious onset and include psychological and psychiatric symptoms and impairments in cognitive functioning. The Scandinavian countries are the research leaders in this field, and in recent years health professionals and industries in the United States and other major industrialized countries have become increasingly aware of the debilitating symptoms that can affect workers exposed to neurotoxins over a long time (Hartman 1995).

The neurological damage resulting from neurotoxins is usually difficult because it tends to be diffuse or may, for example, involve a neurotransmitter imbalance. It is therefore unlikely to be evident on computed tomography (CT) or magnetic resonance imaging (MRI) scans of the brain. A neurological examination may also reveal little (Juntunen 1983), and in many cases cognitive and psychological impairments are the only clear indicators of neurotoxicity. Neuropsychological assessment, therefore, plays a major role in diagnosing chronic OSN. In line with this, the World Health Organization (WHO) and the Nordic Government both require that a neuropsychological assessment be used in the diagnosis of solvent neurotoxicity (WHO and Commission of European Communities 1985; WHO/Nordic Council of Ministers Working Group 1985).

Today, safety standards in industry are constantly being updated as our knowledge and awareness of the effects of solvents and other industrial toxins increase. In the recent past, however, protective clothing was not always worn by workers at risk from solvent exposure, and even today workers may neglect to take the necessary precautions if the clothing makes them too hot or interferes with their ability to do the job effectively (e.g., gloves making it difficult to do fine work). Self-employed workers are particularly vulnerable, as they do not have peer pressure and support to encourage maintenance of safety standards; it is important for them to get through as much work as possible, and protective clothing may slow them down, and the cost of protective clothing may act a negative factor (e.g., the frequent need to replace rubber gloves).

Many victims of OSN do not realize that their chronic fatigue, irritability, poor memory, and other problems may be associated with past or present solvent exposure. Because the symptoms of OSN develop gradually, by the time the sufferer seeks help from a doctor, psychologist, or marriage guidance counselor, the OSN symptoms are likely to be confounded and compounded by other work- and family-related problems. In this sense, chronic OSN is rather like the chronic effects of mild or moderate traumatic brain injury (see Chapter 11). Identifying OSN as the primary cause of the client's problems can therefore be extremely difficult, and proving cause and effect beyond doubt is almost always impossible. That OSN is a significant cause of a person's problems can, however, often be established beyond *reasonable* doubt, provided a number of assessment guidelines are carefully followed, including carrying out a multifaceted assessment that can involve neurologists, occupational medical specialists, psychiatrists, and psychologists as well as neuropsychologists. Other likely causes for the various symptoms must be explored, malingering must be ruled out, and of course the facts about the types, amounts, and years of exposure to solvents must be established insofar as is possible. It is therefore important for health professionals to gain some understanding of the OSN syndrome so they can conduct an informative clinical interview and assessment. In addition, it is important to be aware that some potentially affected clients will have no idea that their problems might be associated with solvent neurotoxicity. Thus, pertinent questions should be asked of clients and patients who present with one or more of the symptoms commonly associated with OSN and who have a history of working in an environment that increases the potential for solvent exposure.

This chapter will focus on the neuropsychological aspects of OSN and on the psychological and psychosocial consequences that can result directly from the effects of the neurotoxicity (e.g., aggressive behaviors, fatigue, irritability) or indirectly as a consequence of the neurobehavioral changes (e.g., loss of employment, marital distress, suicidal thoughts, loss of self-esteem).

Theoretical Background

Causes and Neuropathology of OSN

Ten years or more of exposure to neurotoxic solvents at or above workplace exposure standards is usually necessary before symptoms become apparent (Edling et al. 1990). Accidental intake of solvents into the bloodstream is either via direct absorption through the skin or via inhalation. Solvent abuse via inhalation is also common in young people. Johnson, Bachman, and O'Malley (1979) estimated that 18.7% of high school seniors in the United States had tried solvent-based inhalants. Solvents accidentally or purposefully ingested (e.g., in suicide attempts) are readily absorbed from the gastrointestinal tract. The amount of solvent retained depends on various factors, including the blood and tissue solubility of the solvent, its toxicity, diurnal metabolic cycles of the individual, alcohol use, and possibly obesity (some solvents last longer in fat people than in thin people). The immediate exposure level of the solvent can be measured in urine, blood, or exhaled air.

Some people suffer from acute symptoms of OSN, including nausea, loss of appetite, vomiting, severe headaches, confusion, light-headedness, and dermatitis. The solvent can often be detected on their breath and skin for many hours and even days after they have left the solvent environment. Most of these acute symptoms resolve when they stop working with solvents, but as soon as they come into contact with the solvents again, the symptoms return. People who suffer from acute symptoms do not necessarily develop the chronic syndrome of OSN, possibly because they are so debilitated by the acute symptoms that they stop working with solvents before irreversible neurological damage results. Some workers who develop a chronic OSN syndrome have suffered acute symptoms as well, but others have not.

It is often difficult to demonstrate a clear correlation between deterioration of function and brain damage in chronic OSN. Although some studies have shown diffuse brain damage in persons who demonstrate cognitive deficits as a result of toluene exposure (Cavanaugh 1985; Fornazzari, Wilkinson, Kapur, and Carlen 1983) and in painters who have been exposed to a mix of solvents (Arlien-Soberg, Bruhn, Gyldensted, and Melgaard 1979; Bruhn, Arlien-Soberg, Gyldensted, and Christensen 1981), many individuals who have equally severe cases of OSN do not show central nervous system (CNS) changes on CT or MRI. These inconsistencies in research and clinical findings may be explained in part by the different mechanisms used to damage the nervous system using different toxins, and perhaps using the same toxin in different individuals. In some cases, CNS dysfunction may be caused by the destruction of neurons via the direct toxic effects of the solvent or its decomposition products, and in others by disruption of neurotransmitter mechanisms. Preexisting conditions, including genetic factors, systemic disease, other neurological conditions (e.g., alcohol-related damage, closed head injury), and various physical and psychiatric illnesses may make some persons more vulnerable to neurotoxic effects than others.

Types of OSN

The 1985 International Solvent Workshop (Baker and Seppalainen 1986) postulated, as a working hypothesis, three types of OSN.

Type 1 OSN   The least severe presentation, type 1 OSN is characterized by subjective complaints of fatigue, irritability, depression, and episodes of anxiety. No impairments are apparent on neuropsychological tests. This type corresponds to the WHO classification of organic affective syndrome and is reversible on removal from the solvent.

Type 2 OSN   More severe and chronic than type 1, type 2 OSN requires neuropsychological and clinical assessments to demonstrate chronic symptoms of neurotoxicity and cognitive impairments. The diagnostic features include sustained personality or mood disturbances; fatigue, poor impulse control; poor motivation; impaired concentration, memory, and learning; and psychomotor slowing. Not all symptoms are necessary for the diagnosis to be made. Mild symptoms may be apparent after only 3 years of chronic industrial exposure, but a period of 10 years or more of exposure is usual before symptoms become debilitating. Type 2 OSN corresponds to the WHO classification of mild chronic toxic encephalopathy. Although the term *chronic* indicates long-term changes, in some cases the symptoms may become less severe as the time since the last exposure to solvents lengthens. Recovery may be enhanced by appropriate counseling or rehabilitation.

Type 3 OSN   This type of OSN is a dementia and requires a global and progressive deterioration in memory, other intellectual functions, and emotion. It corresponds to the WHO classification of severe chronic toxic encephalopathy and is irreversible. This level of OSN is uncommon. As safety standards in workplaces improve and self-employed workers become more aware of the importance of safety measures while using solvents, this level of OSN should become rare.

Psychosocial Characteristics of OSN Victims

Typically, people who suffer type 2 OSN are men in their 30s or older who have a family and a mortgage, and who are usually skilled or semiskilled tradespeople (e.g., car and house painters, printers, dry-cleaners, workers in degreasing and extraction industries and in the manufacture of pharmaceuticals and agricultural sprays, leather workers, pest controllers, and agricultural sprayers). It is not uncommon for clients with suspected OSN who are still working with solvents to express reluctance to give up their jobs, even when at times they experience the debilitating, acute affects of solvent neurotoxicity such as nausea, loss of appetite, vomiting, and dermatitis (Arlien-Soberg 1985). This reluctance is understandable in the present economy of many Western countries, where the chance of successfully retraining for and obtaining a job in a new trade that does not involve solvents is low. Thus, the appearance of many potential victims of OSN at a health or counseling agency is often precipitated by a crisis in their marriage or work resulting from their changed personality, extreme fatigue, or significant memory problems rather than by a concern about the acute or chronic effects of the solvents in the workplace.

Physical, Psychosocial, and Neuropsychological Symptoms of OSN

Fatigue, irritability, depression, anxiety, poor concentration, and memory impairments commonly cause problems in the client's daily activities. Depression is a particularly common consequence of the syndrome. For example, OSN from the widely used industrial solvent trichloroethylene (TCE) has been reported to result frequently in severe agitated depression, sometimes accompanied by violent behaviors toward the self and others (White, Feldman, and Travers 1990). The causes of depression, anxiety, and irritability are often difficult or impossible to isolate, but in cases in which OSN seems a likely diagnosis, these symptoms both may be directly and indirectly seen as consequences of the OSN. Indirect causes of depression and anxiety could include a poor memory, lowered sexual drive, fatigue, and low energy levels, resulting in marital stress, hypersensitivity to noise, constant headaches, and other physical symptoms that lower work capacity. Other "psychiatric" symptoms include hallucinations, confusion, inappropriate laughter, suicidal ideation, and emotional lability; these symptoms can occur in various degrees of severity with chronic exposure to some solvents (e.g., toluene), although these symptoms are more likely in cases where the solvent exposure is current as well as chronic (e.g., in toluene abusers).

In addition, the physical symptoms of unwarranted headaches, dizziness, sleep disturbances, poor appetite, alcohol intolerance, heart palpitations, feelings of oppression in the chest, painful tingling in some parts of the body, and excessive perspiring can be present. A client who has these physical symptoms should have a medical checkup to rule out other causes.

Neurological signs, although uncommon in mild to moderate chronic OSN, may be present in more severe cases (Juntunen 1983). In particular, toluene and TCE can cause peripheral neuropathy, and TCE can damage the trigeminal or fifth cranial nerve, which can result in *trigeminal anesthesia* (loss of sensation to the face, mouth, and teeth). This condition may be permanent and can spread to the other cranial nerves (Hartman 1995).

Different neurotoxic solvents can result in different types of cognitive impairment, but a number of deficits seem to accompany type 2 OSN no matter which neurotoxic solvent is causative. In any case, many people who suffer OSN may have been exposed to a mixture of solvents, making it difficult to tailor a neuropsychological test battery to the deficits thought to be caused by a specific solvent. A core battery for the assessment of OSN has been developed by the WHO/Nordic Council (1985), and a number of published studies support the use of similar test batteries (e.g., Cassitio 1982; Hanninen 1982).

The neuropsychological symptoms most commonly found in cases of OSN from any neurotoxic solvent are those associated with diffuse cerebral encephalopathy (Dryson and Ogden 2000, 1993b, 2001b). In this respect, the picture painted by OSN is rather similar to that following a mild to moderate closed head injury in some people (i.e., the postconcussional syndrome). Thus, OSN sufferers are most likely to perform poorly on tests that measure concentration, vigilance, psychomotor speed, reaction time, and memory for new material. Many sufferers also do poorly on complex tests of visuospatial perception and memory, and in more severe (but still type 2) cases, impaired abstract thinking, organization, and planning abilities may also be apparent. These latter deficits are suggestive of possible frontal-lobe dysfunction.

Victims of OSN are unlikely to show impairment on tests of old, overlearned information (e.g., the meanings of words, general knowledge), and their immediate memory span is normally unaffected. Clients who perform erratically or well below expected levels on tests of these abilities may be malingering or attempting to exacerbate their problems so that their difficulties will be taken seriously; additional tests designed to assess these possibilities should be given at a later session.

Case Presentation: Peter

Background

Peter was aged 38 years when he was referred to me for a neuropsychological assessment. He had been a car painter for 22 years and worked with solvent-based paints. The solvents to which he had been exposed included toluene, xylene, and styrene. His referral reached my desk 4 years after he first approached his doctor with complaints of frequent headaches, unwarranted displays of irritability toward his family, periods of depression, and forgetfulness. His doctor had suggested that he was suffering from stress as a result of working too hard and prescribed a holiday. Because it was nearing the children's long summer holiday period, the family decided they would take a longer break than usual and went on a 6-week camping holiday at a beach. It took about 2 weeks for Peter to "wind down," during which time, according to his wife June, "he sat around like an old man, falling asleep in the afternoon." His headaches gradually decreased in severity and frequency, and from the third week on he felt "revitalized," his headaches stopped, and he began to enjoy swimming and fishing with the children. He "even made some of the meals!" Clearly, the doctor was right, and all he needed was a long break from the stress of work.

Within 2 weeks of returning to work, Peter's headaches were back. As his wife said, "He was jumping down my throat at the slightest thing again." He could not afford to take any more time off work, so he struggled on, taking codeine to relieve his headaches and coffee to keep himself awake. Over the next 4 years, at various times Peter was put on a health diet, prescribed antidepressants, and was referred to a psychologist for stress management. He and June also went to a marriage guidance counselor at one point after Peter had, for the first time in their relationship, become violently angry and hit June. None of these interventions seemed to help. Finally, Peter's irritability with his coworkers in the factory and his lowered work output caused his supervisor to become concerned, and he sent Peter to a specialist in occupational medicine. The specialist discovered that Peter rarely wore a mask when spray-painting cars, and because of his other complaints, the therapist felt that Peter's case was highly suggestive of OSN. As a result, Peter was finally referred for a neuropsychological assessment.

I asked both Peter and June to come to the initial interview. It is often helpful to have the views and ideas from family members as well as from the client, especially when memory impairment is one of the problems. Peter was a solidly built man of medium height who looked older than his 38 years. He looked rather worried much of the time, but he and his wife seemed very close and were clearly united in their desire to do whatever was needed to help Peter. They were both very willing to talk openly about their difficulties. As June said, they were desperate to find out what was wrong with Peter. On two occasions, while talking about his problems, Peter became tearful, and June reached over and held his hand. He regained his composure quickly and apologized for his tears, saying he found it upsetting to think of how his health had deteriorated and how he had hurt his wife and children. He had been off work on a sickness benefit for 6 weeks before seeing me and wanted to get back to work as soon as possible because they were finding it impossible to manage on his benefit.

I was interested in learning about Peter's "premorbid" personality and abilities and about the onset and progression of his various symptoms. Fifteen years previously, when he and June had married, he had been a happy, gentle, easygoing person who enjoyed excellent health, played tennis, swam regularly, and lifted weights to keep fit. Their marriage was happy and their sexual relationship satisfying. They shared a love of sports and had regular social outings with a group of couples they had known for years. Until 4 years previously, Peter had always been a good father to his three sons, aged 12, 10, and 7 years, spending time with them in the evenings and weekends. He rarely became angry with them and, in June's opinion, was sometimes too soft on them. Peter smoked about 10 cigarettes a day and had been a social drinker with the occasional "binge" on New Year's Eve, but he gave up drinking 3 years before he saw me because he found he was unable to handle more than a couple of beers without feeling woozy.

June first noticed a change in Peter when their youngest son was about 2 years old. Peter would become moody and depressed for no apparent reason, and their sexual and social life took a turn for the worse. June noticed he often forgot things; for example, he would go outside to the shed and by the time he got there would have forgotten what he went to get. This forgetfulness was the cause of many arguments because he wrongly accused June of misplacing tools and books and forgot plans for social outings, insisting that June had not told him of these plans. June had to drive him everywhere; Peter no longer felt confident that he could remember the route to familiar places. He no longer enjoyed reading or watching television because he would forget the beginning of the book or program before reaching the end. Peter said he was always tired and lacking energy, and his work output had diminished considerably. Often he fell asleep as soon as he got home in the evenings. Yet he suffered from insomnia when he went to bed. When the boys were noisy, he would quickly become irritable, and the noise levels in the factory were often so bad he sometimes had to go outside for half an hour to calm down.

Most worrying of all was Peter's increasing tendency to lose his temper and to shout at and hit the children for trivial reasons. June noticed that the boys were beginning to avoid him as much as possible, which saddened her, as she remembered the fun they used to have together. Peter became visibly upset at this point, but he agreed with June's comments and said he was worried by his inability to control his feelings of aggression and violence at work as well as at home. June said that for some time she had attributed Peter's difficulties and personality change to the fact that he was working long hours not only painting cars in a factory but also working for himself painting cars in the evenings and on weekends. More recently, she had begun to worry that he might have a brain tumor. At this point, Peter broke in and said he often lay awake at night thinking he was going crazy.

Neuropsychological Assessment

Pattern of test results   Peter's assessment was carried out over three sessions to ensure that Peter did not become overtired and was not in an emotional frame of mind that would interfere with his motivation and ability to concentrate. He scored at the low end of the average on the revised Wechsler Adult Intelligence Scale (WAIS-R) subtests of vocabulary and overlearned general knowledge and simple tests of visual perception. Similarly, his score on the National Adult Reading Test (NART), which is designed to estimate premorbid IQ, fell at the lower end of the average range. He left school at age 15 years; so this score is consistent with his level of formal schooling and with his occupation as a painter. On the Performance subtests of the WAIS-R, he was slow, sometimes failing to gain any points because he took too long to complete the test item. This difficulty was particularly apparent on the Block Design and Object Assembly subtests of the WAIS-R. In support of his general slowness, he scored very poorly on the Digit Symbol subtest, a test requiring sustained attention and psychomotor speed. He was able to repeat six digits forward, demonstrating a normal immediate attention span, but he could repeat only two digits backward, demonstrating a problem with sustained attention and manipulating information in working memory. He became confused and irritated when he tried to remember the order of the digits in reverse. Following this test, he seemed distressed and went outside to smoke a cigarette. His wife commented that this was a common pattern for Peter. He became frustrated and distressed when he found he could no longer perform simple tasks that he had once accomplished with ease.

His ability to copy the Rey Complex Figure was also impaired, and he had difficulty organizing his approach, copying the figure in a piecemeal fashion (see Fig. 13-1a). For example, he did not draw the base rectangle as one part; when questioned about the figure at the end of the session, he said he had not "seen" the rectangle, which could indicate a visuospatial impairment or an inability to plan ahead and form strategies, deficits that often signal frontal-lobe dysfunction. On another test of frontal-lobe functioning, the Wisconsin Card Sorting Test, he made numerous errors and was able to complete only two of the six categories. He appeared unable to develop a strategy and became confused and frustrated by his continual errors. The test was abandoned when it became clear he could not grasp what he was meant to do.

On tests of both verbal and visual memory (new learning), he was quite impaired.

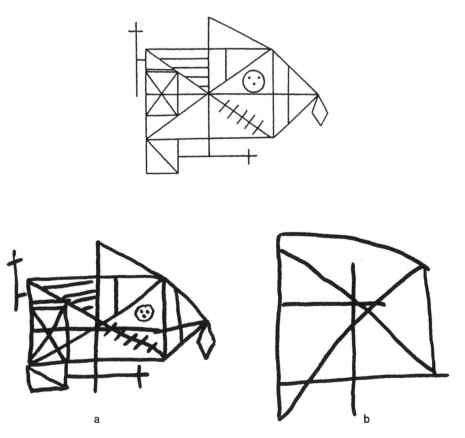

Figure 13-1 The Rey Complex Figure model is in the top row; (a) is Peter's copy of it, and (b) is his recall of it 30 minutes later.

On tests where he had to recall short stories, as well as on tests where he had to learn a list of 12 words over a number of trials, he demonstrated marked difficulties both with putting the new information into long-term store and in recalling words he had managed to store. When asked to draw from memory the Rey Complex Figure he had copied earlier (a nonverbal, visual memory task), he was able to recall only a few details, a markedly impaired performance compared with that of control subjects (see Fig. 13-1b).

Summary and interpretation of the test results   Peter demonstrated a number of cognitive impairments that were consistent with the problems he was experiencing in his daily life. The verbal and nonverbal memory impairments he and his wife reported were supported by his poor performance on formal testing. He was generally slow to think and respond on tests, which fit with his lack of energy, excessive fatigue, and slowed work performance. His poor performance on tests of frontal-lobe function suggests that some aspects of his behavior might also be a result of, or exacerbated by, frontal-lobe impairment. These behaviors include his reduced ability to inhibit aggressive and violent responses and his irritability and depression. Frontal-lobe dysfunction can also result in a lowered tolerance to alcohol (another neurotoxic solvent) and hypersensitivity to noise, both of which were problems for Peter. Overall, his test profile not only is consistent with the reports of his everyday functioning but is also consistent with the literature on the deficits demonstrated by painters with OSN (Dryson and Ogden 1998; Hartman 1995).

The history of Peter's decline in health and cognitive functioning, his very genuine distress about his situation, his frustration at his inability to do some of the tests, and the fact that he scored at estimated premorbid levels on tests that would not be expected to show impairment all signified that Peter was not malingering or exaggerating his deficits. Peter was thus referred for a neurological examination, but this did not show any abnormalities, although the neurologist remarked on Peter's poor performance on simple memory tests and on his slowed response to questions. In view of Peter's young age of 38, a CT brain scan was interpreted as showing signs of a premature generalized mild cerebral atrophy.

Personal and Social Consequences

The emotional, physical, and economic repercussions of OSN on Peter and his family are tragic. Peter has lost his job, and he will also find it difficult to retrain for a new occupation because of his depression and his lowered ability to learn new skills as a consequence of his frontal-lobe dysfunction. His change in personality from a happy, easygoing person to a depressed, irritable, and irrational man has alienated and frightened his children and caused his wife immense emotional suffering. Peter contemplates suicide at times. His children and his wife are in possible physical danger from Peter, and the children are having problems at school and at home. Peter and his family are becoming increasingly isolated from their community because they continually refuse invitations to socialize.

Rehabilitation and Longer-Term Outcome

In Peter's case the most urgent requirement was to ensure the safety of his family from his violent outbursts, which was accomplished with the ready cooperation of both Peter and his wider family. They agreed that whenever there was any indication that Peter was becoming agitated, June would contact Peter's brother, who would come immediately and take him to his home. Peter's brother was unmarried and shared a close relationship with Peter; this strategy proved useful on five occasions over the next 10 months. June, Peter, and their three sons also attended family therapy sessions, but it quickly became apparent that Peter's presence was not helpful. His sons were too afraid to talk freely in his presence, and Peter often found that he could not concentrate on what was happening in the sessions and so emotionally withdrew.

The sessions therefore continued without Peter, and they proved helpful both for the children and for June. The 12-year-old boy had been experiencing a lot of problems at school, and these quite quickly dissipated as he gained an understanding of his father's problems. He learned to predict his father's mood changes and, if necessary, to talk to his mother or telephone his uncle so that he did not have to shoulder the burden of his family's safety. As his confidence grew, he was able to find ways to help his father when he showed signs of depression or frustration, and his love and respect for his father gradually returned. The 10-year-old had reacted by becoming defiant and "tough," which concerned his mother. He, too, was taught strategies to cope with his father's moods but was also encouraged to look at the ways his behaviors were starting to resemble those he disliked in his father. With the help of his two brothers, he found that his father still demonstrated many "good" behaviors: when he had fun with the boys, was loving to their mother, and was sorry for the times when, because he was not well, he hurt them. The 10-year-old son made a decision to banish bad behaviors from the home by increasing his own "good" behaviors and ensuring that his little brother did not learn bad behaviors from him. The youngest child seemed least affected by his father's behaviors and the tension in the family, which his mother felt might be because he did not remember the "old" gentle, happy Peter and was therefore less distressed by the changes. In addition, his brothers usually took the brunt of their father's anger and often protected him.

June's emotional state was greatly relieved by the progress made to help her sons and also by the safety measures that had been put in place. She was not afraid for her own physical safety; Peter had hit her only once and was immediately contrite. Other than her worries about the effects on the family, her major concerns were for Peter's health and well-being, their marital relationship, and their difficult financial situation. She decided to return to work part-time while the children were at school. This not only relieved the financial situation but gave her respite from her constant ruminations about their problems. She rebuilt her social network, which had been reduced considerably as a result of Peter's depressions and continual fatigue.

Peter left his job at the factory with the promise that an effort would be made to find him a new job in another area of the factory, away from paints and solvents, when he was considered well enough by the occupational medical specialist. He attended group sessions in anger management and self-esteem at a community mental health center and had weekly individual sessions with a psychiatrist who was interested in occupational stress and the psychological and psychiatric effects of OSN. Although Peter has found these sessions helpful in a number of ways, his cognitive abilities did not changed over a 2-year period. His headaches resolved once he was away from the solvents, and his irritability and fatigue decreased somewhat as he learned coping strategies. With the help of his family, he was also able to put into practice some anger-management techniques, and he began to feel less guilty about the damage he was doing to his family.

His depressions continued, however, and he remained on antidepressants, which appeared to keep his mood from becoming so low that he could not gain anything of use from his therapy sessions. His low self-esteem remained an enormous barrier to his happiness and recovery. His continuing memory problems, slowed thinking, and difficulty in driving himself around convinced him he would never be able to cope with learning and maintaining a new job. He had suicidal thoughts at times, but his wife's and sons' continuing love and support kept him from making any serious suicide plans for a number of years. However, his wife and therapists were not be able to relax their vigilance over this matter so long as Peter's self-esteem remained low and his depressions continued.

As a result of the permanent damage that had been done to his brain, many of Peter's ongoing concerns about his future were tragically realistic. The family did their best to come to terms with having a husband and father who was likely to remain on a sickness benefit for the rest of his life. Five years after his diagnosis, June and Peter were divorced, after many difficult and painful months of counseling and a trial separation. Only 11 months after their divorce was final, Peter was killed in a car accident when his car, of which he was the sole occupant, crashed through a bridge into a river late at night on a deserted road. A postmortem showed that Peter would have been very intoxicated at the time, and although his death was officially notified as the result of a car accident, June believes it was suicide. June's grief and feelings of guilt about his death sent her back into therapy, and although this, and the passage of time helped, neither she nor her sons have been able to return to the slightly happier times they were beginning to experience when June finally managed to separate from Peter.

The overall outcome of 20-plus years of painting was, for this man and his family, a grim reflection on our past lack of knowledge about solvent neurotoxicity and current less-than-adequate prevention and protection methods. For persons involved in occupations that use neurotoxic solvents, awareness of cases like Peter's should increasingly act as a stimulus to weigh the likelihood that they are damaging their brains and reducing their quality of life, albeit 20 years down the track, in return for a mere 10–20 years of work.

Discussion

On the basis of his chronic neuropsychological and psychological symptoms, Peter would be classified as having type 2 OSN. It is often impossible to say with absolute certainty that cognitive and psychological symptoms are the result of solvent neurotoxicity. By the time the problems are assessed, the client's life may well be in disarray in both personal and work areas, making it difficult to tease apart the organic and psychological causes of many of the symptoms and behaviors. In a situation such as that illustrated by Peter's case, it is easy to assume that many of his emotional behaviors (e.g., depression, irritability, anger, and violent outbursts) are psychological reactions to his cognitive difficulties, fatigue, and headaches; but it is important to realize that all these emotions and behaviors can also be direct consequences of brain damage and, as such, are less likely to be amenable to therapy and rehabilitation programs.

Compared with a number of New Zealand victims of OSN (Dryson and Ogden 1998, 2000; Ogden 1993b), it is clear that Peter's neuropsychological profile is not atypical. The men in our New Zealand studies included painters, printers, leather workers, boat builders, and pest controllers who had been exposed to solvents for periods of 10–40 years. Like Peter, all had been exposed to multiple solvents, and it would have been impossible to tease apart the effects of individual solvents. In industry, multisolvent exposure seems the rule rather than the exception.

Many of the neuropsychological impairments and emotional changes typical of OSN are consistent with the lowered cortical arousal that often follows diffuse brain damage. Poor concentration and an inability to process multiple bits of information selectively and simultaneously result from a poorly aroused cortex, which in turn can lead to psychomotor slowing, difficulties in organizing and planning ahead, and impairments in learning new material. A lowered cortical arousal is synonymous with feelings of fatigue and low energy, and it is not hard to see how a difficulty in processing multiple bits of information and sorting what is important from background noise can lead to irritability in a world where we are constantly bombarded with trivia and noise. Memory, visuospatial, and frontal-lobe deficits could also be results of damage to focal cortical areas caused by the more specific effects of toxins on the brain.

When assessing men with suspected OSN, I have found that, as in Peter's case, it is quite common in the initial interview for the client to become tearful as he tells his story. This occurrence is particularly poignant because most of these men clearly are not accustomed to crying and are often embarrassed by their display of emotion in front of a stranger. True to the stereotype of the New Zealand "working class" man, most tried valiantly to regain their "stiff upper lip" and to continue with the neuropsychological tests. This sometimes worked, but often some preliminary counseling proved helpful, and the neuropsychological assessment was rescheduled for later.

There have been a small number of studies looking at the question of recovery and rehabilitation for sufferers of type 2 OSN. Arlien-Soberg et al. (1979), in a longitudinal study of 26 painters exposed to solvent mixtures for an average of 28 years, found that two-thirds of these men had mild to moderate cerebral atrophy. When they were reassessed neuropsychologically 2 solvent-free years after their first assessment, none of the subjects showed any improvement in their neuropsychological or neuroradiological status. Their conclusion was that a syndrome of chronic solvent exposure did exist and that symptoms were likely to be irreversible once cerebral atrophy or intellectual changes were observed; this seems true in Peter's case. A longitudinal New Zealand study that involved neuropsychological and psychosocial assessments of men at the time of a diagnosis of type 2 OSN, and again some years after the men had given up their work with solvents, supported this conclusion; that is, men diagnosed with type 2 OSN rarely recovered or improved on their neuropsychological scores even after many solvent-free years (Dryson and Ogden 2000).

Although this picture is gloomy, much can be done for individual clients. Obviously, prevention through information, ongoing monitoring of solvent levels in the workplace, and correct use of protective clothing and safety procedures are the most important ways to decrease this syndrome, and it is rarely too late for individuals who already demonstrate some symptoms of OSN to take steps that will prevent further damage (preferably permanent removal from the solvent environment). Strategies can be taught to lessen the effect of cognitive impairments. The proper use of a diary to act as a memory aid is a simple strategy, but it very often fails unless the client is carefully instructed and monitored in its use until it becomes second nature. Problems with planning and organizing can be alleviated with step-by-step instructions for various activities. Because OSN can result in an intolerance to alcohol (also a solvent), and even small amounts of alcohol can further depress the underaroused cortex, thus exacerbating many of the symptoms of OSN, it is important to monitor the intake of alcohol. If it is a problem, an appropriate program aimed at reducing or terminating alcohol intake should be instigated.

As illustrated by Peter's case, counseling and therapy can help the victims and their families with the many psychological problems caused by, or that have built up around, the solvent symptoms. Strategies to fight depression and anxiety, to cope with fatigue and irritability, and to inoculate against stress can all be useful. Anger management is sometimes necessary in cases where frontal-lobe dysfunction causes impulsive and violent behaviors. Environmental adjustments can be made by the family to allow for the difficulties many victims have with noise levels and too many stimuli impinging on them at once. For example, important family discussions should take place in a quiet environment, when the client is not tired, and family members as well as the client may need help to learn to read the signs that signal fatigue, irritability, depression, anger, and aggressive and violent reactions. Such discussions will better enable the family to work together to predict and prevent difficult situations.

Many clients benefit from therapy to help them express and resolve their under-standable anger, resentment, frustration, and grief as they become aware that their occupation has lost them their health, their job, and often their relationships. Marital and family therapy is often essential to help other family members as well as the primary victim. In cases in which a marital separation becomes inevitable, therapy to address the guilt and bitterness that understandably result when a family is torn apart through no fault of its own, and practical assistance to ease the transition to separate lifestyles, can help prevent further distress.

Perhaps most important of all is the task of rebuilding the client's self-esteem. In many cases, this task will include exploring new job and recreational possibilities, ongoing assistance with job retraining, and providing the client with strategies to cope with job difficulties and failures in the future without losing his pride.

14

■

Tomorrow Is Another Day
Living with Multiple Sclerosis

In my early years as a neuropsychologist, I had very little contact with people who had multiple sclerosis (MS), and my general impression was that this demyelinating disease resulted in a range of symptoms that came and went, but that almost inevitably the sufferer became severely disabled and probably ended up wheelchair-bound. I suppose I gained this rather dismal impression of the prognosis for MS sufferers because the few cases I saw were hospitalized in the neurology ward for some sort of treatment or assessment. I gradually built up a more accurate picture of MS as I came into contact with more people with the disease, many of whom remained very capable both physically and mentally, with little or no deterioration over all the years I knew them.

Without doubt, some forms of MS are very debilitating, certainly physically and often mentally, but other forms are almost benign, causing only a small number of episodes in the individual's lifespan when symptoms are obvious for a week or two before completely resolving. In the middle of these extremes is a group of MS sufferers who may become gradually worse over time, but even in this group many remain only mildly disabled into old age. In this sense, taken overall, MS is perhaps the least disabling of the group of disorders that primarily affect the subcortical brain structures. Both Parkinson's disease (see Chapter 15) and Huntington's disease (see Chapter 16) are more disabling, and both more certainly progress to a severe level of disability.

Later in this chapter, I will tell the story of Anne, whose condition falls somewhere in the middle of the MS disability continuum. Although she had to learn to cope with the symptoms of her disorder and plan for an uncertain future in terms of both decreasing mobility and potential cognitive decline, she could live her day-to-day life in the knowledge that she might never become particularly disabled by her form of MS. First, however, I will describe each of the forms of MS and the current wisdom (often, but not always, backed by research) about causes, types of symptoms, treatment, and rehabilitation for this disease.

Theoretical Background

Epidemiology and Neuropathology

MS is an autoimmune inflammatory disease that affects the central nervous system. It is the most common of the nontraumatic neurological disorders occurring in young adults. Overall the prevalence is about 100 cases per 100,000 people (Perkin and Wolinsky 2000). The incidence of the disease does, however, vary across ethnic groups, gender, and geographic locality. Disease onset peaks in the third decade, with less than 10% of sufferers having an onset before puberty or after the age of 55 years of age. The ratio of women to men with MS is 2:1, and some ethnic groups have a much lower prevalence of MS than do others (e.g., Japanese), although this disparity may represent an influence of lifestyle differences more than of ethnicity per se (Martin and McFarland 1993). The incidence of MS for white ethnic groups is twice that of black ethnic groups.

Considerable evidence points to the possibility that the climate experienced before puberty is a factor contributing to MS. More cases are found at the Northern-most latitudes of North America and Europe and the southernmost latitudes of Australia and New Zealand. Children who spend their early years in one of these latitudes and then move to a warmer climate at adolescence continue to have the same risk of developing MS in adulthood as individuals who live all their lives in colder or temperate climates (Kurtzke 1983).

Various lines of evidence indicate that MS is an autoimmune disease that develops following exposure of individuals who may be genetically predisposed to the disease to some environmental factor or virus. Sadovnick and Baird (1988) found that 15% of MS patients had a first-degree relative with MS. Identical (monozygotic) twins have much higher concordance rates for MS than do nonidentical (fraternal) twins. The possibility that a virus or combination of viruses in childhood contributes to the later development of MS has not yet been proven, but it may be a factor (Smith, Samkoff, and Scheinberg 1993).

The neuropathological signs of MS are plaques or lesions that can occur wherever there are myelinated axons within the central nervous system. Because the myelin covering on the axon facilitates the rapid transfer of information along the axons, demyelination slows this transfer. The plaques of MS are commonly found in the periventricular areas of the brain (i.e., around the lateral ventricles; see Fig. 14-1), within the subcortical white matter of the cerebral hemispheres, and along the spinal cord and optic nerves. Plaques vary in stage and type and may be either inflammatory and acute, resolving over a period of days to weeks, or chronic and permanent. The distribution of plaques varies among individuals as well as within the same individual at different times. This is the most likely reason for the variation in symptoms, both across individuals and within the same individual at different times.

Classification of MS Types

MS can be divided into four types as follows.

a. *Remitting relapsing disease* (also known as *exacerbating remitting MS*): This is the most common form the disease takes when the individual first presents with symptoms. Mild symptoms usually come on acutely and gradually increase in intensity over a number of days or weeks before resolving either completely or almost completely over a number of weeks to months. No further acute episodes occur for at least 30 days and often for years. Between episodes the individual may have no neurological symptoms, or if symptoms are present, they will be mild and stable. To be diagnosed with MS, the individual usually has to have experienced at least two such episodes and have evidence of two or more distinct areas of demyelination.

Individuals in a subgroup of those with this type of MS have a benign form of the disease, where episodes are usually restricted to sensory symptoms that resolve completely and the individual remains, at worst, only mildly inconvenienced or occasionally mildly disabled by the disease even after 25 years or longer following diagnosis. Others have a wider range of symptoms, including weakness, ataxia (gait disturbance), and double vision, which also resolve but that in some cases may not resolve completely as the years pass. Nevertheless, these individuals commonly also have only mild disability over many years of the illness.

Typical symptoms in the acute episodes include numbness; a feeling of heaviness in the lower limbs that is sometimes experienced following exercise or when the individual becomes overheated; a disturbance or loss of vision, which usually resolves over a period of weeks; and trigeminal neuralgia. Unusual sensations such as "electric shocks" radiating down the spine into the legs (often induced by neck flexion) or a feeling that a band is tightening around the torso, as well as brief episodes of intense itchiness, can also occur. Sometimes the limbs go into a painful spasm. Numbness usually begins in the lower limbs but may extend to the genitals, buttocks, and upper limbs and torso. Debilitating fatigue is common, as is depression.

b. *Secondary progressive disease*: This common form develops from the remitting relapsing type. Each acute episode may leave the individual with some permanent neurological damage and with permanent symptoms that accumulate over time, between acute episodes, or even in the absence of further acute episodes.

c. *Primary progressive disease*: This occurs in about 15% of MS sufferers and is characterized by the slow accumulation and progression of neurological symptoms in the absence of acute episodes. Spinal cord lesions are often prominent in this type of MS, resulting in lower limb weakness and tightness, an impaired ability to walk for long periods of time, and urinary frequency and urgency.

As the progression of symptoms is gradual, the sufferer may not notice change, and symptom development is usually noted most clearly by asking the individual to assess their level of symptoms and disability on a specific date every year.

d. *Progressive relapsing disease*: This is an uncommon form of MS affecting less than 5% of MS sufferers. It begins as the primary progressive type, but disability is exacerbated by one or more acute episodes of symptoms appearing later in the disease.

Other Symptoms

Epilepsy occurs in about 5% of MS sufferers. Fatigue is a very common symptom and can affect every area of the individual's life if strategies to lessen the effect of the fatigue are not put in place. Depression is common and may be a direct result of the neurological processes underlying the disease, a reaction to the disease, or both (Taylor and Taylor 1998).

Mild to significant cognitive impairments are relatively common and can be demonstrated through neuropsychological assessment in 43% or more of MS sufferers (Demaree, DeLuca, Gaudino, and Diamond 1999; Rao 1986, 1993; Rao, Leo, and St. Aubin-Faubert, 1989; Rao, St. Aubin-Faubert, and Leo 1989; Wishart and Sharpe 1997). Cognitive decline is not uniform, nor are cognitive impairments consistent among MS sufferers who otherwise appear to have a similar presentation. However, as a generalization, deficits in retrieval of new information, poor sustained attention and slowed information processing, impaired conceptual and abstract reasoning, and verbal fluency deficits are the most common symptoms, and mild visuospatial perceptual deficits are also sometimes apparent. In contrast, general intellectual ability, language abilities, immediate memory span, and storage of new memories are usually spared. Severity of cognitive deficits is not strongly correlated with severity of physical symptoms. For example, a wheelchair-bound individual with primary progressive disease and demyelination primarily of the spinal cord is less likely to have cognitive deficits than an MS sufferer with secondary progressive disease who is physically independent, but who has white matter lesions in the brain.

Many secondary symptoms can occur, especially after many years of the disease. Constipation is extremely common, as are urinary problems, both urgency and frequency and, less commonly, incomplete voiding. This latter problem can result in urinary tract infections. Unremitting limb spasticity can result in irreversible shortening of muscles, which results in difficulties of positioning and, if the sufferer is wheelchair-bound, may increase the likelihood of pressure sores. In severe cases, surgical correction of irreversible spasticity may be required. In advanced MS, swallowing problems can develop in a small number of cases and can cause aspiration pneumonia.

Tertiary problems are perhaps the most disabling for many sufferers. These include psychosocial difficulties such as anxiety and stress related to current and potential episodes of MS symptoms and to changes in employment, leisure activities, physical fitness, sexual enjoyment, and living environment as a result of MS symptoms, or of preparation for worsening symptoms. The level of the individual's coping strategies and support networks will often be the deciding factor in how debilitating these difficulties become. People with significant cognitive impairments or marked depression may not be able to remain in employment and may have problems adapting to their changing physical needs.

Interventions

To date, no cure for MS has been discovered. Medical treatments are given in some, but not all, cases of MS to treat the inflammation and loss of immunity that characterizes MS. Corticosteroids are commonly prescribed as they have both antiinflammatory and immunomodulating properties. These can be given orally or by intramuscular or intravenous injection. In relapsing remitting disease, only acute episodes can be treated, and continuous medication should not be given.

Secondary symptoms such as constipation and urinary tract infections are treated as required; for example, with a high-fiber diet and laxatives in cases of constipation, with medications in the case of urinary incontinence, with catheterization in severe cases of incomplete urinary voiding, and with antibiotics for urinary tract infections.

Psychosocial symptoms, including depression, and coping with fatigue and occupational and relationship stress can be addressed by a clinical psychologist. A range of therapy methods including cognitive behavioral therapy may be helpful. Severe cases of depression may require treatment with antidepressant medications.

Physical therapists can assist with gait problems and with better positioning in a wheelchair or bed, and occupational therapists can advise and assist the MS sufferer on the use of a wide variety of aids that will help them remain independent in activities of daily living for as long as possible.

Clearly, good management of MS is a multidisciplinary affair, and an integrated management plan undertaken by a group of health professionals who work from the same location will be of enormous benefit to the person with MS. As physical problems worsen, the stress that results from having to travel to different locations to see different health professionals, and the problems that arise when health professionals do not communicate constructively with one another about that individual's care, can not be emphasized enough.

As with any chronic condition, many new ideas for treatment and an improvement in quality of life frequently arise; sometimes in the research literature, and often in more popular publications. It is an ongoing process for the interested MS sufferer to sift through these ideas and try and sort out the clearly bizarre from those that seem sensible and worth a try. Diet and dietary supplements is one area that has attracted a lot of attention. The jury is still out on whether particular diets will improve MS symptoms and lessen the frequency or severity of symptom flare-ups, but changing to a healthy diet is likely to improve the individual's general health and well-being, regardless of its influence on the neurological symptoms of MS. A book by an Australian medical doctor, George Jelinek, is one such book that many MS sufferers have found inspiring and helpful (Jelinek 2001).

Finally, as with all chronic or progressive illnesses, support groups for the individual with MS and for family members may be of great benefit for some people. Others prefer to utilize support groups for psychoeducational purposes only, perhaps to obtain literature or to borrow useful videos on MS, and some cope better with their MS if they avoid support groups entirely and "get on with their lives" in their own way.

Case Presentation

First Symptoms

Anne, a 50-year-old clinical psychologist, decided to take a weekend break following a particularly busy 6 weeks in the private practice she shared with one other psychologist, Lynn. Anne had been carrying not only her own clinical load but also some of the clients of Lynn, who had been away overseas visiting her mother. On Friday night, Anne drove herself the 200 km to her sister Gael's home. After a lazy Saturday, they enjoyed a casual meal and went out to a party that night. The wine flowed, and the company was good, and by the time Anne and Gael called a taxi to take them home, it was 3 AM, and they were both decidedly merry.

The next morning, Anne woke around 9 AM, and as she began to get out of bed, she noticed that her left buttock and leg felt numb. She pushed aside her fears and told herself that the numbness was probably a result of lying on her left side in an awkward manner. But deep down she knew this was probably not the explanation because she had by this stage also noticed that her genital area also felt numb. She remembered having suffered occasionally from numbness in the past and that she recovered quite quickly from this. She forced herself to go for a walk and managed this reasonably well, although the strange feeling in her leg caused her to stumble on uneven ground. She decided not to worry her sister about her problems, and after lunch she managed to drive the 200 km back to her hometown. By this time she was feeling increasingly concerned as the numbness was not only not dissipating but appeared to be spreading to her other leg and buttock. By the time she got home she was feeling upset and exhausted and went straight to bed.

By Monday morning both buttocks, legs, and feet were numb, and her feet felt like bags of sand she had to drag around. The only positive aspect was that she felt no pain. She phoned her doctor, who made an appointment to see her at 10 AM, and canceled her morning clients. The 10-minute drive to the doctor's surgery was a nightmare, as she realized that she could not feel her foot on the accelerator or brake. By sheer mind-power, she managed to drive herself to the surgery by talking her feet through the motions and going as slowly (if jerkily) as possible.

Her doctor listened to her story but did not examine her. Instead she suggested that Anne's symptoms were the result of the work stress she had been under recently and that she needed to have a rest. Anne was unhappy about this diagnosis, but felt too tired to question the doctor, and managed to drive herself to her rooms so that she could see her afternoon clients. However, when she arrived at her rooms, having tripped and nearly fallen twice on the path to the door of her office building, she found she could not climb the stairs to her office. She was feeling very scared by this point and almost dragged herself into the hairdressers' salon on the ground floor below her own rooms. She phoned her 20-year-old son, Jack, who fortunately answered his work phone immediately, and asked him to come and pick her up as she was unwell and could not drive.

Later that afternoon, after waking from an exhausted sleep, she made an appointment to see a chiropractor in the hope that he could help with the numbness. Jack drove her to her appointment next morning, and after hearing her story, the chiropractor said that he suspected that he was not the right person to help her but that he wanted to consult a textbook and carry out a few tests on her first. After reading for a few minutes, he asked her to walk heel-to-toe across his office (which she could not do) and put her arms out in front of her with her eyes closed. He then said that she should return to her doctor as soon as possible and that he would phone her himself. Anne was now convinced that she either had a brain tumor or MS.

Diagnosis

Anne's doctor saw her later that day, and this time she gave her a full examination. The doctor then apologized for not having taken Anne's symptoms more seriously the previous day and said that she would arrange for a computed tomography (CT) brain scan as soon as possible and a referral to a neurologist. At 5 PM, Jack drove Anne to the hospital for her CT scan, and on Friday morning he drove her to her appointment with the neurologist. By this time Anne's numbness had spread to her arms and up to her lower neck. After examining her, the neurologist said that he would arrange for a magnetic resonance imaging (MRI) scan after the weekend and that, in the meantime, Anne should just rest and try not to worry. He said he suspected MS but could not confirm this without an MRI scan. Anne spent a very long and sleepless weekend trying unsuccessfully not to worry. She phoned her clinical psychologist partner Lynn, who had now returned from her overseas trip, and asked her to come around so Anne could explain what had happened. Lynn was clearly shaken by Anne's story but tried to be positive. Jack called in to see how Anne was; she had not told him the neurologist's preliminary diagnosis of MS but simply said that she should have a better idea of what was wrong with her after her MRI scan on Monday.

Jack left Anne at the Radiology Department on Monday morning and, after an hour's wait, she was finally taken into the scanning suite. She was upset by the rather abrupt treatment she received from the radiology technician, who said that the doctor wanted a full scan of both her brain and spine but that she might only have time to do the scans of her brain, and that Anne would probably have to make an appointment later in the week for her spinal scans. Lying in the scanner she drew on all her knowledge about dealing with stressful medical procedures. One of her specialist areas as a clinical psychologist had been working with clients with intractable pain and with patients and staff in hospices. Being in the bed rather than beside it was certainly a new experience, but she was able to use her relaxation techniques to dissociate herself from the claustrophobic and noisy environment of the MRI scanner. After completing her brain scans, the radiologist disappeared for 10 minutes and then returned to say that they would complete all the spinal scans right now, after all. By this time Anne was sure that the news was bad; clearly her brain was not looking too good given the sudden urgency for the rest of the scans. She was finally released from the scanner and given a package of scans, and the receptionist called her a taxi and told to go immediately to the neurologist's rooms.

Once Anne arrived at the neurologist's rooms, the receptionist relieved her of the scans. After 20 minutes, she was in the neurologist's office. He wasted no time in telling her that she did have MS and that she had almost certainly had it for a long time. He suspected that the periods of numbness Anne had previously experienced, but that were not diagnosed, were earlier episodes of MS. Anne's first feeling was one of relief; at least she did not have a brain tumor, which had remained in her mind as a possibility. She asked the neurologist where the damage was, especially in her brain, and what this would mean for her. Her main concern was about her cognitive abilities—perhaps the difficulty she had been experiencing lately remembering peo-

Figure 14-1 A magnetic resonance imaging scan (a T2-weighted axial image) of Anne's brain carried out when she was first diagnosed with MS. This horizontal section (left hemisphere on the right of the picture, and right on the left, with frontal lobes at the top of the picture) shows extensive signal alteration (whiter areas) indicating loss of density within the *periventricular* (around lateral ventricles), subcortical, and deep white matter of both hemispheres, but occurring more extensively on the left. These changes are typical of MS.

ple's names was not simply the result of normal aging. The neurologist said that he did not think it would be helpful to tell her "where the damage was." As he pointed out, she had been compensating well for any symptoms up until this point, and giving her information about areas of demyelination would only cause her to worry needlessly and perhaps set up expectations that she might have specific problems. But he did emphasize that any damage was diffuse and minor (See Fig. 14-1 for Anne's MRI brain scan).

Anne asked about treatment, and the doctor said that she had two options: He could give her steroids, or she could have no treatment and let the disease heal itself. He explained that her numbness would probably resolve in time, as remyelination occurred, although it may not completely resolve. It may then be years before she had another episode like this, or perhaps she would never have another one. Anne did not even have to think about steroid treatment, given that she was aware that this choice came with potential side effects, and said she would heal herself. She left the neurologist's rooms feeling somewhat calmer and took a taxi home.

Coping and Recovery

Once home, Anne felt so tired she could hardly keep her eyes open. The rest of the day she slept. When she awoke, it was dusk, and she managed with some difficulty to have a bath and some toast and tea. She then took on the task of phoning her sister, Gael, and replying to the phone messages from Jack, Lynn, and her daughter, Stephanie, who had heard about her plight from Jack. She declined all their offers to come around but asked Jack if he would drive her to the clinic next morning and told Lynn that she would come into the clinic next day to see her clients, or at least to reschedule them if she felt she needed some time off. The next morning she saw three clients, but by lunchtime she was exhausted. Her numbness had neither resolved nor gotten any worse. Anne asked Lynn whether she would phone her afternoon clients and cancel their appointments, and she lay down on her couch and slept for 2 hours. On awakening, she spent the remainder of the afternoon phoning all her clients and canceling their appointments for the next fortnight. Lynn agreed to see one client who could not wait 2 weeks between appointments.

The next day, after a disturbed sleep, Anne began her own research into MS. She felt that if she understood the disease process she would have some chance of controlling it, or at least of coping with it. A counselor from the MS Society brought her a number of pamphlets, videos, and books about MS and invited her to the weekly MS meeting. Anne attended one meeting but felt that she did not belong there and did not want to belong. Some of the participants were in wheelchairs; Anne definitely was not ready for this yet. The information she received from the society was helpful, however, and on the whole reassuring.

Armed with her new knowledge, she returned to discuss her situation with her own doctor. This time her doctor was very helpful and again apologized for having dismissed Anne's concerns on her first visit. Together they decided that Anne would

tackle her MS with a healthy diet and with a daily schedule including walking, practicing yoga, listening to a self-healing tape she would make for herself, and lots of
rest. Anne also decided she would have a massage as well as acupuncture at least
once every 2 weeks. Anne's bedroom was upstairs, and it became something of a
challenge each morning and night, getting up and down the stairs. She made a firm
resolution that she would not give into this by moving into the downstairs bedroom.
Her sister, Gael, suggested she come and stay with Anne for a while, so that Anne
could be looked after for a change, rather than being the one who looks after everyone
else. Anne decided that this was a very good idea, but this time she took a plane to
her sister's hometown, as driving was definitely out of the question. Indeed, she was
taken on and off the airplane in a wheelchair, although she could still walk with help.
Gael had been able to take time off from her job, and together they walked every day,
as far as Anne could manage, and Anne slept a lot. One night Gael took her out to
dinner, but as Anne later remarked, "It was pure hell; too noisy and I felt so tired I
could hardly keep my head off the table."

Within a week Anne's numbness had resolved to a state of mild discomfort, and
the dreadful "sandbag" feeling in her feet had also gone. Anne's main problem by the
time she flew back home was a debilitating fatigue. Every now and again she would
notice a "tic" in her tongue or eye, or an unpleasant crawling sensation on her hand
or leg. On occasion she would awake in the morning in a rigid spasm, with a terrible
and indescribable sensation in her left arm, and if she sat up too quickly she would
experience a feeling of vertigo. But with the numbness almost gone, Anne felt much
more positive. During her time with Gael, Anne had been reading books, not only
about MS but also about living with a chronic condition and living positively (e.g.,
Levine 1997). She had decided, with much encouragement from every member of her
family, to employ a locum to take over her clinical practice and to take a 2-month
leave from work. This would enable her to work on her new lifestyle—including a
healthy diet, regular exercise, self-hypnosis, thinking positively, and regular acupuncture and massage. As she commented with some amusement, it was a pretty long list
that almost made her tired just thinking about it, but nevertheless she was determined
to beat the MS, whatever it took.

Anne made herself a tape to help with self-hypnosis and meditation, using imagery
of the body healing itself. As she had made many similar tapes for her own clients,
and had also practiced meditation herself for many years, this was a strategy that was
immediately helpful. Anne also found the fortnightly acupuncture (carried out using
a laser rather than needles) very helpful, in spite of her initial skepticism. Although
it did not stop an episode in progress, it did seem to help with her symptoms, and
especially with her low energy levels. Within 24 hours of each session, she would feel
much more alive. Her massage therapist was very experienced and was used to working with MS sufferers. If Anne was feeling numb in a particular body part, the therapist
would know just how much more pressure to exert so that Anne could feel it. Constipation was an ongoing problem, and massage was also helpful for this. A fiber-full
diet was the other remedy for the constipation. Her massage therapist also helped her

work out an exercise program that she could use daily and added new exercises as different symptoms emerged.

Understandably, Anne also began to think about some of the problems she had experienced in the past but dismissed. In particular she remembered a period about 5 years previously, when she had felt numb around her waist. Her doctor had not found anything wrong, and the numbness gradually resolved. She remembered many times when she dropped things, especially when tired, and now realized this was probably an early symptom of her MS.

After her 2-month leave, Anne went back to work, but she soon realized that she was not ready for it. Her walking was slow, and she continued to suffer from dreadful fatigue. As she commented, "The fatigue would wash over me like a wave, and I had to rest. Trying to push through it did not help. When I occasionally went out in the evening or even to a friend's house for lunch in the weekend, I had to have a sleep before leaving for home. Falling asleep within minutes after getting into the car—especially if driving—was certainly not an option." After struggling on for 2 weeks, Anne decided to reduce her clinical practice so that she could work part-time, seeing clients only on Monday, Wednesday, and Friday mornings. This schedule change enabled her to rest more frequently and to put into practice all her other lifestyle strategies. Although this put her in some financial stress, she had no doubt whatsoever that her health was far more important than money.

It took Anne a long time to learn how to cope effectively with her fatigue, and it was 2 years before she could go more than 3 hours without a rest. She found that one of the most important strategies was to put herself first and to be quite straightforward about her need for rest. If she went to a friend's house for dinner and needed a rest immediately before or after the meal, she would simply say so, and of course she found that this was readily accepted by her friends. Anne was equally firm with herself about her need to take regular exercise, especially first thing in the morning, which she found to be very energizing.

To ready herself for work on Mondays, Anne soon discovered that she needed to spend most of the weekend quietly resting. By Friday, she would often find herself very tired, but a visit to her acupuncturist would result in her feeling "reenergized" within 24 hours. Likewise, a visit to her massage therapist would help relieve her constipation, relax her stiff joints, and provide that all-important touch that we all need for our psychological well-being. Five years after her diagnosis, Anne still goes to her acupuncturist once every 3 weeks and to her massage therapist once a month. As she commented, she would go weekly if she could afford to.

Relapse and Longer-Term Outcome

As the months and years went by, it became clear that Anne had sustained permanent damage to her right foot; the symptoms being a constant sensation of heat along with pins and needles in her foot. When she is tired, her foot drags, although she is usually not aware of this until it happens. On occasion, she will feel "a clenching hand on her abdomen." This unpleasant symptom is the result of the spinal lesions, which earlier in her illness had caused numbness. She does wake with numbness on one side of her abdomen from time to time, which may take from 1 hour to a few days to resolve.

Three years after she was first diagnosed, Anne had her second major episode of MS. In retrospect, she wonders whether it was precipitated by stress, as it came on when she was in her final preparations to travel overseas to visit family and friends. This episode lasted about 7 weeks and was not as severe as her previous episode. Her symptoms this time consisted of clumsiness, poor balance, some loss of strength in both hands, and of course, an increase in her fatigue levels. By this time, Anne had learned a great deal about managing her symptoms, especially her fatigue, and because of this was still able to enjoy her overseas trip. Two years after that trip, Anne made another overseas trip and had a wonderful time with no exacerbation of her permanent symptoms; she was even able to sightsee all day without a rest as long as she went to bed early.

Anne's neurologist has diagnosed Anne's MS as the "Remitting-Relapsing" type, which is undoubtedly a much more positive diagnosis than "Primary-Progressive" disease. Julie, a friend of Anne's, was diagnosed with the "Primary-Progressive" form of MS 2 years before Anne received her diagnosis, and visiting Julie is one of the hardest tasks Anne sets herself. Julie is now confined to a wheelchair and living in a private hospital. She suffers from depression and is failing cognitively, and Anne finds it increasingly difficult to find ways of assisting her. As Anne says, she feels guilty that her MS is so much less debilitating than Julie's, and at the same time, she is a little scared that this might happen to her in the future.

Living with MS

Most of the time, Anne manages to contain her anxious, scared, and fed-up emotions and has fortunately escaped the very common symptom of depression. Once she was over the first "crisis" period of adjustment, she was able to plan her lifestyle changes very systematically. She keeps up with the latest research on MS, mainly by reading a regular newsletter sent out by the MS Society and by reading the many books available about MS and how to cope with chronic illness (e.g., Jelinek 2001). She realizes that the various remedies suggested in self-help books may not be backed up by research, but she figures that as long as they do no harm it will not hurt to try them. Anne has had all the amalgam fillings in her teeth replaced; eats a healthy, balanced diet; takes daily vitamins and omega-3-rich oil; drinks fresh vegetable juice daily; makes sure she gets 15 minutes of sunlight a day (for vitamin D); walks for 30 minutes five mornings a week; and manages her fatigue by carefully planning each day so that she is fully aware of what she is doing and can thus avoid "overdoing it."

Anne is not too proud to make use of her disabled parking sticker when necessary, and she is quite comfortable telling people who need to know that she has MS, but that it is mild and she is in recovery. She believes that the "invisible illness" nature of her type of MS is usually a positive aspect, as most of the people she meets day to day do not realize she has MS and treat her no different than anyone else. She feels edgy about people who do know and insist on taking care of her when she does not ask to be taken care of. Comments such as "You poor thing," and "How are you managing your MS?" put her teeth on edge. Her answer to the latter is likely to be "Well thanks, and how are things with you?" When her close friends and family ask how they will know when she needs help, Anne simply replies that she would (and could) tell them. She is fortunate in that her neighbors are the sort of friends who do not intrude but whom she would have no hesitation in calling on if needed. On occasion she is upset by an insensitive comment, usually from someone she does not know well. Anne gave an example of this: She was getting into the elevator when a work colleague who was walking up the stairs commented "C'mon lazybones, do you good to walk up the stairs." Anne's response was to tell him that she had a chronic illness and was unable to walk up stairs. As she commented later, hopefully this direct approach might result in making him stop and think in the future before making remarks that might be hurtful.

Neuropsychological Assessment

When first diagnosed, Anne considered going to a clinical neuropsychologist for an assessment of her cognitive abilities but decided against this. She figured that as long as she was coping with her work and life she did not need additional worry about possible cognitive deficits. Subjectively, she felt that her ability with numbers and calculation was not as fast as it used to be; that her memory, especially for names, had deteriorated; and that her reaction times were generally slower. Of course, all of these changes may simply have been the effects of normal aging; they were certainly exacerbated by aging, and the comments of her friends of the same age confirmed this as a possibility. She did ask close friends, work colleagues, and family to tell her straight if they thought that she might be losing her cognitive abilities and be unaware of the change. They promised to do so.

Three years after her diagnosis and a few weeks after she had recovered from her second major MS episode, Anne asked her doctor to refer her for a neuropsychological assessment, as she felt that she was now emotionally stable enough to cope with the results, whatever they were. She reasoned that if any impairments were found, she could find strategies to lessen their effect before they became too severe. She was particularly concerned about whether she had any impairments that would make her unsafe to drive. I scheduled her for two 3-hour sessions, 1 week apart, and we spent at least half of the first session just talking about her experiences with MS so far.

Anne found that she actually rather enjoyed most of the tests, with the exception of some of the information processing tests; especially the PASAT (Gronwall 1977), a particularly grueling task requiring sustained concentration while mentally adding sequential numbers under time pressure (see Chapter 11). Most of the other tests, however, she enjoyed, and she felt that she had performed reasonably well. Fortunately, Anne's area of clinical psychology did not include neuropsychology or educational testing, so although she did have some familiarity with earlier versions of the Wechsler Intelligence and Memory Scales from her training 25 years earlier, she had not seen the recent editions of the tests and had little recall of any of the subtests.

A week after her second session, with some trepidation, Anne returned to see me to find out her results. Fortunately, I was able to give her much more good news, than bad. As expected from her educational level and occupation, on the NART-R (Nelson and Willison 1991), a test of premorbid IQ estimate, she scored in the "Superior" range, and on most of the subtests of the WAIS-111 and the WMS-111, she scored in the "High Average" or "Superior" range, indicating no significant impairments of either her verbal or visuospatial abilities. On the timed tests her scores tended to be in the "High Average" range rather than the "Superior" range because she lost a few bonus points for speed; however, her accuracy was not impaired. She did not do quite so well on memory tests, but she still managed to obtain scores in the top of the "Average" range on a list learning test, on recall of stories, on recognition of faces (all from the WMS-111), and on the Rey Complex Figure recall (Rey 1941).

On tests of executive ability, Anne's performance was excellent on the Wisconsin Card Sorting Test (Heaton 1981), but on the Controlled Oral Word Fluency Test (Borkowski, Benton, and Spreen 1967) she scored in the "Average" range, which was moderately impaired for Anne, given her "Superior" Verbal IQ. Anne was not surprised by her performance on this test, as she often experienced word-finding difficulties in daily life and believed these were worse than the word-finding difficulties her friends aged over 50 complained of. Anne's only significant deficits were on tests of reaction time and multiple information processing. She was slower than expected for her age on a computerized choice reaction-time task, and her performance on the PASAT was, as she had feared, moderately impaired, confirming an information-processing deficit.

In summary, she demonstrated a profile often seen in people with remitting-relapsing MS: slightly lowered scores relative to overall IQ on some memory tests (i.e., in the "Average" to "High Average" range in Anne's case), and a moderate impairment on reaction-time tests and tests involving information processing under time pressure. The practical implications of these mild deficits were readily grasped by Anne. Indeed, she had already realized that she should allow more time to complete tasks than perhaps others of her age might require, and she had learned the hard way that carrying out tasks under time pressure resulted in frustration and failure, followed by excessive fatigue. She was relieved to know that if she gave herself sufficient time to think about and complete tasks, she could do them as well as anyone of her age and IQ level. Regarding driving, she decided that she would no longer drive at night or in busy traffic conditions and would also avoid long-distance driving. If she had further episodes of numbness, she would stop driving until she had recovered.

Looking Ahead

Four years after her diagnosis, Anne sold her two-story house with a large garden and purchased a new one-level house with a small, easy-care garden designed specifically for wheelchair access. Anne considered that this was the best move she had ever made, as the new house is low maintenance, spacious, sunny, and quiet, yet close to the city and her workplace. Anne does not think that she will necessarily ever have to use a wheelchair, but figures that if she does, that would not be the time to think about moving. She was gradually able to increase her work hours up to 4 full days a week but made a decision to reduce her hours back to 2 days a week by the time she reached the age of 55, as at that time she could access her superannuation. Her reason for this was not because she felt unable to physically cope with the workload but because it would enable her to do all the other things she wanted to do before she became too old or her MS became worse.

Anne plans on at least 10 more years during which she can travel, spend her money on beautiful things, and retire. A book titled "A Year to Live" by Stephen Levine gave her great inspiration; this book includes Buddhist exercises and asks you to consider what you would do with your life if you had only 1 year to live. Anne has a dual-strategy approach to living: She plans ahead for the big things (such as her house, partial retirement at 55, and trips overseas) but lives life day by day. Once her "master plan" is made, she does not anticipate what she will be doing in 1 year, or 5 years' time, but is highly organized on a daily basis. Anne has learnt to say "no" to invitations she is not really interested in, whether they are for parties which she knows she will find too tiring or for outings with people whose company she does not really enjoy. She has a strong group of close friends and regular contact with her family. She no longer hesitates before buying a painting, book, or CD she really loves if she thinks she can afford it. She hopes to travel the world in stages over the next few years with good friends and her two adult children.

When asked whether she had one positive thought that she would share with others coping with a new diagnosis of MS, she answered "The thing to understand is that remyelination does occur, and so your symptoms will also have a good chance of resolving." Anne is certainly a good role model for anyone with a chronic illness— including perhaps the normal aging process! In a nutshell, her strategy goes like this: Work out what is important to you and then plan your day-to-day life so that you can enjoy as many of those things as possible, even if it means picking and choosing what you do and when, and eat healthily and exercise regularly to ensure you have the energy to live the life you want.

Discussion

Anne's story is a courageous one, and as those of us who work with people who suffer from serious illnesses know, such courage is by no means uncommon. Anne may be "fortunate" in that her MS is not the primary progressive type, but even if she did develop a progressive form, I believe she would remain positive in her thinking and continue to develop strategies that would allow her to live her life to the fullest. How she differs from others in similar situations who do not cope as well with their MS can only be speculative. However, it is likely that depression, a common disorder in MS sufferers, would inhibit rehabilitation. It is likely that for some MS sufferers, depression is a direct neurological consequence of their MS, whereas for others it might be a psychological response to their illness, or they may have a vulnerability to depression independent of their MS. The cause of their depression may never be known for sure, but in every case treatment of the depression is surely important as a first step toward learning to live positively with MS. The treatment might be psychological, psychopharmacological, or both; each person must be assessed carefully so that the best treatment possible for them can be found.

Other important factors contributing to successful coping include psychoeducation; both with up-to-date information about the MS disease process (including positive information on remission and remyelination) and with information about strategies that can support the healthiest lifestyle possible, given the individual's type and stage of MS. Supportive (but not suffocating) family and friends are also important, as of course are health professionals who are willing to work cooperatively with the individual in finding new ways to cope with problems as they arise.

Of course, some MS sufferers do become progressively more physically disabled, and in some cases cognitively impaired. Planning ahead for this possibility will be difficult, especially as MS is usually a disease that is diagnosed in young adults, and much less commonly in adults of Anne's age. It is likely that most MS sufferers who are diagnosed with progressive MS would benefit from counseling or therapy to help them come to terms with their disease and plan for the future as best they can. Given the uncertainty of MS, this is not an easy task. Partners, children, and perhaps even parents may need to become involved in the counseling at some stage.

Research into MS is ongoing, and MS victims and those who love them can hold onto a real possibility that new treatments for symptoms will be found, or even a cure discovered in the near future. Keeping up to date with the current research literature, perhaps through one of the many MS support groups and newsletters, can become an important part of the MS individual's life.

This study can be an enriching and fascinating "hobby" if kept in perspective and not viewed as a deterrent to working on coping strategies to deal with current symptoms. Some people will enjoy volunteering for research projects on MS, even if they realize that the results of the research are unlikely to help them but may help others in the future. For others, a constant emphasis on MS will depress them and serve only to remind them of what they have lost and what they may lose in the future. Encouraging these people to attend MS support groups, read MS newsletters, and become involved in MS research would be counterproductive.

Thus in MS rehabilitation, as for every other neurological disorder, there is not one right way to proceed. Every individual with MS is different and will approach their diagnosis in a different way. Some, like Anne, will face it head on, and others may never learn to accept it, let alone be able to think constructively about ways to overcome the symptoms. It can be difficult living with an increasingly disabled MS sufferer who appears to deny the severity of their symptoms. In a few cases, this denial may be a result of cognitive impairments, particularly executive deficits resulting in a lack of insight. But in other cases, the MS sufferer may not be ready to—or have the psychological resources to—confront their problems. Nevertheless, these people may find other ways of living with MS without seeming to acknowledge it, or may at least be able to talk about it with others. However difficult, it is not for health professionals or even family members to judge but, rather, to be ready to support the individual if and when support is asked for.

15

■

MIND OVER MATTER

COPING WITH PARKINSON'S DISEASE

Recently I read two wonderful novels, both of which included among the central characters a man with Parkinson's disease (PD). When I began the novels I had no idea that they had anything to do with PD or any other neurological disorder—I was planning on reading for relaxation, not for work—but as I became involved in the books, I soon forgot about work, although at one level I was impressed by the accurate and empathic picture each novel painted of a man struggling with PD. In both novels, Jonathan Franzen's *The Corrections* (2001) and Rohinton Mistry's *Family Matters* (2002), PD itself is not the central theme, but the complex effects the symptoms of the disorder have on the victim and on his family are used as a pivot (or perhaps excuse) for family disarray and dysfunction. *The Corrections* centers on an all-American family, in contrast to *Family Matters*, which revolves around an Indian family living in Britain. Although the books are very different, both in style and in content, there are many similarities as these two families from vastly different cultures try to deal with and understand their Parkinsonian relative. The descriptions of the sufferings of the PD victims, often from the point of view of the sufferers themselves, are at times grueling and seem very accurate. Likewise, the struggles and emotions that the different family members go through when trying to empathize and put up with a progressively incapacitated elderly man surely reflect accurately many of the struggles and emotions of families throughout the world who find themselves in this sad situation.

Awakenings (1991), the well-known book by writer and neurologist Oliver Sacks, was first published in 1973 and revised in 1991. It was based on the story of a group of survivors of von Economo's encephalitis, an epidemic of viral encephalitis that began in Europe in 1918. Some survivors developed what was known as "sleeping sickness"—a severe form of PD, the main symptom of which was rigidity. Sack's book dramatized the administration in 1966 of the experimental drug, levodopa, to these sufferers (who had been frozen like statues for decades), resulting in their rapid "awakening" into walking, talking individuals. Sadly, as the effects of the medication wore off, the sufferers returned to their frozen state. In 1990, this book was made into a very successful film starring Robin Williams and Robert de Niro.

It is not unusual for PD to find its way into novels perhaps because it is the second most common of the neurodegenerative diseases, and therefore familiar to many writers, but more likely because many of the sufferers of PD remain intellectually alert (although often with some cognitive impairments) in a disobedient body. Even more common than novels are autobiographical accounts, written by people with PD about their struggle with their disease. Very often the main theme of these books is that of taking control of the symptoms, which is accomplished in many creative ways. Some excellent and often moving and humorous books in this genre are *Ivan: Living with Parkinson's Disease* (Vaughan 1986), as well as various accounts of PD written by medical and paramedical professionals in *Injured Brains of Medical Minds. Views from Within* (Kapur 1997). These autobiographical accounts illustrate the deep involvement, both emotional and scientific, that many PD sufferers develop with their disease.

This level of involvement is also particularly noticeable when one begins a research project on PD. Highly motivated PD volunteers are plentiful, and they often become very involved in the research, beyond the requirements of their enrollment in the study. The numerous Web sites on PD that include support groups, educative material, and the latest research are testimony to this involvement. The fact that PD is a rich and exciting research field does, of course, feed the interest that the disease holds for its victims. Not only are new therapeutic medications and surgical techniques being developed regularly to treat the symptoms, but in the not-too-distant future, a cure, perhaps via gene transfer or genetic engineering, is a real possibility.

PD has in recent years become a high-profile disorder because of the publicity given it by a number of famous PD sufferers. These include the actor Michael J. Fox, the singer Johnny Cash, Pope John Paul II, former U.S. Attorney General Janet Reno, and possibly the boxer Muhammad Ali, although in this last case, multiple head traumas may be the cause of the Parkinsonian symptoms ("pugilist's encephalopathy"). Certainly, Muhammad Ali's severe hand tremor was clearly apparent for the world to see when he lit the Olympic flame at the Olympic Games in Atlanta in 1996.

There is considerable evidence that Hitler was also a PD sufferer and that from 1934, when he was only 45 years old, he had a left-hand tremor. One theory is that he developed Parkinsonism as a consequence of suffering from Economo's encephalitis in 1918 (Lieberman 1996). Ten years later, his symptoms were more marked and included tremor, bradykinesia, postural instability, a wooden facial expression, an increasingly quiet voice, and episodes of severe depression (although there were a number of possible non-Parkinsonian causes for his depressions). It also seems likely that Hitler was becoming severely cognitively impaired, and possibly demented, by the end of his life. The mental inflexibility associated with PD might have been a factor in Hitler's slow response to the D-Day landings in Normandy in 1944, as he was convinced that the Allies would launch their attack at Calais. Hitler's minister of armaments, Albert Speer, wrote of Hitler in 1944, a year before he committed suicide: "Hitler was shrivelling up like an old man. His limbs trembled, he walked stooped with dragging footsteps. . . . His uniform, which in the past he kept scrupulously neat, was stained by the food he had eaten with a shaking hand" (Stolk 1968).

Of course, most PD sufferers are not famous or infamous, and not all have the ability, resources, or motivation to speak or write eloquently about their disease or to enjoy being involved in research. In addition, quite early in the disease process, most PD sufferers do show some specific cognitive impairments, and a small number become demented. A significant proportion of PD sufferers also suffer from depression, which is thought in many cases to be organically based and part of the PD disease process, rather than simply an understandable response to the illness.

The case study later in this chapter follows the progress of Robert, a general medical practitioner, from the time he was first diagnosed with a mild form of PD at the age of 54, to the age of 65, a year after he underwent surgery with the aim of curing some of his Parkinsonian symptoms.

Theoretical Background

Epidemiology and Neuropathology

James Parkinson, a British doctor, first described PD in his 1917 monogram *An Essay on the Shaking Palsy* (Parkinson 1817). At that time, the disease was considered to be primarily a motor disorder with no or few cognitive symptoms. Numerous studies have since demonstrated that although the motor symptoms are certainly the most obvious, most PD sufferers do develop some specific cognitive deficits, and a proportion of sufferers become demented (Loranger, Goodell, McDowell, Lee, and Sweet 1972; Mayeux and Stern 1983). PD is a result of dysfunction of the extrapyramidal system, and in the estimated 10%–15% of cases in which it leads to dementia (Brown and Marsden 1988), it is known as a subcortical dementia, in contrast to the cortical dementia of Alzheimer's disease (see Chapter 17). However, the distinctions between the so-called subcortical dementias (PD, Huntington's disease, and Progressive Supranuclear Palsy) and the main cortical dementia of Alzheimer's disease are far from clear (Brown and Marsden 1988).

PD is the second most common of the neurodegenerative disorders (after Alzheimer's disease) and affects about 1 in 500 people in the population, with approximately 1 in 100 people over the age of 60 years suffering from the disease. The peak onset of the disease is in the sixth decade, but one in seven PD sufferers is diagnosed before the age of 40 years. A slightly higher number of men than women are affected. It is now realized that PD is not a single disease with a single cause, and that it may be more accurately labelled as a syndrome, incorporating the Parkinsonian symptoms of resting tremor, rigidity, bradykinesia, and postural instability. An alleviation of Parkinsonian symptoms in response to levodopa is also considered a factor in distinguishing PD from other disorders. As yet, no definitive cause has been found for most cases of PD (which is therefore called idiopathic or sporadic PD). For a small minority of sufferers, there is a clear genetic factor in the development of their PD, and there have been at least two genetic (familial) forms of PD identified. A range of environmental factors are, however, likely to be implicated for the majority of sufferers. It may be that genetic factors, at least in some PD patients, make the individual more vulnerable to developing PD, but only when exposed to some environmental influence.

Some types of PD are caused by known factors; for example, the postencephalitic epidemic of 1918 resulted in severe PD in survivors, and multiple brain traumas can also result in "pugilistic Parkinsonism." In 1982 a heroin derivative designer drug, MPTP, resulted in the rapid onset of severe PD in a number of young Californian drug addicts, the main symptom of which disease was an akinetic rigid syndrome that could be relieved by the drug levodopa, the drug most commonly used to treat idiopathic PD (Langston, Ballard, and Irwin 1983). This relief stimulated the experimental use of MPTP in animal models of PD.

In the most common (i.e., idiopathic or sporadic) type of PD, the onset of the disease is gradual and the disease progresses in severity over time, although at different rates across individuals and with different clusters of Parkinsonian symptoms across individuals. There is some evidence indicating that people with a late onset of PD are more likely to have a rapid progression of symptoms, with rates of dementia increasing rapidly when disease onset occurs after the age of 70 years (Mayeux et al. 1988). Current treatments have resulted in major improvements of symptoms, but as yet no cure; however, most sufferers will not have a reduced life span as a result of the disease.

The neuropathology of PD primarily involves the basal ganglia—paired groups of subcortical nuclei (or ganglia) that lie deep in the brain at the base of each cerebral hemisphere, and the thalamus—also paired groups of multiple nuclei that lie on either side of the third ventricle at the anterior end of the brainstem. The basal ganglia in each hemisphere include the caudate and putamen (together called the corpus striatum or neostriatum, or "striped body"), the globus pallidus, the substantia nigra, and the subthalamic nucleus (STN). The putamen and globus pallidus are also called the lentiform nucleus, and the globus pallidus is subdivided into the globus pallidus externa and the globus pallidus interna. There are multiple pathways or circuits connecting the various nuclei of the basal ganglia, thalamus, and cortex. In PD there is a loss of dopaminergic neurons in the substantia nigra, which results in dysfunction in two of these basal ganglia–thalamocortical circuits: one direct and the other indirect.

In the healthy brain it is thought that the direct pathway facilitates movements, and the indirect pathway inhibits unwanted movements. Both pathways begin in the cortex, travel through the basal ganglia via the globus pallidus interna, through the thalamus, and back to the cortex. The indirect pathway includes an additional projection from the globus pallidus externa to the subthalamic nucleus, which then excites the globus pallidus interna before projecting to and inhibiting the thalamus. The different parts of these pathways are complex and include both excitatory and inhibitory projections, and descriptions of them are well beyond the scope of this book.

The exact neuroanatomy of these pathways and how the loss of dopamine results in the various Parkinsonian symptoms is not yet fully understood, but one simplified hypothesis is that because of the loss of dopaminergic input to both pathways, the direct pathway becomes less active (thus resulting in impoverished functional movement), and the indirect pathway becomes more active (thus resulting in more unwanted movements because of the loss of inhibition of such movements). Another common neuropathological finding in PD is the presence of Lewy bodies in the substantia nigra. These are cytoplasmic inclusion bodies found in neurons in the brains of sufferers of many neurological illnesses, including Alzheimer's disease and Down syndrome. It has been hypothesized that in PD these Lewy bodies are responsible for neural death in the substantia nigra, but this theory is controversial, as some studies have found evidence that refutes this (Calne 2003).

Symptoms of PD

Motor symptoms   The main motor symptoms of PD are *tremor, muscle rigidity* (in severe cases resulting in a "frozen" state), *bradykinesia* (a slowness of movement), and postural instability. About 70% of PD sufferers have tremor, which usually begins on one side of the body and progresses to the other side. Tremor is most common in the hand and in the resting (rather than action) state. However, tremor can involve all parts of the body, including the head. Rigidity is a common early symptom of PD and can result in the patient becoming "stuck" in his chair or when turning around, turning over in bed, or making fine finger movements such as fastening buttons. The individual's posture can become stooped (as in Pope John Paul II) and his or her face stiff (masked face), so that it appears to lack expression. Cogwheel rigidity refers to the stuttering nature of the movement when, for example, a rigid arm is passively moved by the doctor examining the patient. Body rigidity can cause considerable discomfort and muscular pain for the patient.

Bradykinesia results in slowness to initiate movements and slowness in carrying out motor tasks. Rapid limb movements are slowed, and coordination is impaired. Walking often becomes impaired, with stride length shortening such that the patient takes small, shuffling steps. Sometimes their gait becomes unbalanced, and to compensate, their shuffling gait becomes faster and faster and not entirely under their control. Some of the descriptions in the book *Ivan* (Vaughan 1986) provide graphic illustrations of this. Many sufferers learn tricks to help overcome their slowness in initiating movement. For example, they may need to swing their arms back and forward a few times to begin walking, and sometimes lines drawn on the floor, like railway sleepers, seem to provide the external visual stimulus they require to initiate their stride (see an example of this in the film *Awakenings*).

Once movement is initiated, often with great difficulty, movement sometimes becomes fluid and automatic for a brief period, as long as there is no interruption to the flow, either by the individual consciously thinking about what he is doing or by someone or something else distracting him. Ivan Vaughan illustrates this in his autobiography (Vaughan 1986), in which he describes his early-morning runs (which he often has to terminate by colliding with a wall) and his ability to swim as long as he is not tired.

Bradykinesia also contributes to the expressionless face, which, of course, can result in social difficulties if others do not realize that the person's face is unable to express their emotions. Patients with bradykinesia of the hands show a change in their handwriting; as they move across the page, their writing becomes smaller and more cramped (*micrographia*).

A loss of balance (postural instability) resulting in falls is a symptom that usually occurs later in the disease. Dystonias, which are persistent muscle spasms of body parts, not only look very awkward but are often very painful and may be a complication of medication or, in some cases, a symptom of the PD itself. Some sufferers experience varying degrees of unusual skin sensations such as an electrical tingling sensation in the limbs. Constipation is common and is a result of the reduction in the ability of the bowel to contract. As in most neurological disorders, fatigue is an ongoing problem and is exacerbated by the motor dysfunction the patient suffers, such as tremor and muscle rigidity; these symptoms cause physical fatigue, as they would for anyone constantly on the move or who holds their body in awkward and stiff positions. As one patient I assessed commented, "At least I should be fit; by the end of every day I feel like I have run a marathon!"

Psychological and cognitive symptoms   Depression occurs in about 40% of PD sufferers; however, only about 25% of PD sufferers have a depression severe enough to be classified as major depression (Brandstadter and Oertel 2003). In many cases the depression is considered part of the organic disease process, as it often begins before any other symptoms are apparent—and before anyone is aware that they have PD (Mayeux, Stern, Rosen, and Leventhal 1981)—and is not necessarily correlated with disease severity. One hypothesis is that reduced dopamine function leads directly to depression, and another is that there are reduced levels of a metabolite of the neurotransmitter serotonin in the cerebrospinal fluid of depressed PD sufferers, but not in nondepressed PD sufferers, and that these levels are related to depression (Mayeux, Stern, Cote, and Williams 1984). Of course, depression may also be an understandable response to having PD. In any case, it is important to treat the depression using psychological therapy techniques where these work, and medication where appropriate.

It has been apparent since the early 1970s that PD does result in a range of cognitive impairments (Loranger et al. 1972; Mayeux and Stern 1983; Mohr et al. 1990) and that almost all PD sufferers will demonstrate at least mild deficits of some cognitive skills quite early on in the disease. Executive or "frontal lobe" impairments seem to be most common, although these are usually quite subtle. As the basal ganglia have rich connections with the prefrontal cortex, such impairments are not surprising. In particular, PD sufferers may have difficulties with organizing and planning ahead, switching mental set, and carrying out cognitive and motor plans (Sullivan, Sagar, Gabrielli, Corkin, and Growdon 1985; Taylor, Saint-Cyr, and Lang 1986), but only when they have to rely on their own spontaneous internal strategies. When external visual cues are given, the executive difficulties do not seem to occur (Brown and Marsden 1988, 1990).

One family of deficits that has also been linked to frontal executive dysfunction is that of sequencing, temporal ordering, and recency discrimination. A number of studies have demonstrated that some PD sufferers have more difficulty (compared with matched age controls) putting past public events (e.g., assassination of John Kennedy, Watergate, and explosion of the *Challenger* space shuttle) into the correct temporal sequence, although they have normal recall of the content of those events (Sagar, Cohen, Corkin, and Growdon 1985). A difficulty in changing from one mental set to another certainly seems to be associated with PD; sufferers often have impaired scores on the Wisconsin Card Sorting Test (Owen et al. 1993; Taylor et al. 1986) and on other tasks that involve mental set shifting (Cools, Van den Bercken, Horstink, Van Spaendonck, and Berger 1984; Flowers and Robertson 1985).

Impairments on some visuospatial tasks are also common (Loranger et al. 1972; Martin, Loewenson, Resch, and Baker 1973; Ogden, Growdon, and Corkin 1990) and can be quite marked even in sufferers at the very earliest stage of the disease who have only mild motor symptoms (Ogden et al. 1990). Figure 15.1 shows the impaired copies and recall drawings of the Rey Complex Figure for a group of people with PD who were generally high functioning. However, it is important to note that executive dysfunctions of planning and organizing will also influence scores on the Rey Figure, and a number of researchers have hypothesized that impairments on visuospatial tasks are often a consequence of more generalized executive impairments, such as an inability to plan ahead without the assistance of external cues, rather than a problem with visuospatial functioning per se (Brown and Marsden 1990).

PD sufferers tend to have impairments on memory tests that require spontaneous recall, but not on recognition memory tests (Flowers, Pearce, and Pearce 1984; Taylor et al. 1986; Weingartner, Burns, Diebel, and LeWitt 1984). As recognition memory by definition involves external cues to "jog" memory, but recall memory requires free recall without external cues, this dissociation also fits the hypothesis that PD sufferers have a generalized difficulty with tasks that require the use of internally generated strategies. Another hypothesis is that PD individuals do have a difficulty with working memory, which is the limited-capacity memory system in which incoming information is manipulated and worked on before being processed into a longer-term memory store. Alan Baddeley has proposed a "Central Executive" limited-capacity attentional system that oversees or "supervises" the working memory process and that is a frontal-lobe function (Baddeley, Bressi, Della Sala, Logie, and Spinnler 1991), and this Central Executive may be compromised in PD (Dalrymple-Alford, Kalders, Jones, and Watson 1994; Owen et al. 1993).

Bradyphrenia, or slowed thinking, has also been postulated as a symptom of PD. Certainly PD individuals often take longer than age-matched controls to complete neuropsychological tests, such as the Block Design subtest of the Wechsler scales, but if given more time, they will perform normally. In this case it is likely to be the motor impairments (tremor, rigidity, and bradykinesia) that have resulted in the slowed performance, and not slowed thinking. Thus, to assess bradyphrenia in a PD population, a task that does not require a motor response is ideal, but such tasks are hard to find. Alternatively, two tasks are given, both of which have the same motor component,

Figure 15-1 The Rey Complex Figure model is at the top. The eight drawings below are the copies of this figure (labeled A) and the 45-minute delayed recall drawings (labeled B) for four subjects with PD (designated 1, 2, 3, and 4, respectively). 1A and 1B are the drawings of Robert, the case presented in this chapter, when assessed at age 58 years, a few months after his formal diagnosis of PD. Subject 2 is a 71-year-old woman with a 9-year history of stage II PD, subject 3 is a 67-year-old man with an 18-month history of stage I PD, and subject 4 is a 71-year-old woman with a 2-year history of stage I PD. (Reprinted from Ogden 1990, p. 133, with copyright permission from Lippincott Williams & Watkins.)

and one of which has a higher cognitive demand and requires more information processing. Comparisons with control subjects are also necessary, as cognitive complexity often results in longer response times in healthy people. Results have been inconsistent, and at best only some subgroups of PD sufferers (e.g., elderly PD sufferers) have demonstrated some tendencies toward "bradyphrenia" (Wilson, Kaszniak, Klawans, and Garron 1980). Thus, it appears that slowed thinking per se may not be a valid or common symptom of PD (Brown and Marsden 1990).

A small number of PD sufferers become demented (Bentin, Silverberg, and Gordon 1981; Chui et al. 1986; Pirozzolo, Hansch, Mortimer, Webster, and Kuskowski 1982), although these cases may be atypical forms of Parkinsonism (Facca and Koller 2003). There is no substantial evidence that in idiopathic PD, dementia is tied closely to progression of motor symptoms. In clinical practice one comes across many people with PD who are wheelchair-bound and who have some of the specific cognitive deficits described above, but who are very definitely not demented. I recall one woman in her mid-70s who was wheelchair-bound, had difficulties swallowing, and spoke in such a quiet voice that she was very difficult to understand, but who continued to play bridge, the card game, at a high level, often winning games against local champions. At the other end of the spectrum, a PD patient who suffers some motor symptoms but who is still physically relatively independent may obtain scores in the demented range on tests of dementia such as the MMSE (Folstein, Folstein, and McHugh 1975) or the Blessed Dementia Scale (Blessed, Tomlinson, and Roth 1968).

Assessment of PD

The assessment of PD is usually carried out by neurologists who specialize in motor disorders, as there are a number of disorders that can be confused with PD. In 1967 a classic article was published in *Neurology* by Margaret Hoehn and Melvin Yahr, based on their careful observations and assessments of over 800 sufferers with Parkinsonism, and from which they defined categories of Parkinsonism and proposed a 5-point scale of severity. The most common category was Type A, or true PD, of unknown cause (i.e., idiopathic). Other types included Parkinsonism resulting from known causes such as encephalitis. The authors' 5-point scale, known as the Hoehn and Yahr Scale, remains in use today, more than 35 years later. This is a fine illustration of the immense value of careful observational and descriptive clinical research. The Hoehn and Yahr Scale (1967) is follows:

Stage I: Unilateral involvement only, usually with minimal or no functional impairment.

Stage II: Bilateral or midline involvement, without impairment of balance.

Stage III: First sign of impaired righting reflexes. This is made evident by unsteadiness as the patient turns or is demonstrated when he is pushed from standing equilibrium with the feet together and eyes closed. Functionally the patient is somewhat restricted in his activities but may have some work potential, depending on the type of employment. Patients are physically capable of leading independent lives, and their disability is mild to moderate.

Stage IV: Fully developed, severely disabling disease; the patient is still able to walk and stand unassisted but is markedly incapacitated.

Stage V: Confinement to bed and wheelchair unless aided.

These stages refer to the motor symptoms of PD only, as in 1967 cognitive and psychological symptoms were not widely recognized. It has been found that the motor stages do not correlate well with cognitive symptoms (Mortimer, Pirozzola, Hansch, and Webster 1982); some sufferers may reach stage V but have only mild to moderate cognitive impairments, whereas others may be classed as having dementia as early as stage III.

A broader and more extensive scale, the Unified Parkinson's Disease Rating Scale (UPDRS; Lang and Fahn 1989), has since been developed to assess gross intellectual impairment (primarily memory), mood, activities of daily living, and complications of therapy as well as motor functioning (including a modified version of the Hoehn and Yahr scale). These are now the standard measures used in research studies of PD.

Specific cognitive functions require additional assessment using a neuropsychological test battery, as symptoms vary from individual to individual and over time. As described in the section on cognitive symptoms, executive difficulties appear to be the most common problems and often result in poor performance on other cognitive tasks, especially visuospatial and memory tasks. Thus, interpretations of the neuropsychological assessment results must be cautious, especially when standard tests are given without carefully controlled alternative tests also being given to tease apart, for example, a problem with utilizing internal strategies rather than a visuospatial or memory problem per se.

Medical and Surgical Treatments for PD

Treatments for PD are aimed at increasing dopaminergic input to the two basal ganglia–thalamocortical circuits described earlier, and this is currently possible via a number of methods. Medication is the first treatment of choice and is usually effective in reducing symptoms for a number of years. As dopamine does not cross the blood–brain barrier, medication is in the form of a precursor of dopamine, levodopa (L-dopa), which does cross the blood–brain barrier. Carbidopa is often added to the L-dopa, as it inhibits the peripheral conversion of L-dopa to dopamine and allows more of the drug to cross the blood–brain barrier before it is converted where it is needed— in the brain. At present, the most beneficial drug for PD is Sinemet, which combines L-dopa and Carbidopa. Carbidopa has the added advantage of reducing some of the side effects of L-dopa such as nausea and vomiting. There are many other drugs that treat various PD symptoms, including Amantadine, an antiviral agent that potentiates the effect of dopamine, and catechol-o-methyltransferase (COMT), which is a monoamine oxidase inhibitor that can prevent dopamine being broken down. Although the main aim of drug therapy is to reduce the movement disorders of PD, there is some evidence that the drugs can also affect some of the cognitive symptoms (Owen et al. 1993).

Many sufferers become intolerant to levodopa after 5–10 years of L-dopa therapy and experience an ON/OFF syndrome. During the ON phase, they suffer side effects of too much dopamine and suffer from severe dyskinesias (involuntary movements of the limbs), rather like the motor symptoms of Huntington's disease (see Chapter 16). The ON phase usually occurs not long after the patients take their medication and is called "peak-dose dyskinesia." In some cases, the dyskinesias are diphasic and occur twice while the drug is in its effective state: once not long after taking the Levodopa, and again just before the medication finally wears off (after about 2 hours). In this case, the dyskinesias may be more likely to take the form of dystonias, which are painful flexions or extensions of the limbs, usually the foot. As the drug wears off, both types of patients experience an OFF phase, in which their Parkinsonian symptoms become very severe and they have severe rigidity, akinesia, and tremor. PD sufferers with peak-dose dyskinesias often "prefer" the dyskinesias of the ON stage to the rigid and "frozen" state of the OFF phase, although from the observer's perspective, the dyskinesias are often more disturbing and can give rise to an uninformed belief that the PD patient is "crazy."

Some PD victims who reach the point at which a drug regime that satisfactorily controls their symptoms without severe side effects can no longer be found may be candidates for surgical intervention. At present, available surgical procedures include using stereotactic functional neurosurgery to place a tiny radiofrequency lesion unilaterally in either the ventrointermediate nucleus (Vim) of the thalamus (thalamotomy) or the globus pallidus interna (pallidotomy). Thalamotomy was first introduced in the 1950s and is used for the relief of tremor on the side opposite the lesion. Pallidotomy can reduce akinetic symptoms and dyskinesias, bradykinesia and rigidity, and to some extent, tremor, and it is probably the more common operation of the two in current practice. In some cases, both operations may be carried out during the same procedure on the same side, and some PD sufferers may have a second operation on the opposite side after an interval of 3–6 months or longer. With carefully selected, nondemented PD individuals who no longer respond well to drugs, these operations can result in a dramatic and immediate cessation of symptoms, which can last for at least 2 years. Pallidotomy requires further longitudinal studies to assess the very long term alleviation of Parkinsonian symptoms, the effects of carrying out a second pallidotomy at a later stage on the other side of the brain, and possible unwanted side effects including permanent (if subtle) cognitive deficits, especially in older patients (Lang, Lozano, Montgomery, Tasker, and Hutchison 1999).

A new procedure is Deep Brain Stimulation (DBS). A multielectrode lead is implanted into the ventrointermediate nucleus of the thalamus and is connected to a pulse generator that is surgically implanted under the skin of the upper chest. The PD individual passes a handheld magnet over the pulse generator to turn it on and off. When the generator is on, the thalamus is electrically stimulated, which results in a blocking of the tremor. The battery (which is very expensive) requires replacing about every 5 years, and this requires another small operation. Most sufferers turn the stimulator off overnight or when their tremor is not a problem for them. This relatively new technique is promising, but some sufferers may experience side effects including tingling in their head and hands, depression, a slight paralysis, slurred speech, a loss of balance, and a loss of muscle tone. A deep brain stimulator can also be placed in the globus pallidus interna or the subthalamic nuclei, with promising experimental results, including reduction of akinesia, bradykinesia, tremor, and dystonia, but as yet only stimulator placement in the thalamus is approved by the Food and Drug Administration in the United States.

Other exciting therapeutic advances are in the experimentation stage. These include the implantation of dopamine-producing cells, in the past harvested from the adrenal medulla, and more recently from the human fetal substantia nigra. The ethical issues involved in using human fetal material for implants have resulted in considerable slowing of this research and have prompted a search for other less controversial transplant tissue. Research currently in the early stages includes the use of human stem cells in transplantation (Lindvall, 1999). Xenotransplantation, which is the transplantation of tissues from one species to another (as opposed to allografts, which refers to same-species transplants) must overcome rejection by the recipient of donor tissue and has the potential for transference of viruses from the donor animal species to humans. The pathogen-free pig is considered a possible candidate, and clinical trials are in progress in which PD sufferers in the advanced stages of the disease receive fetal pig neural cells.

In the future, it is likely that genetic engineering will play a major role in the treatment and, in time, in the cure of PD. Designer cells producing dopamine, other neurotransmitters, and neurotropic factors relevant to PD are likely to be developed over the next few years. Genetically engineered neurotropic factors that can prevent the degeneration of dopaminergic neurons may be able to be injected into the person with PD or drip-fed via implantable pumps, possibly into the cerebrospinal fluid in the ventricles of the brain. In the surgical field, further refinements of gamma knife and proton radio surgical devices may make this less invasive alternative to stereotactic neurosurgery for thalamotomy and pallidotomy a viable option. At present, however, these procedures are complex, and the resulting lesions not able to be clearly defined. Ablation of tremor and other symptoms also takes months, rather than minutes, when these nuclear techniques are used.

Psychosocial Aspects of PD

The slow and progressive nature of PD has both positive and negative aspects for the PD sufferer. On the positive side, it allows for the gradual adaptation to and acceptance of the disease, as well as preparation for later disability. It also encourages hope for better treatments of symptoms, and possibly even a cure in the individual's lifespan. On the negative side, the inexorable and unavoidable decline and worsening of symptoms must be disheartening, to say the least, for both the victim and her family members. The physical symptoms of PD often result in discrimination by outsiders who do not know the person suffers from PD (and who thus perhaps appears to be drunk, for example), or who believe that PD renders the person incapable of normal functioning. Employers who believe that PD causes significant intellectual decline, in the absence of assessment of the specific PD sufferer, may well choose not to employ them on the basis of this faulty perception (perhaps without making their reasons explicit, and thus risking being accused of discriminatory practices). The book *Ivan* (Vaughan 1986) demonstrates vividly the resourcefulness of one PD sufferer (a college lecturer) in the manipulation of his medication to maximize the possibility that his drugs would be at their most effective when he was scheduled to give a lecture or perform some other social role.

It is important for people with early PD to delay taking Levodopa or other Parkinsonism medications for as long as they can, as once started, the medication gradually loses its effectiveness. PD sufferers vary in how long they can remain medication-free and put up with their Parkinsonian symptoms; this often depends on their lifestyle and employment. A 70-year-old woman who lives at home and does not work may be quite undismayed by a hand tremor and bradykinesia, whereas a 50-year-old woman employed in the public arena may feel embarrassed by her tremor and slowness. Many PD sufferers learn strategies or "tricks" to help overcome their physical symptoms; for example, swinging their arms to begin walking or when stuck while turning. Learning strategies to allow them to remain independent with respect to daily living activities is of utmost importance. If driving is important for their employment or for their independence, every effort should be made to ensure they can continue to drive for as long as safely possible. It is, of course, likely that restrictions on when and where they should drive need to come into force at some point. Likewise, personal toilet requirements and sexual activity, as well as less intimate activities such as housework and cooking, should all be continued independently for as long as possible.

The rigidity of PD is the most devastating symptom for many PD sufferers. The helpless feeling of being unable to move is, for them, far more disturbing than the tremor, slowed movements, and dyskinesias they may suffer. The masked face that some PD sufferers show to the world as a result of their bradykinesia or rigidity causes a social barrier and can result in a reluctance to interact with others apart from their family and close friends. Learning simple ways to explain this symptom to new friends may reduce the anxieties they experience about socializing.

Given that most PD sufferers do not become demented, a continued involvement in intellectual activities is of utmost importance. As PD usually does not make itself apparent until the age of 60 years or older, advancing old age per se will also have its effect, and research has shown that the more physical and mental activities that the healthy elderly are involved in, the less likely it is that they will decline intellectually or develop dementia (Dustman, Emmerson, Steinhaus, Shearer, and Dustman 1992; Dustman et al. 1984).

The depression that accompanies PD in about 40% of cases is one of the most disabling symptoms and may make it more difficult for the individual to utilize other physical and psychological strategies to assist them in coping with their disease. Even though the depression may be organically based, psychological therapies as well as antidepressant medications may be worth trying to see whether the depression can be modulated, if not entirely dispersed. Anxiety is also common, and hallucinations can occur later in the disease, often as a result of long-term levodopa treatment. Hallucinations are usually visual rather than auditory, as in schizophrenia, and appear to be fairly innocuous and often not frightening or upsetting for the PD individual. However, if they do become disturbing, medications such as serotonergic agonists may provide relief (Goetz 1999).

Sleep disorders are extremely common, with insomnia being an issue for about 60% of PD sufferers (Larsen 2003). Other sleep problems include frequent awakenings, difficulties with falling asleep, and early awakening. Depression is the most common correlate of sleep problems, so treating the depression is a priority. Motor manifestations of PD such as being unable to turn over in bed, dystonia or painful cramps, and arousal from the dopaminergic drugs may all be causal. A careful assessment of the sleep problems is therefore necessary before the most effective solutions can be found. Psychologists or medical professionals who specialize in sleep disorders may be of assistance here.

As the PD progresses, regular reviews of medications by a neurologist who specializes in motor disorders is important, and can lead to a change in medications or a change in the balance of current medications as time goes on. Information about surgical and other non-drug treatments can be provided as they become available, as well as information about research projects that the PD individual may wish to become involved in. Physical and motor difficulties including pain and stiffness can often be alleviated by exercises suggested by a physical therapist, and for some, a regular body massage may offer relief. A visit to an occupational therapist may result in helpful changes to the home or workplace. Sessions with a clinical psychologist who has experience with the PD population can assist with finding ways to cope with or overcome the many psychological problems that go hand in hand with chronic illness generally, and PD in particular. These include depression, poor self-esteem, loss of confidence, and difficulties in personal relationships. Couples therapists and sex therapists with a special interest in physical disability or chronic illness and sexuality may be particularly helpful in addressing the sexual difficulties that can arise from the Parkinsonian symptoms, as well as from the medications, and from a loss of self esteem and confidence resulting from the PD sufferer's perceptions of how he or she may have changed physically. For many individuals with PD, a collaborative relationship with therapists and doctors is often empowering; together they may come up with effective ways of "tricking" the symptoms, dealing with social and workplace discrimination, and sometimes even finding humor in some of the situations PD individuals find themselves in.

Case Presentation

Dr. Robert Jacobs, MD, first admitted to himself that he had some anxiety about the slight tremor that only occasionally plagued his left hand following a lecture he gave to the local Medical Historical Society. This was a group of doctors and other interested health professionals who met monthly to listen to a lecture, usually given by one of the group, on a medical topic or medical figure of historical interest. Robert's lecture was on James Parkinson, the doctor who first described PD in 1817. Robert was strongly left-handed, and during his lecture, he became acutely aware that his left hand was shaking to the extent that he was too embarrassed to hold his laser pointer in it, for fear that his tremor would be transposed to the point of light on the projection screen. As a result, he used the pointer awkwardly in his right hand. On a couple of occasions, however, he forgot, and to his surprise, when he picked up the laser pointer in his left hand, his hand stopped shaking. During the wine and cheese supper following his lecture, he noted that his left hand still shook at times and that he was obliged to bury his hand in his jacket pocket and hold his glass in his right hand.

Driving home later that evening, Robert began to consider the awful possibility that perhaps he was one of the sad cases of "shaking palsy" that James Parkinson had so aptly described and that he himself had spoken about that very evening. On the other hand, he argued with himself that he was only 58 years old, surely somewhat young for PD to strike, and that his tremor, which seemed to have abated by this time, was probably caused by anxiety at having to perform in front of his colleagues. Possibly it was simply a benign familial tremor; he vaguely remembered that his father (who died some years previously) had experienced a problem with a shaking hand. Robert dismissed any possibility that he might have PD and went on with his busy life as a general practitioner, husband, and father of two adult sons.

Nevertheless, every now and then the anxiety would creep back as the spasmodic tremor returned. He noted that it usually occurred at the end of a busy day and, indeed, was usually most apparent when he was not using his hand. About 4 months after his lecture to the Medical Historical Society, his son Peter, who had graduated from Medical School himself 2 years previously, and who was working as a registrar on the neurology ward of the city hospital, joined him one Sunday for a friendly round of golf. Neither man was a serious golfer; they played more to force themselves to take some exercise and to spend some father–son time together. At the ninth hole, Peter broached his concern about his father's tremor. He told Robert that he had been aware of the tremor for some months now and that his mother had also been concerned about Robert. She had told Peter that when she mentioned to Robert that he should perhaps get a check-up, he "bit her head off." Because of his status as a doctor, Peter had been given the short straw and had agreed to raise the issue with his father. As Peter said to his father, he realized that the tremor was probably nothing to worry about and was just another sign of advancing age, but that both he and his mother, Lillian, had also noticed that Robert was a good deal slower in his movements at times than he used to be.

Robert made an effort to listen to his son and not dismiss his concerns, and he said that he would go to his own general practitioner for a check-up when he had time. Peter then played his trump card and said that he had mentioned his concerns to Dr. Bracken, the Senior Neurology Consultant on the ward he worked on, who had a specialist interest in Motor Disorders. Dr. Bracken had suggested that Robert drop into his private rooms the following evening after he had finished his clinic for the day; indeed, he had made an appointment for 7:30 PM, and Robert need only phone in if he really could not make it. Robert was decidedly annoyed by this "going behind his back" but reluctantly agreed to keep the appointment. Peter offered to go with him, but Robert firmly declined that offer.

That evening, after Peter had left, Robert and Lillian had an emotional argument in which he accused her of treating him like a child by talking about him to Peter (and everyone else, he supposed), and Lillian became upset when trying to tell him that he had been snappy and unkind to her lately and that she had had to talk to someone (only Peter) because she was becoming increasingly worried about Robert. An uneasy truce was finally reached, and Robert promised he would pass on everything the neurologist said when he got back from his appointment.

The next evening, he duly showed up at Dr. Bracken's rooms following a reminder call from Peter (which, as Robert told him, he did not require). Robert had meet Dr. Bracken on a couple of occasions in the past but did not really know him. Fortunately, Dr. Bracken had a very easy and relaxing manner and treated Robert more like a colleague than a patient. He began by asking him about his own observations of his tremor and any other symptoms he was aware of and asked what hypotheses Robert had about these symptoms. Robert found himself admitting that he had wondered about early PD but thought that he was too young for this, and that anyway his symptoms were too mild to be used to diagnose PD even if, in time, this is what it turned out to be.

Dr. Bracken agreed that this was a reasonable approach but commented that although 58 years old was quite young for PD, early symptoms could certainly begin to show then. He suggested that even if it were too early to diagnose PD, deciding it might be a possibility could be helpful in a number of ways: It would allay the anxiety attached to trying to suppress his concerns, it would certainly allay his family's anxieties somewhat to know that he was being monitored, and it would allow him to take careful observations of any symptoms, given his own expertise as a doctor. Thus, if it did turn out to be PD, then they could utilize every possible treatment when necessary, but not before necessary. Finally, as a doctor, he would want to be extra careful that he was on top of his job, as PD did result in some cognitive problems in most people. Although this was obviously a worry for Robert, being aware of potential problems would allow him to monitor himself and to do what he could to compensate for mild cognitive deficits if they developed.

Dr. Bracken suggested that he conduct an examination, and then they could discuss his findings. The examination began with a standard neurological assessment of the 12 cranial nerves and Robert's reflexes. Dr. Bracken then assessed Robert's walking and turning both during normal gait (to assess arm swing and stride length) and then walking heel to toe, as well as his standing with eyes closed, to see whether he lost balance when pushed gently on each shoulder (to assess postural stability). Dr. Bracken then asked Robert to close his eyes and hold his arms and hands out steadily in front of him, and then with his eyes open to use the index finger of each hand in turn to touch his own nose and then Dr. Bracken's finger (which he moved to different positions) as fast as possible (to assess tremor and bradykinesia). Dr. Bracken then moved Robert's arms passively back and forth from the elbow (to assess cogwheel rigidity) and asked him to write a few sentences across a page (to assess bradykinesia and micrographia). Robert was finally asked to place pegs in holes in a board as fast as possible, first with the right and then with the left hand (to assess bradykinesia).

By the time the examination was over, Robert was feeling tired and glum, as he could see for himself that all was not normal. Dr. Bracken was straightforward in his summing up and told Robert that he appeared to have Parkinsonian signs restricted to his left side. He had a resting tremor of the left hand, some minor rigidity of his left arm, and a slowed left arm swing when walking. He was considerably slower at placing pegs in the holes with his left hand than with his right hand, even though he was left-handed. On the positive side, Robert had no signs of postural instability or micrographia. Thus, it would appear that he had three of the signs of Stage I PD; that is, unilateral tremor, bradykinesia, and rigidity.

Robert had to agree with Dr. Bracken's conclusion and bravely asked what the next step was. Dr. Bracken said that he thought it best to delay starting medication for as long as possible, but that given Robert's occupation, he would need to monitor his symptoms carefully so that medication could be started if the symptoms began to interfere with his practice. He also suggested that for Robert's peace of mind, and again because of his occupation, he should have a baseline neuropsychological assessment. This would show any obvious cognitive problems that may be of concern for Robert's practice as a doctor but, more important, would also act as a baseline for future assessments.

Robert said he needed time to think about all this and to talk it all over with Lillian and Peter, and that he would get back to Dr. Bracken in a few days and let him know whether he wanted to go ahead with the neuropsychological assessment, as well as his decision about whether he should start his medication now or later. Dr. Bracken agreed that this was a sensible plan and said that Robert should take all the time he needed, that his condition was not such that Dr. Bracken considered there to be any urgency at all.

Robert drove home in a daze and, to his embarrassment, was unable to prevent himself from crying when later that evening he received a very sympathetic hearing from Lillian when he described what Dr. Bracken had found. By the following day Robert felt calmer, but he did become upset again when both his sons came around and he told them of his diagnosis. He waited until the following week before contacting Dr. Bracken and agreeing that he should have a neuropsychological assessment and informing the doctor that he would then decide whether he should begin medication.

The neuropsychological assessment was incredibly difficult for him; though not because he could not do most of the tests quite well—indeed, he thought he performed normally on most of them. The clinical neuropsychologist was a young woman who seemed extremely competent and professional, but nevertheless, she was young enough to be his daughter, and he was acutely aware of his extreme anxiety and that he was profusely perspiring throughout the 2-hour ordeal. His tremor constantly betrayed him, and on one occasion he simply froze and could not complete the simple block design task. When he was asked to copy a complex figure, he lost his way in the maze of lines and became very confused about which line ended where, and he could see by the end that he had made a right muck of his drawing. He felt even more disheartened following his miserable attempt to draw the figure from memory later in the assessment (see Fig. 15-1). He felt happier when given some verbal memory tests, as these did not involve using motor skills, and he felt that he performed reasonably well on these tests. On a test on which he had to sort a stack of cards according to secret and changing rules, he did well for the first few categories but then became increasingly frustrated, as whatever he did the neuropsychologist told him he was wrong. He began to think that it was a trick test designed to see whether he could cope with frustration rather than a test of any cognitive skill. As he said to the neuropsychologist at the end of the session, he felt that many of the tests were hardly a fair test of his thinking abilities, as his tremor and slowness prevented him from demonstrating his cognitive abilities. She agreed that this was an issue and said that when she scored and interpreted the tests she would take this into consideration, and in some cases the test scores would probably be unhelpful. She said that she should be able to get a report written and sent out to him and to Dr. Bracken within a week.

It was a long week for Robert, and he did not feel much better when the report arrived and he read it. It was clearly written and emphasized his very high IQ and excellent cognitive abilities in many areas, especially on what the neuropsychologist called "verbal" subtests. However, the report said that even when the confounding factor of the tremor was taken into consideration, Robert did have some mild impairment on some "Performance" tasks, mainly because he was slower than other people of his age and general intellectual ability. On a test on which Robert had to copy a complex figure, his performance demonstrated that he had possible visuospatial perceptual deficits as well as "executive" deficits, including poor organization and forward planning. This was certainly no surprise to Robert, as he knew he had done badly on that test. Apparently on the card sorting task, also a test of executive functioning, he was unable to change mental set as well as he should be able to. On verbal memory tests, he had performed reasonably well for his age. The neuropsychological report concluded that his mild deficits were consistent with a diagnosis of PD and that his mild to moderate executive difficulties, although probably not a major problem now, should be monitored very carefully over time, given his high-level occupation. The neuropsychologist suggested that it would be wise to consider whether he should continue to work as a sole practitioner and to think about taking on a partner that he could consult with over any difficult or unusual cases.

After discussing the neuropsychological report with Dr. Bracken, Robert decided he should begin L-dopa treatment, as his tremor was beginning to be a problem. This turned out to be the right decision: His symptoms rapidly improved, and he felt much happier about continuing in his practice. With encouragement from Peter, he advertised for a partner, and within 2 months a pleasant young woman doctor joined his practice. As the months went by, Robert became accustomed to the fact that he had PD, and most of the time never gave it a thought. He had a check-up with Dr. Bracken every 3 months, and over the next 4 years, apart from some changes in his medication, felt he was on top of his disease. He learned exactly when he needed to take his L-dopa to perform at his best. He made a decision not to stress himself by giving any more lectures to the Medical Historical Society, but he still enjoyed attending the meetings. He continued to play golf for a few years and actually found that swinging his golf club back and forward helped him overcome his rigidity. He found that family, friends, and colleagues were very understanding and did not make a big issue of his condition. He chose not to go to the local PD support group, as he felt that would only depress him, and he was able to keep up with new research on PD via the Internet and the Medical Library and through Dr. Bracken. His son, Peter, who now worked as a general practitioner in a large community practice, had also developed a special interest in PD, primarily as a result of his father's illness.

A year after his diagnosis, Robert's symptoms had spread to his right side. To control his increasing bradykinesia and rigidity, his medications had to be increased. Robert went through times when he felt depressed. He had been taking Prozac for some years, and this did seem to relieve his depression. A follow-up neuropsychological assessment 2 years after his diagnosis showed to his relief that his visuospatial and executive impairments had not worsened significantly and that his verbal memory was still within normal limits. However, he did give up driving soon after his diagnosis, on finding that he sometimes had difficulty changing traffic lanes when he should. Dr. Bracken had suggested this might be a result of his difficulty in changing mental set.

Robert had ongoing problems with sleeping, mainly because of his inability to move into a comfortable position in bed. He often got stuck in one position and was unable to turn over, or even get out of bed if he needed to in the night. As a result, he occasionally ended up wetting the bed, much to his embarrassment. He and Lillian decided to sleep in separate rooms, so that she could get some sleep, and they had an alarm system installed so that if necessary, Robert could push a button attached to the side of his bed within easy reach of his left hand, and a buzzer would sound in Lillian's room. Lillian coped remarkably well most of the time, although, as it took a lot of strength sometimes to pull or push Robert into a position in which he could start moving again, especially first thing in the morning, before his first dose of L-dopa, she became very tired at times. She also had to suffer considerable frustration when Robert became irrational and illogical during some argument, usually when he was tired. This was a complete "personality" change for Robert, who had previously been a very nonjudgmental person, always ready to listen to the other side of an issue. Dr. Bracken thought that this new inflexibility was also a result of executive problems.

Three years after his diagnosis, Robert and his practice partner took on a third part-time doctor so that Robert could reduce his hours to only 3 hours in the mornings, when he felt at his best. Their receptionist/practice nurse became very skilled at finding out what patients were coming in for and ensuring that Robert saw only those who had straightforward illnesses like colds and flu, or who needed a basic check-up or a repeat prescription for a chronic illness. By this time, his voice had become very quiet, and when he was writing his words became smaller and smaller, until they could hardly be read. Fortunately, writing that was almost impossible to read is fairly standard for doctors, and the local pharmacist was able to interpret most of his scripts.

Of course, Robert knew that this "honeymoon" period of being able to keep his Parkinsonian symptoms under control to a reasonable degree would not last forever, and sure enough, 5 years after his diagnosis, he began to experience one of the worst side effects of L-dopa treatment, the "ON/OFF" syndrome. Some 30 minutes after taking his medication, his arms and head would begin to writhe; these dyskinesias would go on for about 30 minutes. If he were lucky, he would then enjoy about an hour of relative normality, but then his Parkinsonian symptoms would take over, and he often found himself stuck immobile in his chair if he did not take his next dose in time. At this point, he could no longer work as a general practitioner. By now he had reached the age of 63, and because he and Lillian had made considerable efforts to put in place some additional investments when he was diagnosed with PD, he was now in a good financial position to retire. The part-time doctor in the practice was delighted to be able to buy Robert's share of the practice.

Robert was relieved to have the responsibility of the practice off his shoulders, and he now felt able to concentrate on coping with his ever-increasing disability and trying to ensure that he and Lillian also continued to enjoy some social life, as well as enjoy time with their grandchildren. He followed a careful and healthy diet and made an effort to go for a walk every morning before breakfast. Unfortunately, this became increasingly difficult because of his rigidity in the morning, and he found he needed to wait 1 hour after his medication until his dyskinesias abated; he could then go for his walk before his rigidity took over. His walk was more of a shuffle, and often he would end up shuffling faster and faster until he either fell over or collided with a wall. If he were particularly unlucky he would then freeze and have trouble getting up. This resulted in his second son, Jack, joining him every morning for his "walk." By this stage, Robert's interest in surgical treatments for Parkinsonian symptoms began to take dominance in his thoughts.

Dr. Bracken agreed to enroll him in the assessment program for pallidotomy, and to Robert's relief, he was pronounced a suitable candidate. After being on the waiting list for 6 months, his day in the theater finally came, and a right-sided pallidotomy was performed. The results were excellent: Robert's left-sided bradykinesia and rigidity were much reduced, and he was able to reduce his medication so that his ON/OFF syndrome was significantly reduced. Though his voice remained quiet, to Lillian's delight, the operation also improved Robert's ability to show facial expressions; he had had a very wooden face for the last 3 years. Robert now had a slightly lopsided expression, but Lillian thought it very attractive when compared with his previous bland one. To celebrate Robert's newfound mobility, Lillian and Robert embarked on a 2-month trip to England and Ireland, where they visited relatives and, on the whole, had a good time.

One year after the pallidotomy, Dr. Bracken asked Robert whether he would like to try DBS on the left side of his brain to see whether this would reduce his right-sided symptoms. Dr. Bracken was involved in a research trial of DBS of the subthalamic nuclei, which meant that the operation, including the pulse generator and battery, would be funded through the research project. Robert was excited by this, and felt sure that he would be a suitable subject. He gladly underwent the numerous research tests, including another of the dreaded neuropsychological assessments, which demonstrated some worsening of his previous cognitive deficits as well as a new deficit: a mild difficulty with new verbal learning. Fortunately, his cognitive deficits were not considered bad enough to make him ineligible for the research trial, and he soon had his second day in theater. He was well aware that he might suffer some side effects from the DBS and that it might take him a while to get the hang of it. Indeed, he did find that his speech became a little slurred when he turned on the pulse generator, but this was a minor price to pay for the ability he now found he had to "turn off" his tremor and to reduce the bradykinesia and rigidity on his right side simply by waving a magnet (or "magic wand," as Robert called it) across his chest, where the pulse generator was implanted.

Robert was well aware that the positive effects of his two surgical interventions may not last forever and that, in time, his illness would probably result in him becoming wheelchair-bound. However, he felt blessed by the fact that at age 65 years, 7 years after his diagnosis, his cognitive impairments, although certainly more marked than previously, were still largely restricted to visuospatial and mental flexibility problems, with his verbal memory being, in his opinion, not much worse than the memory of many of his friends of advancing age. As far as Robert was concerned, he had not lost the abilities most important for his quality of life: He was still able to enjoy reading, listening to music, playing with his grandchildren, and with careful planning of his medication, even occasionally making love to his wife. And on that positive note, we will leave Robert enjoying his retirement.

Discussion

In my experience, Robert's intelligent and constructive approach to his disease is not uncommon in the PD population. Certainly, as a researcher, PD patients are rewarding to work with. Cutting-edge research on neurosurgical, neural transplant, and genetic engineering techniques designed to alleviate Parkinsonian symptoms and even produce a cure for PD are amongst the most exciting developments in neuroscience today.

There is, of course, a much darker side to PD, as graphically illustrated by the character of Alfred in Franzen's novel *The Corrections* (2001). The unrelenting and ever-worsening symptoms the largely elderly group of people with PD suffers on a daily basis places an enormous burden on families, PD support groups, and health services. The disease is relatively common in both men and women over age 60 years, and thus the enormous effort and substantial funding that is spent on research into finding a cure or at least long-term symptom relief is certainly worthwhile. One does not need a crystal ball to predict that dramatic advances in the treatment and cure of PD will be one of the great medical success stories of the twenty-first century.

In the meantime, less dramatic therapies and rehabilitation strategies have an essential role to play in assisting PD patients in coping with their symptoms. This might involve finding innovative ways to "trick" the mind so that the body performs more fluently, adapting the environment to make living easier, or providing psychological therapy to help patients climb out of depression and find the will to look once again for small pleasures in their daily lives.

PD patients are often distressed by their inability to use their minds to control their bodies. In observing their struggle, we become aware of the beautiful and effortless mind–body synergy in those of us fortunate enough to be in good health. It is easy to understand the feelings of triumph in PD sufferers like Ivan (Vaughan 1986) when they find ways of using their mind to "trick" their body into performing normally. The task of neuroscientists and medical researchers of PD is to reconnect the mind and body and, perhaps in doing so, to discover another piece of the puzzle that, when complete, will tell us how our mind/brain works.

16
■

HUNTINGTON'S DISEASE

A FAMILY CHALLENGED

Huntington's disease is the focus of one of the most remarkable stories of discovery in medical history. In 1872, George Huntington, a North American general practitioner, published the first unambiguous description of this unrelenting neurodegenerative disorder in *The Medical and Surgical Reporter* (Huntington 1872). The title of his article was simply "On Chorea," and his description of this type of chorea as a specific hereditary disorder became quickly and widely accepted and became known as *Huntington's disease* (HD). HD is a chronic, progressive hereditary disease, usually of adult onset, and is typified by a number of motor abnormalities, most obviously the excessive, spontaneous irregular movements called chorea, but also other motor disorders such as rigidity. Accompanying these motor disorders is a range of psychiatric, behavioral and cognitive disturbances and a progressive decline to a severe dementia is almost inevitable if the patient lives long enough.

Huntington's description classified HD as a disorder fitting the criteria for Mendelian autosomal dominant inheritance, although Mendelian genetics, first published in 1866, went unnoticed until 1900. Autosomal dominant inheritance is marked by a number of criteria as follows: equal incidence in both sexes, equal transmission by both sexes, 50% of the offspring of an HD parent will become affected if they live long enough, offspring who do not develop HD by old age will not pass on HD to their descendants. HD generally fits these criteria, although as more is discovered about the genetics of this disorder, and especially about borderline cases, in which an individual carries an intermediate allele, it has become apparent that there are slight variations.

One of the pivotal reasons for the rapid advance of knowledge about HD is the genuinely collaborative research effort spanning, in particular, the United States, United Kingdom, and Europe. This collaboration resulted in the identification and isolation of the HD gene and mutation and in the ability to predict, with a high level of certainty, which asymptomatic members of a family with HD will go on to develop the disease. The continuation of these collaborative research efforts will undoubtedly result in better treatments for HD symptoms, the ability to delay the onset of the disease in those who carry the HD mutation, and ultimately a cure or an ethically and culturally acceptable means of preventing the disease from continuing its destructive path down through the generations.

In common with a number of other medical conditions, the stimulus for setting up research and support institutions came initially from individuals who had themselves been personally affected by HD. *The Hereditary Disease Foundation* was initiated by Dr. Milton Wexler after his wife died from HD. This foundation, which promotes research into HD, was continued by Milton Wexler's daughter, Dr. Nancy Wexler. The foundation has played a central role in the remarkable Venezuela project. The study of the large HD population living by the shores of Lake Maracaibo in Venezuela is the best example of how quickly a dominantly inherited genetic disorder can take over a small, isolated community; in this study, stemming from one ancestor with HD, there are about 7000 members in the genealogy, with 100 living members symptomatic for HD. This detailed and unique geneology was a crucial factor in locating and isolating the HD gene and mutation. A book giving the background to this project and describing the activities of the Hereditary Disease Foundation from the Wexler family perspective has been written by another Wexler family member, Alice Wexler (Wexler 1995).

Some 10 years after the gene involved in HD was initially localized by a Boston research group led by Gusella, and including Nancy Wexler (Gusella et al. 1983), the HD gene and mutation was isolated by Gusella and his colleagues, and their findings were published by the Huntington's Disease Collaborative Research Group (1993). This group was a collaboration of six U.S. and British research teams, and although Gusella's team isolated the gene, the credit was rightly given to the entire collaborative group, as the research leading to the gene isolation was an essential aspect of the discovery and a truly collaborative effort (Harper and Morris 1996).

HD is more than a gene mutation: It is a family matter that challenges families in every way. Not only do all family members have to live for many years with the knowledge that they might develop the disease, they must also watch and care for their grandparents, parents, and sometimes their children as they struggle through the stages of HD. The physical, psychological, social, and economic stresses on all members of an HD family are enormous and unrelenting. The experience of these stresses had a major effect on Marjorie Guthrie, the wife and later the widow of the iconic American folk singer, Woody Guthrie, who developed HD symptoms around 1952 and died in 1967 at the age of 55 years. Following Woody's death Marjorie Guthrie founded the *Committee to Combat Huntington's Disease* (CCHD) in 1967. The aim of this American committee was to promote services for families and to promote education and research. In 1978, it led to the formation of the *International Huntington's Association*, which now includes at least 27 member countries (Harper and Morris 1996).

Theoretical Background

General Characteristics of HD

HD is equally common in men and women. The mean age of onset of HD is between 35 and 44 years, although diagnosis is frequently 8–10 years after onset. In 5%–10% of cases, onset takes place before the age of 20 years and can occur as early as 4 years of age. This is called Juvenile HD and it usually includes, from the early stages, rigidity, hypokinesia, and seizures, as well as choreic movements. Juvenile HD can occur within a typical HD family. Death in the more common midlife onset cases usually occurs around 50–60 years of age, so survival length after onset is about 13–17 years. In about 20% of cases, the onset of HD is after 50 years and can happen as late as 84 years of age (Brinkman, Mezei, Theilmann, Almqvist, and Hayden 1997), and very late onset cases often present with chorea only and relatively little other disability. These patients may remain reasonably intellectually intact and with minimal motor disability until their death.

HD can be divided into three clinical stages, each lasting about 5 years. In stage 1, the patient develops neurological or psychiatric symptoms. Chorea is more prominent than other motor symptoms, and the effect of these symptoms on the individual's independence is minor. The main burden on the family at this time is likely to be a result of psychological or psychiatric problems, if the individual suffers from these. Death is rare, other than suicide. In stage 2, the motor disorder becomes more generalized, with major physical disability usually including rigidity as well as chorea, and the individual becomes dependent on others for many activities. The physical strain and psychological distress suffered by family and caregivers during this stage can be great and are largely a consequence of the physical and psychiatric problems displayed by the patient. Deaths during this stage are not uncommon and usually result from apparently unrelated causes (e.g., accidents, other health problems). In Stage 3, the patient is severely physically disabled and demented and is, thus, totally dependent. Death may occur at any time and is often the result of a combination of weight loss, immobility, a tendency to aspirate food, and an increased vulnerability to pneumonia, cardiovascular disease, and other diseases.

Molecular Genetics of HD

Every cell in the human body has 35,000 genes that instruct the cells to make specific proteins. In about 9999 people out of every 10,000, the Huntington's gene fulfills a useful purpose, but in 1 out of 10,000 cases, the gene carries a mutation that results in the production of a toxic protein in the striatum, which kills the cells of the striatum. Detailed descriptions of the genetics of HD are well beyond the scope of this book, but following is a simplified summary of the current knowledge of the main genetic research findings.

From the original description of Huntington in 1872, it was clear that HD was an autosomal dominant hereditary disorder. Careful pedigrees of generations of HD families around the world confirmed this and demonstrated that 50% of the children of a parent with HD would develop HD if they lived long enough. (See Fig. 16-1 for a typical HD genealogical family tree, or *genogram*). This occurs because each child inherits one copy of a gene pair (each gene of the pair is called an allele) from each parent, and in most cases the HD-affected parent carries the HD mutation on only one of the alleles of the pair of genes (i.e., the parent is heterozygous for the HD gene mutation). Thus, each child has an equal or 50% chance of inheriting either the gene with the HD mutation or the normal gene. If the HD gene and mutation are inherited, the child will also be heterozygous for the HD gene and mutation, will inevitably develop HD if she lives long enough, and will in turn have a 50% chance of passing on her HD gene and mutation to her own child. That is, HD appears to be close to 100% penetrant, given that penetrance is defined as the proportion of individuals with a specified genotype (e.g., the HD gene and mutation) who show the expected phenotype (e.g., the symptoms of HD), under a defined set of environmental conditions (e.g., living the normal expected life span). In rare cases, there may be individuals who are homozygous for the HD gene; that is, they carry two alleles of the HD gene and mutation, and thus always pass one allele with the mutation onto their children. A number of homozygous HD individuals are found among the Venezuela HD community, in which interbreeding between people with HD has been occurring for many generations. Interestingly, the homozygous individuals' HD symptoms and disease progress appears to be no more severe than the disease of the more common heterozygous HD individuals (Wexler, Young, and Tanzi 1987).

Before the HD gene and mutation itself was localized, there was a major research breakthrough in 1983, when a genetic marker for the HD gene was discovered (Gusella et al. 1983). A genetic marker is a gene located close to the HD gene on the chromosome, which therefore has a much higher than 50% chance of being coinherited, along with the HD gene, by the offspring. The marker, G8, was a functionless piece of DNA, detecting several "restriction fragment length polymorphisms," and was found first in a group of American families with HD and was confirmed by the finding that it was also present in the much larger Venezuelan HD group (Gusella et al. 1983). This discovery of a close linkage to HD led to the possibility of presymptomatic testing of asymptomatic members of an HD family and to prenatal diagnosis of at-risk pregnancies.

Following a great deal more collaborative work, a mutation in the form of a trinucleotide CAG repeat (i.e., a triplet code of the three bases of cytosine [C], adenine [A], and guanine [G]) on a novel gene in the IT15 region of chromosome 4 was identified. The CAG repeat also showed variation of repeat length in the normal population, but what was of significance was the discovery that all patients with HD showed expansion of the repeat CAG sequence, indicating that this expansion on this gene was the causative mutation involved in HD. This historical finding was published, under the leadership of Gusella, by the Huntington's Disease Collaborative Research Group (1993). This research and further research since have demonstrated that in people without HD, the CAG repeat ranges from 6 to 35, with 99% of this group having fewer than 30 repeats. In people with HD, CAG repeats generally range from 36 to 66, with some repeats up to 100 or more in cases with juvenile onset. A small number of individuals who are at risk for inheriting HD and who have CAG repeats falling in the borderline range of 36–41 (labeled an *intermediate allele,* as carriers might or might not go onto develop HD) are problematic for diagnostic testing. In this range, it appears that penetrance is less than 100%, with penetrance increasing as CAG repeat-length increases, such that penetrance is less than 90% for 39 CAG repeats and 99% for 41 CAG repeats (Brinkman et al. 1997).

Analysis of a large cohort of over 1000 HD-affected and asymptomatic at-risk people demonstrated that as the CAG repeat length increased, there was a significant increase in the probability of onset by a certain age, with the median age of onset decreasing by 3.4 years for each CAG length increase in the 39–50 repeat range. As an example, 50% of people with a CAG repeat length of 40 will be affected by the age of 59 years, whereas the age of onset will be 37 years for 50% of people with a CAG repeat length of 45. The individual with 46 CAG repeats has a 100% chance of onset by age 45 years (Brinkman et al. 1997). However, as the range of age of onsets for a specific CAG repeat size is broad (Brinkman et al. 1997), and CAG repeat length accounts for only half the variance in age of onset (Andrew, Goldberg, and Hayden 1997) it is recommended that these figures not be used to predict the age of onset for individual patients. However, these data could provide asymptomatic people who carry the HD mutation with estimates of the amount of time they might reasonably expect to have before the onset of symptoms. In addition, these data might be used as a measure of success of future clinical drug trials aimed at delaying onset of HD symptoms.

Another problem for predictive diagnosis using molecular genetics is that the number of CAG repeats can increase or sometimes decrease when passed onto the next generation. Thus, very rarely, a parent with only 40 CAG repeats may never develop HD, but the HD gene inherited by his or her child may mutate to 42 repeats, a CAG repeat size with 100% penetrance, meaning that the child will, at some point, develop HD.

Neuropathology of HD

Before the availability of a specific molecular genetics predictive test for HD, neuropathology was the accepted gold standard for its firm diagnosis. The primary anatomic finding is a generalized shrinkage of the brain with preferential atrophy of the caudate nucleus and putamen, structures in the corpus striatum (Folstein 1989). There may also be atrophic changes in cerebellum and thalamic nuclei, as well as cortical changes, especially as the disease progresses. Neurotransmitter level alterations accompany the basal ganglia degeneration, including reduced levels of the inhibitory neurotransmitter, GABA (gamma aminobutyric acid) (Folstein 1989), and an increase in excitatory neurotransmitters, which can have a neurotoxic effect at concentrated levels (Nutt 1989). In addition to the severe motor disorders resulting from the striatum cell loss, an important consequence of these neuropathological changes is that fronto-striatal circuits are damaged, which results in various disorders of executive functioning, such as difficulties in switching mental set. As the disease progresses, so does the damage to these fronto-striatal circuits, and in addition, cortical atrophy, especially to the frontal lobes, results in ever-worsening executive impairments.

As HD patients with the typical neuropathological changes almost invariably have the HD gene mutation, the molecular predictive test offered to asymptomatic people at risk of HD can be considered highly accurate; that is; if the individual has the HD gene and mutation of 42 CAG repeats or more, he has a 100% risk of developing HD. Conversely, if he has 35 or fewer CAG repeats, he will not develop HD, nor can he pass HD on to his descendants.

Epidemiology

The prevalence of HD varies from country to, country and even within countries, and ranges from a low level of 0.38 per 100,000 population in Japan (Kishimoto, Naka-mura, and Sotokawa 1957) to 10 times that in most populations of European origin. In the United Kingdom, prevalence rates vary depending on the locality, with, for example, high prevalence figures for south Wales and northeast Scotland (8.85 and 9.95 per 100,000 population respectively), around 4.6 to 5.5 per 100,000 for much of the United Kingdom, but with a prevalence as low as 2.5 per 100,000 in Essex in the southeast of England (Harper 1996). In the United States, prevalence rates again differ depending on locality. One of the most reliable studies reports rates of 5.15 per 100,000 in Maryland, with white Americans having a slightly lower prevalence (4.94) than black Americans (6.37) (Folstein, Chase, Wahl, McDonnell, and Folstein 1987). Interestingly, it appears that HD in American blacks is long-standing and can rarely be traced back to the admixture of Caucasian genes; rather, it may be largely of African origin in this population (Folstein et al. 1987; Harper 1996). As described earlier, in the large HD population living by the shores of Lake Maracaibo in Venezuela, there are about 7000 members in the HD pedigree, with 100 living members symptomatic for HD.

All cases of HD worldwide are the result of the same mutational mechanism: an identical type of CAG repeat expansion. It seems likely that all cases of HD arose originally from the small proportion of individuals who carry the intermediate allele; that is, a borderline number of CAG repeats. The length of these repeats gradually increases over many generations, until the number of repeats falls within the clinical range and results in overt HD. Once the HD gene and mutation is in the population, it can be spread by migration of HD carriers to other localities. There is, however, no requirement to use migration as the explanation for the distribution of HD across the world (Harper 1996).

Neurological Symptoms of HD

Chorea is the most common and prominent symptom and is usually among the earliest symptoms to develop. Lakke (1981), on behalf of the World Federation of Neurology, defined it as a state of excessive, spontaneous, random, and abrupt movements, with a range of severity from restlessness with mild, intermittent exaggeration of gesture and expression; fidgeting movements of the hands; and an unstable, dancelike gait, to a continuous flow of disabling, violent movements.

Other motor abnormalities include dystonias, which are sustained muscle contractions, that often cause twisting and repetitive movements and abnormal postures, and muscle rigidity, as seem in Parkinson's disease (PD)(see Chapter 15). Rigidity is a major feature of advanced HD and also appears early in juvenile HD. Bradykinesia (a slowness of movement), one of the main symptoms of PD, is frequent later in the course of the illness but also can be observed early in the disease, even when the main sign is chorea. Freezing can occur in HD patients with bradykinesia. Gait abnormalities are obvious in patients who have had HD for some years. Those with chorea have a wide-based staggering gait.

Eye movement abnormalities occur early in disease in the majority of patients and gradually worsen. Patients have difficulty in initiating saccades within the field of vision and a decrease in saccade velocity. They are often unable to suppress blinks and head movements during saccades, and the accuracy of saccades is also impaired, resulting in undershooting of the target.

Dysarthria (speech distortion) is common, and early in the disease, the rate and rhythm of speech is often abnormal and worsens until speech becomes unintelligible. Some patients become mute before their motor disability is very severe.

Dysphagia is another distressing and common symptom, and can involve multiple abnormalities of ingestion, including inappropriate selection of food and inappropriate rate of eating, retention of food in the mouth after swallowing, regurgitation, choking and asphyxia.

In the later stages of HD, serious weight loss and loss of muscle bulk occurs in spite of an adequate diet and feeding. This is not the result of the hyperkinesia (excess movement) and appears to be an integral aspect of HD, the cause of which is not understood.

Choreic movements largely cease during sleep. In the later stages of HD, the patient may be sleepy during the day and wakeful at night. About 20% of HD patients become incontinent in the terminal stages of the illness. Epilepsy occurs in 1%–3% of adults with HD, and at a much higher frequency in juvenile HD.

Psychiatric Symptoms

Nearly all patients with HD experience psychiatric symptoms, with some research as well as anecdotal reports indicating that in up to 79% of patients, such symptoms may precede chorea and other motor symptoms (Morris 1991). Rates of depression are very high in HD patients, varying from 9% to 44%. Depression is especially prominent in the early stage of HD, when the patient is fully aware of his condition and of his grim and unalterable prognosis, and there is some evidence that depression may precede the symptoms of HD. However, other studies do not support depression as a predictor of HD (Morris and Scourfield 1996). Suicide rates are higher than in the healthy population; around 5.7% in one U.S. study, compared with 1.5% for the healthy population (Morris and Scourfield 1996).

Many other psychiatric and behavioral problems are common, with one study of 52 HD patients finding that 98% of the cohort had exhibited at least one such symptom in the previous month (Paulsen, Ready, Hamilton, Mega, and Cummings 2001). Dysphoria, agitation, irritability, apathy, anxiety, disinhibition, and euphoria (in order of decreasing frequency) were experienced by 30%–69% of HD patients. Delusions, aberrant motor behavior, and hallucinations were found in only 1.9%–11.5% of patients. Interestingly, the dementia severity, chorea severity, and disease duration were not significantly correlated with any neuropsychiatric symptom. Another study of 82 HD patients (Thompson, Snowden, Craufurd, and Neary 2002) does not entirely agree with the findings of the Paulsen et al. (2001) study. In Thompson et al.'s (2002) study, depression and irritability did not correlate significantly with functional capacity, motor impairment, or cognitive impairment, but the measure of apathy did. As the authors point out, it is not surprising that apathy correlates with cognitive function, given that apathy can be viewed as an executive disorder, or at least as exacerbating some of the common executive problems seen in HD. For example, reduced activity and initiative could influence forward planning and goal-directed behavior. Most studies do concur with the finding that depression and irritability, both common features of HD, do not develop in a linear fashion as the disease progresses. It may be that other factors, including premorbid personality characteristics, also contribute to the presence and severity of affective symptoms. In addition, as the patient becomes more demented and loses insight, apathy may increase and depression decrease.

Other symptoms that cause concern for families, and that probably often arise from the psychiatric symptoms already mentioned, include moodiness, aggression, violent behaviors, hypersexuality, paranoid suspicions, lying, stealing, a loss of interest in personal appearance, marked self-neglect, and mutism.

Cognitive Impairments in HD

A review article by Brown and Marsden (1988) examined the neuropsychological evidence for HD and for PD with dementia, belonging in a category called the "subcortical dementias," in contrast to Alzheimer's disease, which should fall in a separate "cortical dementia" category. Brown and Marsden concluded that the three disorders shared many characteristics in common and that, although each pair of disorders displayed some similarities and some differences, the similarities between PD and HD did not outweigh the similarities between any other pairs. However, the review was based on the accumulated evidence of a large number of studies with different methodologies, and in which the participants were in different stages of their disease progression. It is perhaps not surprising that HD overlaps with both PD and AD because, although it begins with primarily a subcortical atrophy, as the disease progresses, generalized atrophy of the brain and especially the frontal lobes occurs. Brown and Marsden (1988) did emphasize the similarities between PD and HD with respect to some of the executive difficulties they experienced, as well as some differences in HD, including a deficit in skill learning–not found in PD–and severe memory deficits, which are more similar to those seen in AD rather than PD.

The damage to fronto-striatal circuits in HD supports the finding that the earliest and most prominent cognitive impairments are frontally mediated executive problems and problems associated with basal ganglia dysfunction. In early HD, a pattern of impairments including a difficulty in planning ahead, difficulty in switching mental set, impaired pattern recognition memory (Lawrence et al. 1996), and impaired facial recognition (Jacobs, Shuren, and Heilman 1995) has been found. The two latter impairments are thought to be caused by damage to the ventrocaudal striatum, whereas the impairment in switching mental set is likely to be a result of dysfunctional fronto-striatal circuits.

The cognitive impairments worsen and gradually extend to affect many areas of cognition as the atrophy of both subcortical and cortical structures becomes more widespread. Neuropsychological testing becomes increasingly difficult, and probably pointless, as the motor symptoms, and psychiatric and behavioral problems, especially apathy, increase. Thus even by stage 2, neuropsychological testing may be limited to gathering a gross measure of deterioration with the use of dementia scales, and by stage 3, the patient is severely demented and may remain so for 5 or more years, until released by death.

Behavioral Assessment of HD

Motor abnormalities, psychiatric symptoms, cognitive impairments, and functional capacity (activities of daily living) require assessment at regular intervals to plan and provide the best treatment possible. Motor impairment can be assessed using the motor examination from the Unified Huntington's Disease Rating Scale (UHDRS; Huntington Study Group 1996), which allows standardized ratings of oculomotor function, dysarthria, chorea, dystonia, gait, and postural stability.

Psychiatric problems can be assessed by instruments used more generally for assessment of psychiatric patients, or an instrument specifically designed for HD can be used. An example of such a scale is the Problem Behaviors Assessment for Huntington's Disease (PBA-HD) (Thompson et al. 2002). This semistructured interview includes 40 items covering a wide range of behaviors and is scored in a similar way to the UHDRS, with each item given a separate severity and frequency rating. As it covers a wider range of behaviors than the behavioral assessment section of the UHDRS, the interview can be used instead of this section of the UHDRS. The items can be categorized into three subscales, Apathy, Irritability, and Depression, which cover the main problem areas experienced by HD patients.

Functional capacity can be assessed by any number of activities of daily living scales, or again by an instrument designed specifically for HD patients. One such scale is the HD Functional Capacity Scale (Shoulson and Fahn 1979), which yields scores in the range of 0–13, with lower scores indicating greater impairment.

Cognitive assessment should be carried out by a neuropsychologist and, in the early stages, should include a broad battery such as the Wechsler scales, with additional executive function tests. Dementia screens commonly used include the Mini-Mental State Examination (Folstein, Folstein, and McHugh 1975) and the Mattis Dementia Rating Scale (Mattis 1976).

Genetic Counseling and Predictive Tests in HD

Genetic counseling has been a central aspect of the management of HD for many years. Well before it was possible to predict whether an individual member of a family carried the HD gene and mutation, some asymptomatic family members wanted to know what their chances were of developing HD. With the isolation of the Huntington's gene and mutation, and the development of an accurate molecular genetic predictive test, genetic counseling has become extremely important (Harper, Houlihan, and Tyler 1996; Smith et al. 1998). Various bodies have established (and revised) guidelines to assist professionals with the complex processes and decisions that must be made when deciding whether or not to go ahead with predictive tests for HD when some of the family members who will be affected disagree with the person asking for the test (International Huntington Association and World Federation of Neurology 1994; Smith et al. 1998).

Counseling ideally involves two or more interviews spread out over a number of weeks or months to ensure that the individual has plenty of time to carefully consider all the implications of predictive testing (Harper, Soldan, and Tyler 1996). In the interviews, the counselor must ascertain that the at-risk individual's reasons for wanting the predictive test are acceptable, as well as feel confident that the implications of taking a predictive test are fully understood. For example, if the at-risk person is likely to be at risk of suicide, severe depression, or some other mental illness if the result shows that he has the HD gene mutation, then predictive testing is unlikely to be carried out. The individual must understand that if he is found to have the HD gene and mutation, there is no cure currently—or in the foreseeable future—and he will go on to develop HD.

Some laboratories will only test people with a 50% risk; that is, people who have one parent with clear HD symptoms. To establish level of risk, a careful genogram must be established, which is sometimes difficult if parents and grandparents have died before HD being diagnosed, or cousins do not want to be involved, or the at-risk individual was adopted. Most individuals who want predictive testing are asymptomatic children of a parent with HD, who want to know whether they carry the gene so that the risks for their children, already born or as yet unborn, may be estimated. On occasion parents want to have their young children tested for the gene, but many genetic laboratories decline to do this, as it would remove the ability of the child to decide for himself, when older, whether or not he wishes to know his status. Social workers may also request testing of children of HD families who are available for adoption, but for the same reasons, many genetic laboratories refuse to do this. Adolescents who request predictive testing should be given extensive counseling, as a test result that is positive for HD could be more devastating to them than living with a 50% risk of developing HD—but perhaps not until late middle age—would be. In many cases, counseling and support might be all the adolescent requires, given the knowledge that at a later stage he or she could request predictive testing.

Prenatal predictive testing can be carried out at 9–12 weeks on the unborn fetus, usually because the parents wish to be fully informed before deciding whether to abort the fetus, which they consider they would almost certainly do if the fetus were found to carry the HD gene and mutation. If the fetus tested positive for the HD gene mutation and was not aborted, this could cause an ethical dilemma, as the child would grow up without the right not to know his HD status. A recent development in preventing the birth of babies with the HD gene mutation is to inject a number of the father's sperm into a number of the mother's eggs in a laboratory and to test each resulting embryo immediately. Those carrying the HD gene mutation are discarded, and an embryo without the HD mutation is planted in the mother's womb. This technology is controversial given criticisms that it could lead to "designer babies," although as the advocates of this technology for preventing HD point out, in predictive HD testing of embryos, neither the sex of the embryo or any other genetically mediated characteristics are tested for.

Counselors need to ensure that the individual requesting predictive testing has not been coerced into this by other well-meaning relatives. For example, parents or grandparents may believe that young adults at risk should establish their HD status before marriage or having children. Many young adults do not want to risk knowing their status and possibly constraining their future prospects in relation to marriage, children, employment, health insurance, and psychological well-being.

Test results should be given at a face-to-face meeting, preferably with a support person also present and at a prearranged meeting time, so that the individual is not on tenterhooks waiting for the telephone call or letter announcing that the result is in. One or more follow-up meetings some weeks or even months after the predictive test results have been given to the individual are essential, as this be a difficult time not only for those who have the HD gene mutation but sometimes also for those who find they do not carry the gene. In both cases, a major adjustment is necessary, from living with terrible uncertainty, to living with the knowledge that either you will or will not develop HD, while other family members remain at risk. This latter situation can lead to survivor guilt and a heavy involvement with the affected relatives, sometimes to the serious detriment of the "lucky" individual's own life style. Some individuals who find they do not carry the HD gene mutation suffer a loss of identity with their extended family, where many members either have HD or are at risk of developing it.

A difficult situation can arise when an individual with a 25% risk requests predictive testing. This could be the grandchild of an HD grandparent, whose own parent has not yet developed HD but may do in the future. The parent may not want to know whether she carries the HD gene mutation, but if her child is found to carry it, this will mean that the parent also carries it. Such cases need to be treated on a case-by-case basis, as often careful counseling of both generations including full explanations of the implications will gradually resolve the issue one way or another. (Fig. 16-1 is a *genogram* that includes individuals with different levels of risk of HD.)

A compromise is to carry out exclusion testing by genetic linkage. In this situation, the individual at 25% risk (which could be a fetus) is tested to see whether the gene linked to the HD gene received from her at-risk parent comes from her affected HD grandparent or from her unaffected grandparent. If the latter is the case, then her risk of developing HD is negligble, whereas if she has the linked gene from her affected grandparent, her risk increases from 25% to 50%. Her parent's risk remains at 50%. This, of course, does not mean that she has the HD gene and mutation, as she may have inherited the normal allele from their affected grandparent (as may her parent), but at least this does not alter the risk from 50% for the parent who does not want more information, and of course, for the third-generation party, it may result in the new and welcome knowledge that she almost certainly has not inherited the HD gene and mutation from her affected grandparent.

Confidentiality is of utmost importance in predictive testing. Some individuals do not want anyone to know, not even their partner or doctor. Clearly, there are possible implications of knowing one has the HD gene and mutation that affect employment and health insurance.

Management and Therapy

There is no cure for HD, and where necessary, pharmacological treatments are used to manage the various symptoms, such as chorea. For chorea, a range of neuroleptic drugs which block central dopamine receptors may be used; haloperidol in low doses is effective for many patients. However, drug treatment should be avoided for as long as possible because of its considerable side effects, including rigidity. There are few studies on drug treatment for rigidity in HD. Depression is often alleviated by SSRIs (Selective Serotonin Reuptake Inhibitors) that selectively block the reabsorption of the brain chemical serotonin. These drugs are preferred by many experienced HD clinicians over the tricyclic antidepressants, as the SSRIs have fewer side effects. Wherever possible, psychological therapy and supportive counseling should be tried first (or in tandem with drug therapy). HD patients who become acutely psychotic should have a full psychiatric assessment carried out before any antipsychotic drugs or other drugs are prescribed. Delirium, which can be misdiagnosed as psychosis, can occur in HD, and needs to be excluded as a diagnosis.

There are no medications that have been proven to be effective for the memory and other cognitive impairments of HD. As is the case for other neurogenerative conditions, memory aids can be helpful, as can behavioral techniques to assist with executive problems of disorganization, disinhibition, and physical aggression. For severe behavior problems common in HD, the appropriate medication in the appropriate dosages can sometimes make an enormous difference. For example, antiepileptic medications carefully titrated and monitored by a neurologist with expertise in HD treatment can sometimes result in an agitated, violent, disinhibited patient becoming calm, happy, and clear-headed, whereas medicating the patient with antipsychotics might reduce the difficult behaviors but result in an apathetic and "drugged" patient.

Whether at home or in an institution, a stable environment with regular routines, reduction of environmental stimuli, avoidance of direct confrontation, and clear, simple explanations of activities and changes in routine can all help the patient manage his or her problematical behaviors. Physiotherapists, dietitians, speech pathologists (for help with communication problems), and occupational therapists (for help with activities of daily living) can all assist in disease management.

HD individuals may be able to remain at home for longer periods of time with the assistance of outreach HD workers with expertise and long experience working with HD families. This is especially important for families living in towns and rural areas without ready access to HD specialists. Home care attendants, meals on wheels, adaptations to the home environment as physical disabilities worsen, day care programs, and time out for the family by admitting the HD individual to a respite nursing home for short stays on a regular basis are all helpful. Volunteer HD support groups can provide information and support for the HD sufferer, at-risk family members, and caregivers. An empathic and knowledgeable general practitioner can be a very important member of the HD sufferer's support team. In large cities, families should ensure they find a neurologist with specialist knowledge of HD, as this is a rare disorder, and general practitioners and even most neurologists will have had only limited opportunity to learn about and keep up-to-date on the complex requirements of patients with this disorder.

Many HD families become involved in research, which can provide them with stimulation, information about the latest studies, and even personal support. For many families, to participate in the amazing HD research endeavors that have continued for many years now is one of the few positive aspects of living with this tragic condition. The best example of this must surely be Nancy Wexler, who has become a major figure in HD research. As a young woman with a 50% risk of developing HD, she became a central figure in the Hereditary Disease Foundation and the remarkable Venezuela research project, started by her father, Dr. Milton Wexler. She must surely be the ultimate example of a person who turns a personal tragedy into a fulfilling and magnificent ambition (Wexler 1979; Wexler 1995).

Research to find a cure for HD focuses on trying to find a way (perhaps a drug) to turn the mutant gene off and stop it producing the toxic protein that kills off the striatal cells. Other research avenues include looking at ways to inject growth factors into the brain to block the toxic protein's effects and inducing stem cells to divide and grow into new striatal cells that can then be used to replace the cells that have been lost.

Case Study

Background

I have known Christine, her husband Stephen, and her three children for more than 25 years. At 58 years of age, Christine still has the same clear olive skin she had at 30 years, her face remains unlined, and her brown eyes and warm smile convey a sense of serenity and well-being. She is physically fit, swimming and walking most days, and she and her husband fit their many and varied social and recreational activities around their busy working professional lives, Christine as a general medical practitioner, and Stephen as an architect.

Thus, if you met Christine, you would be excused for thinking she must have enjoyed a good life with little to worry her. You would be very wrong. Christine is the daughter of a father who died of HD and the elder sister of two brothers, both of whom died from the complications of HD before they reached 50 years of age—her youngest brother dying less than a year ago. Christine and her younger sister, Sara, have shown no signs whatsoever of HD as yet, and as they get older, they perhaps allow themselves to feel a little more hopeful that they do not harbor the HD gene. For Christine, with three adult children of her own, her concern is for them rather than for herself, especially as they form long-term relationships with decisions of their own to make about whether to have children. (See Fig. 16-1 for a genogram of Christine's family.)

Christine does not talk to friends about her experiences with HD, as she discovered early on that few people can really comprehend this dreadful disease and the sword it suspends above every member of the family. She and her family cope by putting enormous energy into those aspects of their lives not controlled by HD and, as a consequence, have traveled widely and had many amazing adventures. When Christine heard I was revising this book and planned to include a chapter on HD, she spontaneously and very generously offered to share her painful experiences of HD with me. As she said, although she did not want to write her story herself, she has had 40 years of personal experience of HD as well as becoming a "walking encyclopedia" on the medical aspects of the disorder, and if her story could help readers understand a little better how HD affects families, that would be worthwhile.

Hearing her painful story was a humbling experience, and it is not possible to do it justice in a short case study. Rather, I have tried to convey some of the most salient aspects of her story illustrated by "incidences" that, as Christine said, are very typical

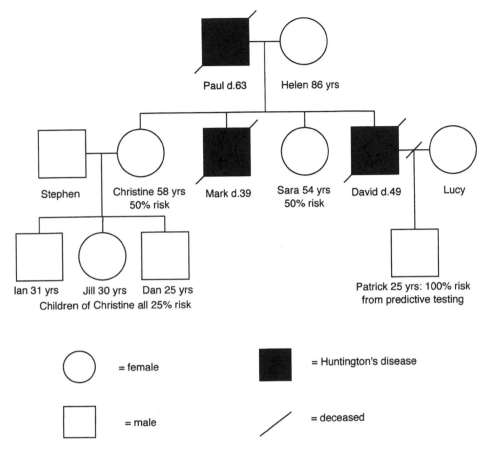

Figure 16-1 A *genogram* (genealogical family tree) of Christine's immediate family, showing members who have died of HD and the risk levels for their descendants.

of the experiences of many HD families. Of course identifying details have been changed, but I have retained Christine's profession as a medical practitioner, as it is clear that this has allowed her to understand the medical aspects of HD better than a layperson might, and it has also enabled her to cope with the many medical emergencies that are part and parcel of HD.

Christine's Family

Paul   Christine's father, Paul, was born in 1915, the eldest of four brothers. When Paul was 16 years old his father, who was still only in his early 40s, died from malaria that he had contracted as a young man working in New Guinea. In retrospect, at the time of his death there was some indication of possible neurological problems, but his death certificate gave malaria as the cause of death. The family was poor, and

Paul's widowed mother struggled to bring up four boys. Paul soon became the bread-winner and the surrogate "father" for his younger brothers. He trained as a teacher while working part-time to support his mother and brothers, and when he was 25 years old, he married Helen, a trainee teacher at his school. When World War II was declared, he went to war and was invalided out in 1943 with a badly damaged leg. Paul and Helen's first child, Christine, was born in 1945, followed by the births of Mark in 1949, Sara in 1951, and David in 1954.

On returning from the war, Paul decided to retrain as architect, which he did by attending university part-time while still working as a teacher. By the time Christine was 8 years old, Paul had earned a reputation as one of the most sought-after architects in the large Australian city where they lived. The family's lifestyle had improved rapidly, and they now lived in a beautiful home with large gardens overlooking a river. Helen remained at home to care for the four children, and Paul was a wonderful father. Christine's memories of her childhood are, to this day, very precious, not only because of the happiness she remembers but also because of the normality of her childhood. Paul had an enormous love and knowledge of the wilderness and would take his whole family camping and hiking in the Australian bush for 3 weeks of every year. The family also traveled to England and Europe on two extended trips. At home, Paul was well ahead of his time; cooking meals in the weekends, washing dishes, and taking his wife away for a week of golfing or skiing at least once a year. Christine remembers him as the rock of the family, emotionally very warm and loving, free-spirited, and full of energy and joy.

When Christine was about 17 and her father was in his late 40s, Paul's personality began to change. He became increasingly solitary and began to withdraw from his friends and even from his family. Most obvious and upsetting were his sudden explosive rages, precipitated by trivial things that previously would not have concerned him at all. For example, Christine recalls a time when one of the children used the last of the milk at breakfast so that there was not enough for his cup of tea. He smashed the milk bottle on the table in front of them. He would quickly return to his normal, stable self, leaving the family shaken and upset. David, the youngest, at 9 years old still occasionally wet his bed at night. If this occurred when his father was tired or stressed, Paul would sometimes take a belt to his son; physical punishment was previously unheard of in this family. The marriage was now under serious strain, and Helen often took the brunt of Paul's rages. Looking back, it is clear to Christine that these rages occurred at times when her father was working long hours and was very tired.

All four children were very academic and did exceptionally well at school. Christine entered medical school at age 18 years, but when she was 20, the family's financial situation changed dramatically. Fortunately, the family home was in Helen's name, but Paul had complete control of the family finances and only gave Helen a weekly allowance for domestic spending. Thus, it came as a shock when Helen was contacted by their bank with the news that they were deeply in debt. After some investigation, it became apparent that for the past 3 years Paul had earned no income, and his costs to run his architect's office, as well as the family's costs, had been coming out of their savings. Every day Paul had been dressing in his suit and driving to his office, where he sat all day, doing nothing. He had dismissed his secretary, and nobody had realized his predicament. At this point, Paul decided to retire at the age of 52. He had two children in university and two still at school. As the house was in Helen's name, the family was able to remain there for a time. Helen tried to find a teaching position or any other work but was blocked by Paul.

To add to the stress, Paul was at this time diagnosed with a lymphoma that was treated successfully with radiotherapy through his neck. His behavior continued to worsen, however, and his moods fluctuated from his normal, affectionate old self, to apathy and withdrawal, to violent rages that included physical attacks on Helen. Throughout, he stubbornly refused to see a doctor or get any help. Following a dreadful scene when he tried to strangle Helen, Christine called the psychiatric crisis team, but when they arrived at the door, Paul sent them away telling them they were trespassing. At this point, Helen moved out for her own safety. She rented an apartment and was finally able to go back to her teaching and start building a new life for herself. She never saw Paul again after this, which enabled her to recover some quality of life but left her with feelings of guilt, especially as her children now took on the full burden of Paul.

Left to himself, Paul did nothing in the house or garden, and it became a hovel. Christine, now married to Stephen, and with their first baby, moved in for 3 months to try and tidy it up. Paul continued to bar anyone else from entering the property and continued to refuse to see a doctor or go into hospital. Christine thought that he must have sustained some brain damage when he received the radiation treatment for his lymphoma but was unable to get this checked out. Around this time, when her father was 55 years old, Christine noticed that he had a tremor, but again she thought this must be a consequence either of his radiation therapy or perhaps secondaries from his lymphoma.

By the time Paul was 60 years old, Christine was feeling very concerned about his true diagnosis, especially as her brother Mark had also been diagnosed with a serious psychiatric disorder. She managed to get her stubborn father, now suffering from choreic movements as well as tremor, to spend some time with them where they now lived, in another town. While he was there, she had him surreptitiously diagnosed by a neurologist friend who came to their home for dinner. He had no doubt that Paul was suffering from HD and that this would also explain Mark's illness. Paul continued to refuse any formal examination or tests and denied that he had a problem. He returned home and lived in his own mess, allowing only his children in to attempt to clean the house or him. No maintenance workmen were permitted entry. On the positive side, Paul spent most of his time sitting in a chair in the garden, looking at the river. Finally, when he was almost bedridden, his children were forced to have him committed, and this scared and stubborn man had to be forcibly removed from his house into an ambulance by the police. He spent 3 weeks in a ward for chronic psychiatric patients, where he continued to refuse all help. He then suffered a stroke and was transferred to a nursing home. He refused to eat and died 6 weeks later at the age of 63 years. A postmortem showed the brain pathology typical of HD.

Mark   Academically, Mark was the most exceptional of the four children, with his IQ being assessed at the very top of the "Very Superior" range at school. When he was 18 years old and in his first year at university, he gained exceptionally high marks in all his courses. In his second year, Helen, who at this point was still living with Paul but was on the verge of leaving, received a letter from one of Mark's tutors telling her that his essays were "gobble-de-gook" and that she should try and find out what was going on. Helen took Mark to a psychiatrist, who diagnosed him with paranoid schizophrenia, admitted him to a psychiatric hospital, and told Helen that she could not see him or contact him for 6 months, as his schizophrenia was rooted in a dysfunctional relationship with her.

Christine, now with two young children and working as a general practitioner, visited him regularly, as did his other two siblings. Mark improved somewhat on medication, and after 6 months he was transferred to a halfway house. Although he coped reasonably well some of the time, he became a regular user of marijuana and alcohol. His good friends began to fade out of his life as his behavior worsened. However, one good friend found him a small apartment close to a biscuit factory, where he was able to obtain a simple job. The routine of walking to the factory every day and working kept him on a reasonably even keel for 2 years, although by this time he was an alcoholic. He was finally thrown out of the apartment when the owner saw the mess spilling out the door, and he went back home to live with his father. Given his father's state of health and the state of the house, this was an even greater nightmare for Christine, as they were incapable of caring for themselves or each other. On one occasion two men broke into the house and sexually abused Mark. Around this time, as a result of his father being diagnosed with HD, it became clear that Mark also suffered from HD.

When Paul died, Helen was able to sell the house and buy a small apartment for Mark close to an outpatient psychiatric facility. He went daily to therapy sessions there and also to Alcoholics Anonymous, although he was never able to remain sober for long. He was helped by the social worker at the psychiatric unit, as well as by a music therapist with whom he established a good relationship. Finally, this too failed as his behavior became increasingly erratic and motor problems began to show. Helen, now in her late 60s, took him into her apartment to care for him. Mark was 6 feet 2 inches tall, and although he was extremely thin and by now very weak, he was very difficult for Helen to handle. However, her apartment was close to a beach that he loved, and he would spend long hours swimming and sunbathing in the sand dunes. Mark still retained much of his witty sense of fun, and when he was feeling relaxed and not plagued by the dreadful fatigue that is so debilitating for HD patients, he almost seemed like the old Mark.

At this point, Christine was desperately trying to find a nursing home who would take him, but with no success. HD patients have very specific nursing needs, and none of the nursing homes had the appropriately trained staff or facilities to cope with relatively young mobile patients with psychiatric problems whose severe motor problems put them in constant danger. The HD Association worked with her to find a suitable nursing home, and finally, after years of struggle, they were able to set up a special ward in a single-storied building in the grounds of a general hospital. Mark spent the final 3 years of his life in here, going to stay with Christine or his other sister for 3 days of every week. Christine felt these visits were essential for his well-being, but they were very difficult for his family, as Mark was up all night, incontinent, and had to be fed with pureed food.

In the last year of his life, Mark was mute, blind, and wheelchair-bound. At this point a very difficult decision had to be made about whether to insert a feeding tube directly into Mark's stomach. The purpose of this was to enable the nurses to feed the patient easily and quickly with a high-calorie substance, as feeding him by mouth at this point with sufficient pureed food to keep him alive took about 3 hours a day, which was clearly not possible for busy nurses to achieve. The negative side of the feeding tube is that it prolongs life long past the time when the patient has any quality of life, and indeed has been reduced to a vegetative state. Patients in the final stage of HD die from choking (which is why they must be fed with pureed food or gel); from respiratory illnesses such as pneumonia, as they become increasingly emaciated and weaker; or from malnutrition and heart failure. The family made a joint decision that their HD family members would not have feeding tubes inserted, so that they could die naturally and not have their lives prolonged as the result of being maintained via artificial feeding. So, for the last years of his life, Mark's mother visited twice every day to spend 90 minutes carefully feeding him with pureed foods. Mark died of pneumonia when he was 39.

David   David was an adventurer and a journalist. He was very close to Mark and spent long hours with him throughout his illness. His job as a journalist enabled him to work overtime for 9 months of the year and then take 3 months off to travel the world. He had good friends and a girlfriend or two, although once it became clear that the family had the HD gene girlfriends tended not to hang around. He did form one serious relationship, and when Mark was 25 his girlfriend became pregnant. Lucy, a devout Roman Catholic, decided to go ahead and have the baby, although she was aware that the baby could carry the HD gene. Lucy and David's relationship was over before Patrick was born, but right up until David's death, David saw him on a regular basis, and he and Patrick developed a strong father–son relationship over the first 12 years of Patrick's life.

It was not until David was 35 that Christine first became aware that he had not escaped the HD gene. She was looking at a video taken that Christmas of David mowing the lawn and playing with her children. On the video, his movement disorder, though subtle, was clear. David, deep down, was also aware that he was having trouble with tremor and choreic movements, especially when tired. Of course, he knew that he must have HD, and he was devastated. His symptoms worsened rapidly, but he managed to hang onto his job for another 3 years. He stubbornly refused to stop driving in spite of numerous minor accidents because he relied on his car for his independence. His executive functions rapidly deteriorated, and his ability to organize himself and to plan ahead became severely impaired. Indeed, at one point he obtained a copy of a book that gave instructions for committing suicide, but his executive functions were so poor by this time that he was unable to work out how to put these instructions into practice.

Yet, like Mark and his father when they were severely disabled, if he was interested in a topic and he liked the person talking with him, David could converse at a high level on current affairs, politics, and journalism. He retained his sense of fun and his wit, but he also retained his stubbornness, a trait no doubt inherited from his father. He did not want to live with his mother and so remained alone in a fourth-floor apartment. He refused any help, including meals on wheels, help with housekeeping, or visits by social workers. If his sisters brought him prepared meals, he would refuse to open the door, and when they had gone, he would retrieve the meal and throw it in the trash. On the positive side, unlike many HD victims, including his brother, David did not try and alleviate his suffering with alcohol or drugs, although he smoked heavily—an ongoing danger in his filthy apartment stacked high with old newspapers.

Christine talked to David and tried to convince him that he must live with either her or her sister for his own safety and their peace of mind. His response to this was to lock himself in his apartment for 3 weeks, after which time Christine was convinced he must have died as no amount of knocking and calling to him resulted in any sound. The family were forced to take out a guardianship bond that would allow the health authorities to remove him (if he were still alive) to a psychiatric ward for 4 days once a month so he and his apartment could be cleaned up. This involved a very public procedure of using a cherry picker crane to get a fireman and a male psychiatric nurse in through his window on the fourth floor. He was brought out alive, but kicking and screaming and accusing his sister of letting him down, while she was in tears below on the street.

Once a month this scene was repeated. On his second stay in the psychiatric ward, David escaped and hitchhiked 15 km back to his apartment, which was being sprayed with pesticide. The sprayer told him he could not stay there, as the fumes would do him in. David's reply—that he would just sit in the apartment while the spraying continued—resulted in the sprayer leaving and yet another "HD crisis call" to Christine. Once again Christine had to rely on her partner in her medical practice to see her patients, and on her husband to take care of their children, so that she could catch a flight from her hometown some 250 km away to sort out the situation.

A nursing home was finally found for David as he became demented and less mobile. The HD ward that Mark had been in had been shut down by the local government, who needed the land for further development. This had caused a great deal of anguish for the HD Society, whose members, including Christine and her sister Sara, had put a great deal of time, money, and care into the facility and into the gardens surrounding it, as well as into training the staff in the specialist skills required to care for HD patients.

From the age of 39 to 49 years, David was unable to care for himself, and he spent his last 2 years immobile on his back, mute, choking on food, and able to use only his eyes to follow his carers' movements. This "locked in" state was agony for his family, as it was impossible to know how much he could understand, whether he was in pain, or how they might be able to help him. As she did for her eldest son, in his final years Helen visited David twice a day to sit with him and fed him with gel. He died from pneumonia when he was 49.

Neuropsychological and Psychosocial Consequences

The sad stories of Paul, Mark, and David are very typical of the stories told by HD families everywhere. Neuropsychologically, the most common and debilitating impairments are the executive deficits of poor organization and planning, difficulty in initiating behaviors and putting plans into action, disinhibition and lack of self-control, and poor ability to foresee the consequences of one's actions. These deficits can become apparent very early in the disease. As the dementia worsens, the individual becomes less aware of the state they are in. This increasing lack of insight can exacerbate characteristics such as stubbornness, which is apparent in a refusal to accept help. Alcohol and drug use, perhaps started to dull the psychological and physical anguish of HD, can quickly become addictions, as the individual does not have the executive powers of self-control to be able to stop these destructive behaviors. The alcohol and drugs further dampen the frontal lobes and exacerbate the frontal-lobe deficits. In time, alcohol abuse will result in further permanent frontal-lobe damage. Labile emotions and explosive rages are also associated with the frontal-lobe atrophy that is typical of advanced HD.

The enormous difficulties Christine and her sister and mother had trying to help their HD family members was largely a result of these frontal-lobe problems. Of course, the very debilitating motor problems, including the unsteady gait, rigidity, choreic movements, dysarthria, incontinence, and not being able to swallow, make the physical care of HD patients very tiring as well. Although they become very emaciated, they can still be difficult to lift, especially if they are very tall, as Mark was, and are unable to help themselves if they fall, or cannot get out of the bath.

Christine can recount numerous examples that illustrate the executive difficulties that typify HD. For example, her sister would put David on the train to Christine's hometown when he was still able to walk. On one occasion when Christine went to the station to pick him up, she arrived just as the train was pulling away from the platform. David was nowhere to be found. Then she noticed a battered bag lying open on the platform with clothes spilling out, which she recognized as David's. She drove speedily to the next station and just managed to get there before the train arrived and was able to get David off. He had known his stop was coming up but thought, incorrectly, that he had time for a cigarette. When the train stopped and everyone got off, he continued to smoke but then as the train engines fired up again he finally realized he had to get off, so he hurled his bag—not done up—through the window, and then tried to make it out the door. It closed before he could get out. This is a very clear case of a poor ability to plan and put those plans into action.

Rehabilitation and Family Support

Rehabilitation is not a long-term option for people with HD, of course, but there are many strategies that Christine found to be helpful for her family members. For example, as for all people with dementing disorders, and especially those with executive problems, it is important that they live as long as possible in a place with which they are familiar. Fatigue exacerbates both the motor disorders and the emotional and psychiatric symptoms of HD sufferers. Fatigue is a direct consequence of the neuropathological changes of HD and is also an understandable consequence of the enormous energy required for constant choreic movements. To add to this problem, most HD people have trouble sleeping soundly at night. Thus, Christine emphasized the importance of frequent rests during the day. Keeping to a very stable routine is also important, and it helps if each new activity is first explained carefully and repeated often. Instructions—for example, to make it easier to transfer from a wheelchair to a bed—should be simple, frequently repeated, and convey one movement at a time. Whenever the HD individual is involved in an activity that requires concentration (i.e., everything in the middle to latter stages of the disease), care should be taken to do only one thing at a time. HD patients cannot "multitask." For example, while eating, they cannot listen to a conversation. Throughout, it is important (although difficult) to avoid sounding patronizing or treating the HD individual like a child, even though in many respects he may need to be treated like a child. By the time Christine's brothers were in nursing homes, they had to be told firmly that they must have their faces washed and that they could not have a ham sandwich, because it would choke them.

HD is like no other disease because its victims are often relatively young and mobile in the early stages but are constantly in danger of hurting themselves because of their motor disorders and executive problems. They often retain their intelligence while losing their executive abilities, and as a result, they can become very frustrated when they cannot perform what they know should be an easy task, or when others treat them as imbeciles.

No amount of theory, or even working with other debilitating diseases or dementias, can prepare a caregiver for the challenges of caring for HD patients. For Christine and her family, a woman neurologist who had dedicated her 25 years of working life to HD patients and their families gave them the strength and knowledge to cope. She remained tranquil in the midst of the chaos of HD, and her very presence calmed HD sufferers and family members alike. Her knowledge of the effects of different medications on HD symptoms and behaviors and the care she took to find the right dosage of the right drug for each individual patient resulted in almost miraculous improvements in both Mark and David's difficult behaviors at times. She led a team of nurses and social workers who took their skills and knowledge into the community and into towns and rural homes. Likewise, nursing staff who have many years of specialist experience caring for HD patients are worth their weight in gold, and genetic counselors with years of HD experience are of immense value to families grappling with the complex ethical and personal issues intrinsic to HD.

For families and HD patients alike, the HD Association and HD support groups can also be a lifeline. Often local branches of these are run by one or two dedicated people, usually family members of HD victims, who devote their lives to helping HD families cope, raising funds for HD facilities and research, and raising public awareness of HD. Just being able to share "HD crisis" stories with other families lifts the burden and reassures families that they are not alone.

Most important of all for Christine is the unconditional love and support Stephen has given her. As she said, it is almost impossible for her to comprehend how he could have stayed around through 30 years of coping with and cleaning up her father and brothers, as well as coping with her constant absences to deal with HD crises and supporting her emotionally. For Christine, one of her deepest regrets is that, because of the dominating presence of HD in their lives, her children's needs have sometimes been neglected. As an outsider looking in on this vibrant, loving family, it is difficult for me to believe that these now adult children would feel that they had been neglected, but then, I have never asked them.

I asked Christine whether she could see any positive outcomes at all from her long and painful HD experiences. After some moments of contemplation, she replied that she thought her experiences had made her a very good doctor. She went on to tell me about an incident that had occurred when she was a 19-year-old university student. Frightened by her father's increasingly violent rages and personality change, in desperation she had telephoned a professor of psychiatry at her university to ask his advice. She did not know this professor personally but had attended a lecture he gave in which he showed a therapy video of himself with a psychiatric patient. His compassionate attitude on the video had impressed Christine, and thus she was distraught when he responded to her initial explanation about her situation with an abrupt statement that he had not time to discuss personal problems with students and rudely terminated the conversation. As Christine said, he could at the very least have given her the name of a health professional she could contact. Christine never forgot that feeling of being pushed aside and left alone, and in her own practice she always takes all the time she needs to listen very carefully to what her patients or their families are telling her and takes special care with adolescents, trying to find out what is really going on for them and give support. This is surely a lesson that all health professionals, especially those who are busy and important, could well take notice of.

Social and Economic Implications

The HD individual who is wracked by choreic movements and facial grimaces can seem scary and crazy to the uninformed public. This can result in prejudice and painful experiences for families with HD. Christine told of an occasion when she, Stephen, and their two small children took Paul, not long before his death, for a weekend at the coast. Shortly after their arrival at the motel on the beach, Paul fell through the plate glass window, cutting himself, though fortunately not too badly. Christine cleaned and stitched up his wounds, but Paul was very upset and insisted that they could not stay there. They put their bags back in the car and went to the motel office to check out, explain about the broken window, and give the proprietor a check that would more than cover the replacement cost. In front of Paul and the children, the proprietor let fly with abusive language, shouting at them that he knew he should never have let them stay in the first place with their crazy father. The family drove off with Christine in tears, Stephen angry, and the children upset.

In an attempt to pacify the children, after about an hour's drive, they stopped at a café (where they had never been before) in a small town so that the children could have a milkshake and ice cream. On entering the café, Carrie, the sole woman running the café, greeted them warmly and asked them if they would like some lunch. Christine explained that her father had a motor disorder that prevented him from eating any food that was not pureed. On hearing this Carrie sat down with Paul and asked him what his favorite foods were. He replied (with some surprise no doubt) that he loved liver pate, whereupon Carrie bustled out to the kitchen and made him a delicious pureed liver pate, as well as pureed fruit salad to follow. She then sat down with them and chatted away to the children while Christine concentrated on feeding Paul, and then talked to Paul while the family ate their lunch. Paul had severe dysarthria (difficulty in speaking resulting from poor muscle control), but Carrie concentrated on what he was saying and managed to carry on a perfectly normal conversation with him. The family left warmed by this other side of human nature and knowing that their memories of this abbreviated weekend break would no longer hold quite so much pain. After her father died, Christine returned to the café to thank Carrie. The memory of Carrie's compassionate and normal interactions at a time when they were desperately needed still brings a lump to Christine's throat more than 25 years later.

The prejudice against people with HD is not restricted to the uninformed public. It is common for the police to pick up HD individuals assuming they are drunk. Mark was frequently picked up by the police, and at times the family spent 24 hours or more searching for him before they discovered him in a police cell. The worst occasion occurred when he was arrested for armed robbery after his car was found abandoned in a seedy part of town. It was some days and a court appearance later before fingerprints at the scene of the crime were found to belong to a known violent offender and Mark was released.

Probably most HD families become involved in research on HD at some point, and this can be rewarding. Researchers in this area are usually clinically astute, compassionate, and very sensitive, but this is not always the case, and some researchers may forget that, for the family, there is a loved person behind this exciting research opportunity. Within an hour of Mark's death, Helen was shaken by a telephone call from someone she had never spoken to before, asking her without any prior discussion or warning whether she would release Mark's body parts for research purposes. Hopefully researchers and clinicians today are no longer this irresponsible and take care to explain research projects at an appropriate time and in a sensitive manner, with unlimited time given for the HD patient or family to consider whether they wish to be involved.

One final sad story concerning Paul illustrates the family stress that is caused by the social restrictions and prejudices associated with an ignorance of HD. The incident occurred at a relatively early stage of Paul's illness, when he had only very subtle executive deficits and was still quite mobile, although with a wide-based gait and quite significant dysarthria that made it difficult for people he did not know well to understand him. Christine and Stephen and their two children, aged 1 and 3 years, had just returned from a year overseas. On arriving home, their father, who was still a very doting grandfather, asked whether he could take the children for a stroll in their double push-chair. The house was in a very quiet street, it was a beautiful day, and the push-chair helped Paul's stability, so they agreed this would be helpful and give Christine and Stephen a chance to wind down and unpack. When Paul had not returned in an hour they went out to find him, but to no avail; he had disappeared. After searching for their lost father and babies for a number of hours and telephoning hospitals and police, a police sergeant who knew their father recognized him as the man being held in their suburban police station. It transpired that the police had seen him with the push-chair in the small bush park at the end of their street and had thought that he was drunk. He and the children had been held in a suburban police station while they attempted to find out who Paul and the children were. Because of Paul's dysarthria, they could not understand him when he tried to explain who he was. Apparently, communication between suburban policing centers in this large city was not very efficient: While police were out searching for him in one area, Paul was locked up as a drunken vagrant in another. Of course, at this time the problems associated with HD were still very new to Christine and Stephen, and their learning curve was steep. After that, they knew to check out the police stations when any of their family members disappeared.

HD is fortunately a rare condition and affects only a tiny proportion of the population. This rarity does, however, have its down side, as it is not a "vote winner" like heart disease or cancer, and it is an ongoing struggle for families to attract state funding for the specialist facilities needed to care for their family members. Thus, the personal financial cost to families is enormous. Each of Christine's brothers stayed with her regularly so that they could enjoy the stimulation of a different environment and time with the family, but neither could be left alone in the house while Christine and Stephen worked, and a male psychiatric nurse on a high hourly rate had to be employed to care for them during working hours. When David became immobile, the family purchased a special leather bed that was designed to help prevent bed sores and could be wheeled from room to room so that even in his last months he could look at a different ceiling and hear different sounds. Medical insurance is not available to family members who are at a high risk of developing HD, and most insurance companies will not even insure the houses of HD sufferers. As Christine commented, all members of HD families are forever treated as second-rate citizens.

Genetic Counseling

Christine's first two children were born before the family knew it carried the HD gene. At that time there was no predictive test for HD, and by the time a test that did not require samples from family members who had HD did become available, the children were growing up. After thinking all the issues through and discussing it with her mother, husband, and sister, Christine, as well as her sister Sara, decided not to have the test at that time. The possibility of either one being found to have the HD gene was too painful, and the family thought that coping with the thought of this being in their future would be unbearable on top of caring for Mark and David. When the children reached their teens, Christine offered to have the predictive test so that they would have more certainty on which to base their own decisions about having children of their own. They felt that coping would become impossible for them if they found out that their mother was going to develop HD, and they would rather not know.

All three children have grown up with HD relatives and were always very accepting and natural with their grandfather and their uncles, visiting them in their nursing homes right up until their deaths. As Christine said, this Christmas was the very first of their lives that was not spent with an HD family member. To balance this, for Christine and Stephen, it has been important to live as normal a life as possible, and as a result their children do not concern themselves unduly with worrying about what might be. Every member of this family lives life to the full; perhaps a result of harboring the "free-spirited" gene that seems dominant not only in Christine's gene pool but also in Stephen's.

Christine's cousin Patrick did make the difficult decision to have the predictive test. His risk of contracting HD was 50%, as his father David had HD, whereas for Christine's children the risk is 25%. Sadly, Patrick's test came back positive, increasing his risk to 100%. Since that time, Patrick has been in counseling and has struggled with depression as well as with high-risk behaviors, including one major car accident, when he crashed into a wall on a straight road. Whether this was a suicide attempt is not clear.

As Christine and Sara approach their 60s and are still symptom free, their risk of getting HD decreases. However, Christine's family history does not give her too much peace of mind. Her father's first symptoms were psychiatric and appeared when he was in his late 40s, and he died 15 years later demented and dysarthric, but not immobile. Her brother Mark's first symptoms were also psychiatric and appeared when he was only 19 years old. He died 20 years later, mute and immobile. David's HD lasted 14 years. His first symptoms were motor, first becoming apparent when he was 35 years old, but he quickly deteriorated, spending his last years demented and immobile until death released him at age 39 years.

For Christine, the fact that all three immediate family members showed symptoms by the age of 47 at the very latest holds little comfort. Her father had three younger brothers, and one brother, Jack, who was also a medical practitioner, showed the first signs of HD at the age of 72 years. His symptoms were primarily motor: tremor, bradykinesia, and mild chorea. He had the genetic test with a result of 36 CAG repeats;

at the lower limit of the borderline range of 36 to 41 CAG repeats that might or might not cause HD. Jack died of cardiac failure only 8 years after his first signs emerged. His four married children, all with children of their own, now live with the sword poised over their heads. Paul's other two brothers, now ages 82 and 84 years, are very alert and physically fit and seem extremely unlikely to carry the HD gene.

For Christine and Stephen, even though they are now free from the stress of caring for Christine's brothers, the shadow of HD is ever present. Their three adult children have inherited their parents' intelligence, wit, and adventurous spirit, but instead of feeling uncomplicated joy whenever one of them does something free-spirited, a part of them wonders whether this is a first sign of a changing personality and all that implies. To friends who know their children, they are as stable, normal, healthy, energetic, and successful as any parent could wish for, but of course living with the challenge of HD can only be understood from personal, painful experience.

Christine's son Ian now lives in Canada and recently announced that he and his Canadian partner were planning to marry the following year. The pleasure this brings Christine and Stephen is shadowed by her still unknown HD status, and she is once again contemplating having a predictive test. If she does, she plans to do it without her family's knowledge, so that if she is so very unlucky to have a positive result, she has time to get used to this before sharing this knowledge with her husband and children. In the meantime, she plans to fly to Canada so that she can talk through the HD issues with Ian and his partner. She wants to know how Ian now feels about Christine having a predictive test and to talk through the options the couple might have if her status remains unknown, or if she should she obtain a positive result. With her medical knowledge of HD, Christine is well placed to explain about the option of predictive testing of the fetus, should they decide to have children while Ian still carries a risk. Given that predictive testing of a fetus implies a willingness to abort any fetus carrying the HD gene, this may be a significant issue for his partner, who is Roman Catholic. Also of importance is the fact that, if Christine does carry the HD gene, Ian will have little hope of securing health or home insurance unless he too has a predictive test and is found to be negative. And so this dreadful disease continues to color the lives of every family member in every generation.

Discussion

HD has some similarities to Parkinson's disease (PD); both are progressive neurodegenerative disorders causing atrophy to parts of the basal ganglia, and both have motor abnormalities as primary symptoms. Rigidity, bradyphrenia, and freezing in particular are found in both disorders. However, the two disorders perhaps have even more differences than similarities. The primary motor disorder in PD is tremor, whereas it is chorea in HD. HD inevitably progresses to a severe dementia, whereas only 10%–15% of PD patients become demented. Executive deficits, found in both disorders, are more marked and more debilitating in early HD than in PD, and cognitive impairment is generally more severe at all stages of HD. Most significant of all is the etiology of the two diseases. Although a genetic factor has been found in a small number of familial types of PD, for most cases environmental factors (including viruses) are likely to be causative, at least in part. Indeed, there appear to be numerous causes of PD. In stark contrast, HD is a clear case of autosomal dominant inheritance.

One might surmise that the known cause of HD should make it simpler to treat or cure in comparison to PD, where the causes are multiple and in most cases not well understood. This has not, as yet, proven to be the case. In PD, drug and surgical treatments have allowed sufferers to enjoy a reasonable lifestyle for many years in spite of the ongoing progression of their disease, and research on a cure or at least a slowing of the disease progression (e.g., via transplant of dopamine-producing tissue) is quite well advanced. In contrast, the drug treatments for the symptoms of HD are less effective (and less effective at correcting specific and known neurotransmitter imbalances) than for PD. Research to find a cure for HD is certainly very vibrant, but at this time a cure for HD appears to be a long way off.

For advocates of voluntary euthanasia, HD must provide a clear case for careful consideration. Some individuals at risk of developing HD or who are in the early clinical stages of the disease might welcome the legal right to request euthanasia when they have reached the final stage of the disease. The problem is, of course, that they could not be considered mentally fit to make this decision when they are in the final stages, and thus the decision would have to be made well in advance.

Such a right to have their lives ended with some dignity might relieve some of the psychological stress and anxiety at-risk and HD individuals must surely suffer as their disease progresses. This could be one way to reduce the incidence of premature suicide and "accidental" deaths in the HD and at-risk-for-HD populations.

Although few asymptomatic family members would be willing to admit to themselves or others that they too would be relieved if euthanasia for their affected family members were legal, nevertheless it seems likely that many family caregivers would prefer this alternative to the current situation of watching their loved ones struggling on through the final stages of HD. These complex ethical issues are of course bound up in moral, religious, spiritual, and cultural beliefs, which serves only to highlight the point that decisions about euthanasia must be made freely and autonomously by the HD sufferer early in the disease course or before symptoms emerge.

The research on HD is exciting and advancing rapidly, and there is hope that in the future this disease might be treatable and that, with predictive testing of the fetus available, it will be more frequently prevented from passing down through the generations. But in the meantime, HD families could well take Woody Guthrie's classic blues "Hard, Ain't It Hard," as their anthem.

17
■

DEMENTIA

A FAMILY TRAGEDY

In most Western countries, the proportion of elderly to young in the population is increasing rapidly because of the dual factors of improving health care, leading to longer life expectancy, and decreasing family size. The incidence (number of newly diagnosed cases) of dementia rises with increasing age and exceeds one new case per 100 in the 70–80 age group and two new cases per 100 in the over 80 age group. As patients with dementia tend to live for a number of years, the prevalence (total number of sufferers in a specified population at any one time) is higher than the incidence. The prevalence of dementia doubles every 5 years after the age of 60 years. In the age bracket 60–65 years, 1% have dementia, and in the age bracket 85 years and older, 35%–40% suffer dementia (Hendrie 1998). Therefore, the number of elderly people with dementia that the population must support is increasing dramatically (McLean 1987a). In 1999, the World Health Organization estimated that there were 20 million people suffering from dementia (of all types) worldwide, a figure estimated to reach 40 million by 2025, and that 66% of these dementia victims live in developing countries (Richter and Richter 2002; Walker and Salek 2002).

A great deal of money and effort is currently being poured into research on the causes and treatment of the dementias, and especially Alzheimer's disease (AD). The annual treatment costs of AD in the United States are estimated to be about US$100 billion, and as the majority of this cost goes to support the institutionalization of AD sufferers, even a small delay in the cognitive and functional decline of patients would reduce these costs massively (Brookmeyer, Gray, and Kawas 1998). Thus, identifying and reducing risk factors for AD, and developing drugs to delay progression of the disease, thus allowing AD sufferers to remain in the community for longer, are of international economic importance as well as of importance to the patients and their families.

More than half of all dementias are AD, which is the fourth most common cause of death after heart disease, cancer, and stroke (Mortimer 1983; Tomlinson, Blessed, and Roth 1970; Walker and Salek 2002). There are, however, about 50 other disorders that result in *dementia*, a general descriptive term for a brain disorder that produces widespread deterioration of mental functions and social capabilities. Dementia is a chronic condition and is usually progressive, although the term can also be applied to static conditions. Whereas AD and many other forms of dementia are irreversible, some dementias can be reversed with the appropriate treatment. The correct diagnosis is therefore of utmost importance.

The second most common dementia is Vascular Dementia (VaD), which accounts for 15% or more of all dementias (Funkenstein 1988). A differential diagnosis between AD and VaD is by no means always clear-cut, and not only may both forms of dementia be diagnosed in the same patient but some researchers have speculated that there may even be a causal relationship between the two. Both disorders share a number of vascular risk factors, and vascular lesions might play a role in the development of AD, or at least exacerbate the cognitive and functional impairments in a patient with AD (Gold, Giannakopoulos, and Bouras 1998; Kokmen, Whisnant, O'Fallon, Chu, and Beard 1996). Other rarer forms of dementia include Frontotemporal Dementia (FTD), which includes a rare form of dementia called Pick's disease; Dementia with Lewy Bodies; Binswanger's disease (a type of vascular dementia), Creutzfeldt-Jakob disease; and Kuru, a form of dementia found only in New Guinea. These latter two dementias are caused by a slow virus. Progressive supranuclear palsy (PSP) is not a dementia per se, but dementia occurs in approximately 60%–80% of patients with PSP.

Some forms of dementia, such as Huntington's disease (HD) and Parkinson's disease (PD), primarily affect the extrapyramidal motor system; that is, the motor pathway from parts of the deep brain structures called the basal ganglia to the spinal cord. This extrapyramidal pathway parallels the pyramidal or corticospinal pathway from the motor cortex in the frontal lobes to the spinal cord. Because of their association with the basal ganglia, HD and PD are sometimes classed as subcortical dementias. Dysfunction of the extrapyramidal tract results in motor abnormalities: either too little motor activity, such as the profound decrease of spontaneous movement (*akinesia*) characteristic of PD, or too much motor movement, such as the involuntary rapid jerking of the limbs and facial grimaces (*chorea-form movements*) characteristic of HD. Both disorders also involve cognitive impairments, in part because the basal ganglia have rich connections with the higher cortical areas, particularly the prefrontal cortex, and in part because of the reduced cortical metabolism or cortical atrophy sometimes observed in PD and HD. Only about 10%–15% of PD sufferers become demented (Brown and Marsden 1988), but HD invariably progresses to severe dementia accompanied by chorea-form movements. Chapters 14 and 15 describe PD and HD in detail.

Down syndrome individuals are born with three copies of chromosome 21 instead of the usual two (trisomy-21), and 50% or more develop a classic AD if they live to over 30 or 40 years of age. This is thought to be related to the genes encoding the amyloid precursor protein (the APP genes) on chromosome 21. A rare autosomal dominant early-onset familial form of AD (Familial AD; FAD) has also been linked to heterozygous mutations in the APP genes on chromosome 21q. Research into the role of this gene in AD is ongoing.

Correct assessment of dementia is extremely important because although dementia includes psychiatric symptoms (Assal and Cummings 2002), many other physical and psychiatric conditions can present as dementia. Overdiagnosis and misdiagnosis are serious problems (McLean 1987a, 1987b). *Pseudodementia* is the term used for psychiatric conditions confused with dementia, and depression is the psychiatric condition that is most commonly confused in this way. Obviously, to diagnose someone who has a psychiatric condition as being demented will result in incorrect treatment in addition to causing the sufferer and family extreme anguish. Physical illnesses that may have dementia-like symptoms as a secondary complication include nonprogressive or treatable neurological conditions, such as strokes, tumors, and meningitis, and severe respiratory, cardiac, gastrointestinal, and endocrine disorders, which may result in depression, poor concentration, confusion, and personality changes.

A deficiency of thiamine (vitamin B), often associated with alcoholism, can damage the mamillary bodies and thalamus bilaterally, causing Korsakoff's dementia. The main symptom of this disorder is amnesia for new material (anterograde amnesia) and a loss of memories for a number of years before the onset of dementia. There is a temporal gradient to the retrograde amnesia, such that the most recent past memories are less able to be retrieved than earlier memories. Thus, childhood and early adult memories are often readily accessible to the Korsakoff's sufferer. Although Korsakoff's is not progressive once the damage has been done, it is usually not reversible, although if picked up in the early stages the damage may be minimized by giving the sufferer large doses of vitamin B.

Missed diagnoses of dementia are not uncommon, and various reports have demonstrated that general practitioners do not recognize many cases of dementia (Berkowitz 1981; Williamson, Stokoe, and Gray 1964), confirming the complaints of many relatives that doctors are not interested in their elderly relatives' memory loss and confusion (McLean 1987a).

This chapter focuses on Sophie, a victim of AD. The assessment process, many of the symptoms, and the effects of the illness on the victim and the family are similar whatever the type of dementia; therefore, the problems Sophie and her family had, and the interventions attempted to alleviate some of the stress, are common to all dementias. The multidisciplinary assessment process that is often necessary before making a diagnosis of AD (or any other form of dementia) is outlined in some detail in the case presentation. The greatest emphasis is on the clinical neuropsychological and clinical psychological (or psychiatric) aspects of the assessment, but the medical aspects are of equal importance, especially when ruling out other physical causes for the symptoms. Although an extensive and detailed assessment is particularly important when diagnosing possible dementia, it provides for the clinical neuropsychologist and clinical psychologist a model of assessment that can be applied to many other neurological conditions.

Theoretical Background

Diagnosis of Dementia

The diagnostic criteria for the common dementias are listed in the *Diagnostic and Statistical Manual of Mental Disorders*, 4th edition (American Psychiatric Association 1994, pp 133-155), which is appropriate given that psychiatrists and other mental health professionals are often involved in the assessment and management of people with dementia. The NINCDS-ADRDA definitions of dementia (McKhann et al. 1984) also provide guidelines for the clinical diagnosis of AD.

The neurobehavioral and clinical criteria for all types of dementia (Cummings and Benson 1986; McKhann et al. 1984) include an impairment in the ability to learn new material (anterograde amnesia) or evidence of impairment of past memories (retrograde amnesia), along with impairment of one or more higher cognitive functions. For example, the patient may develop *aphasia* (language disturbance), *apraxia* (impaired ability to carry out motor activities despite intact motor functioning), *agnosia* (failure to recognize or identify objects despite intact sensory function), or a disturbance in executive functioning (i.e., planning, organization, sequencing, and abstracting).

These impairments must be severe enough to interfere significantly with the patient's work, usual social activities, or relationships (functional impairment). Neither the DMS-IV nor the NINCDS-ADRDA criteria allow for early dementia where there may be sufficient cognitive decline to satisfy the dementia criteria, but there is no documentation of concurrent functional impairment in daily living (Knopman and Selnes 2003). Thus, many early cases will be missed, as it is common for family members to "cover" or show reluctance to recognize functional impairments in their loved ones until the AD is quite advanced.

Other causes for the symptoms must be excluded; for example, delirium (i.e., when the state of consciousness is clouded). A careful history, physical examination, and laboratory tests should be carried out to assess whether a specific organic factor is present that is judged to be etiologically related to the specific type of dementia. In the absence of such evidence, it is important to establish that no other nonorganic mental disorder (e.g., depression) could account for the cognitive disturbances. It should, however, be noted that a significant percentage of elderly people with clinical depression and no symptoms of dementia can go on to develop frank dementia. A study by Reding, Haycox, and Blass (1985) found this to be the case in 57% of a group of 28 depressed elderly people who had no symptoms of dementia at initial assessment.

AD: Diagnosis, Etiology, and Neuropathology

The particular neurobehavioral hallmark of probable AD is a gradual onset and continuous cognitive decline. All other specific dementias, such as vascular dementia, should be excluded by the history, physical examination, laboratory tests, and brain imaging. AD fits the criteria for primary degenerative dementia. In a small proportion of cases, its onset is between age 40 and 65 years, and this form is sometimes labeled presenile AD, or early-onset AD. In some cases this is an inherited form of AD called FAD, which is related to mutations of the APP gene on chromosome 21. Other genes have also been identified as causative factors for early-onset AD. The great majority of cases of AD are diagnosed at 65 years or older (senile or late-onset AD). Some studies demonstrate that patients with late-onset AD have fewer neurofibrillary tangles than those with an early onset (Berg 1988). Most researchers, however, believe there is insufficient pathological or behavioral evidence to distinguish between early and late onset AD (Lezak 1995).

The time from diagnosis to death ranges from 3 to 20 years, with an average survival of 7 years. Death is not a result of the AD per se, but of other illnesses and infections to which demented people are more susceptible. AD affects men and women equally, but because the ratio of women to men increases during old age, women are more likely to be affected. AD creeps up on the sufferer gradually and is often quite advanced before the victim is first seen by a doctor or other professional. There is some autopsy evidence emerging that the neuropathological changes of AD may develop very gradually over five decades (Ohm, Muller, Braak, and Bohl 1995).

AD, when diagnosed in the living person on the basis of cognitive impairments and other behaviors typical of AD, and even when supported by brain scans, until quite recently was often labeled Dementia of the Alzheimer's type (DAT). The DAT label recognized that a certain diagnosis of AD could be made only following a brain biopsy while the victim is living (a rare occurrence), or more commonly after death when the brain was autopsied. Today, specialist dementia or memory units are more confident in making a reasonably firm diagnosis of AD if the patient fits the inclusion criteria for the disease, and other possible causes for dementia are excluded. Increasingly sophisticated laboratory tests can be used to exclude other causes for dementia, and magnetic resonance imaging (MRI) brain scans taken every year or so can measure whether the progression of cerebral atrophy is greater than would be expected for normal aging. Single-Photon Emission Computed Tomography (SPECT) measures regional cerebral blood flow, and perfusion defects in the bilateral posterior temporal and parietal regions in a patient with memory deficits and the other cognitive and behavioral symptoms of AD is highly predictive of AD. Of course neuropsychological assessments demonstrating the progressive, gradual cognitive decline in memory and other cognitive abilities remains an essential aspect of the diagnosis of AD.

Risk factors   The cause of most cases of AD is not known, although a number of causes have been suggested. In addition, a number of risk factors have been identified that, although not causal per se, may increase the potential for developing AD in vulnerable individuals. The main hypothesized "causes" and risk factors (with no priority attached to their order) are as follows.

A slow virus: As in Creutzfeldt-Jakob Disease.

Neurotoxins: A small proportion of people who suffer from organic solvent neurotoxicity following very long or intensive exposures to occupational or environmental neurotoxins go on to develop an irreversible dementia that continues to progress even after exposure to the neurotoxins ceases (See Chapter 13 of this book). The International Solvent Workshop (Baker and Seppalainen 1986) defined this as "type 3 OSN". This form of dementia is decreasing in prevalence as knowledge about the effects of exposure to neurotoxins increases and safety standards in the workplace improve, and it is unclear whether type 3 OSN is indistinguishable from AD. However, it does raise the possibility of neurotoxins as a factor in the development of AD.

Oxidative stress with the formation of free radicals: This has been shown to cause brain damage. Abnormally high levels of aluminium and iron have been found in AD patients in brain tissue susceptible to degeneration. These metals may be the cause of chronic oxidative stress and thus a causative factor in AD (Schneck, Reisberg, and Ferris 1982). Aluminium injected into animals causes memory loss and abnormal behaviors and neuropathological changes similar to those found in the brains of AD patients. Not all AD patients, however, have elevated aluminium or iron levels, and there is no definite proof that these metals play a role in dementia.

A history of traumatic brain injury: This has been reported in AD patients in a number of studies (e.g., Chandra, Kokmen, Schoenberg, and Beard 1989; Graves et al. 1990; Mortimer, French, Hutton, and Schuman 1985; Mortimer et al. 1991), and the "punch drunk" syndrome or "pugilistic dementia" suffered by some boxers has been found to show similar pathological changes to AD at autopsy (Jordan et al. 1997; Roberts, Allsop, and Bruton 1990). One hypothesis that might explain the link between head injuries and later dementia is that frequent concussions break down the blood–brain barrier and alter the immune system, allowing viruses and toxins that might cause dementia to enter the brain (Mortimer and Pirozzolo 1985).

A genetic predisposition to the disease: First-degree relatives are four to seven times more likely to develop AD than are people without a family history. The apolipoprotein E (ApoE) genotype is associated with both early-onset AD and other forms of dementia. The Alzheimer precursor protein (APP) gene on the twenty-first chromosome is associated with both early-onset FAD and the AD that develops in Down syndrome. Genes on chromosomes 1 and 14 are also associated with early-onset dementia.

Different alleles of ApoE appear to either protect or predispose their carriers to late-onset AD. Whereas nearly 80% of Caucasians carry the ApoE3 allele, only about 15% carry ApoE4, and 7% ApoE2. The ApoE2 allele appears to be underrepresented in the AD population, and it thus may be a potential protective factor. The ApoE4 allele appears to be overrepresented in patients with late-onset AD. Having two ApoE4 alleles produces a fivefold increase in the risk of developing AD and an earlier onset of the disease (Richter and Richter 2002). Carrying these "risk" genes does not, however, predict AD, and patients with these alleles may never develop the disease. Thus genetic screening based on these alleles is not recommended, as it could cause unwarranted concern for many people who have them, yet may never develop AD. There appear to be no consistent clinical differences between early-onset or FAD, and late-onset AD, in spite of the apparent genetic differentiation.

A "new" disorder labeled Mild Cognitive Impairment (*MCI*): This disorder is emerging as a potential risk factor for AD, as a significant proportion (15% or more) of people assessed as having MCI go onto develop AD (Fabrigoule et al. 1998; Peterson et al. 1995). This is in contrast to people without MCI, as only 1%–4% (depending on age) of this group go on to develop AD. MCI is not easy to assess, but it does appear to be correlated with smaller hippocampi, probably as a result of atrophy. Although there is no agreed criteria for assessment of MCI, one suggestion is that such patients should have normal daily functioning and normal nonmemory cognitive functioning but demonstrate an impairment of delayed free recall in the range that would fit with AD (Peterson et al. 1995). This definition is being used to select very early or potential AD sufferers for clinical trials of medications developed in the hope of delaying the onset of AD (Knopman and Selnes 2003). The diagnosis of MCI and its predictive value for later AD might also be linked to the finding that individuals with high levels of linguistic ability when young are less likely to develop AD than those with low levels of linguistic ability, as described " "next.

Cognitive ability: Various lines of research suggest that people who are highly educated or physically and mentally active into old age are less likely to develop AD (Stern et al. 1994; Mortimer and Graves 1993). A fascinating long-term study by Snowden and his colleagues (Snowden et al. 1996) carried out on 93 white American nuns from the School Sisters of Notre Dame religious congregation demonstrated that the density of ideas expressed in brief handwritten autobiographies written by the nuns when they were in their early twenties predicted whether or not they would develop the cognitive impairments typical of AD in old age. Those with the lowest density of ideas were much more likely to demonstrate severe cognitive impairment 58 years (on average) later. As the findings were the same for a subset of 85 college-educated nuns whose occupation was teaching, it seems unlikely that either education or occupation were relevant factors. In a subset of nuns who died (14 nuns from the main study and a further 11 nuns from another similar convent who had also written autobiographies as young nuns), low ideas density in their autobiographies at age 22 (on average) predicted the number of neurofibrillary tangles in the hippocampus and neocortex, and thus neuropathologically confirmed AD. Low ideas density in early adulthood was present in 90% of the 25 nuns who had neuropathological evidence of AD, and only 13% of those without AD.

As all of the nuns had lived in a very similar environment from young adulthood, Snowdon et al. suggested that the relationship between poor linguistic ability in early adulthood and impaired cognitive performance in later life was likely to be associated with cognitive ability in early life and not with environmental, health, or educational factors in adulthood. One hypothesis put forward by Snowdon et al. (1996) was that the nuns with a high density of ideas as young adults had a higher "neurocognitive reserve capacity" and would therefore be less vulnerable to the later neuropathological changes of AD. To support such a hypothesis, it would be expected that some nuns who had a high ideas density in their twenties, and who did not demonstrate severe cognitive impairments in old age, would nevertheless demonstrate the pathological changes of AD on autopsy. Only one of the 25 nuns who died and was autopsied showed this pattern, and thus Snowdon and his colleagues concluded that the "neurocognitive reserve" hypothesis could not be supported.

An alternative hypothesis is that low linguistic ability in early life is an early expression of later AD. In support of this theory Ohm et al. (1995) demonstrated in an autopsy study of individuals aged 20–100 years that the neurofibrillary tangles and neuropil threads characteristic of AD develop over five decades.

Protective factors   Potentially protective factors for AD are currently thought to include the ApoE2 allele, higher linguistic ability, possibly a higher educational level, the use of vitamin E and other antioxidants, the use of anti-inflammatory agents, and the reduction of "bad" cholesterol (LDL) with the use of statins (Poirier 2002).

A cautionary note must be attached to studies that find positive correlations between certain factors and a lower incidence of AD, and conclude therefore that those factors are potentially protective. The recent publication of results from the large Women's Health Initiative (WHI) trial of more than 16,000 women aged 50–79 years who took hormone replacement therapy (estrogen plus progestin) over a 4–5-year period, showed that, contrary to earlier reports, the HRT group had an increased risk not only of cardiac disease and breast cancer but also of ischemic stroke (Wassertheil-Smoller et al. 2003). A subset of over 4000 women from the trial who were over 65 years and took HRT had double the risk of probable dementia when compared with the control group, and the risk of developing mild cognitive impairment was no different between the HRT and placebo groups (although the HRT group demonstrated a nonsignificant tendency toward a higher risk for MCI) (Rapp et al. 2003; Shumaker et al. 2003).

Previous preliminary results from this trial and from other smaller trials had suggested that HRT might reduce the risk of stroke and dementia and delay age-related cognitive decline. Publicity about these findings encouraged millions of women to embark on HRT not just in the short term to ameliorate the debilitating symptoms of menopause that some women experience, but over many years in the hope that the HRT therapy would act as a protective factor against diseases of aging and normal age-related cognitive decline. The subsequent results from the trial and the early termination of the study because of the negative findings provide a grim lesson in the dangers of jumping to conclusions based on small numbers of participants, methodologically flawed studies, the rapid publication of preliminary data analysis of major epidemiological studies, and in some cases, studies funded by drug companies that may contain dangerous biases. Although large numbers of women have stopped using HRT, no doubt drug companies will continue their efforts to find a drug that will delay one of most feared "diseases" of the Western world: normal aging. As most of us realize, we all have to die sometime of something, and once over 85 years of age, dementia is perhaps one "normal" way to go.

Neuropathology   The neuropathology of AD, which can only be confirmed by biopsy or autopsy, includes the presence of neurofibrillary tangles and amyloid or senile plaques. Neurofibrillary tangles are strands of axonal material that displace normal neurons; although these tangles are present in normal elderly persons, they occur in much larger numbers throughout the brains of AD patients and especially affect the functioning of the hippocampi. The density of these tangles correlates with the degree of psychological disturbance before death. Given the importance of the hippocampi for memory (see Chapter 3), it seems likely that the high number of neurofibrillary tangles either in the hippocampus or in structures connecting the hippocampus to other important structures relate directly to the severe memory deficits that are one of the hallmarks of AD. Amyloid plaques are degenerated nerve cell material with an amyloid-filled core. They occur in small numbers in the normal elderly but in large numbers throughout the cortex and deeper structures of the brains of AD victims as well as in other dementias, including Kuru and Creutzfeldt-Jakob disease. The brains of AD victims also have large numbers of granulovacuolar organelles (small clusters of dead brain cell material that collect in the neurons). These are particularly dense in the hippocampi. At the biochemical level, AD is characterized by a reduction in the enzyme used in the production of the neurotransmitter choline acetyltransferase, which provides some basis for developing treatments that increase the activity of the cholinergic system (Corkin 1981; Wimo and Winblad 2002). Other neurotransmitter abnormalities (e.g., reduced dopamine, serotonin, and noradrenaline concentrations) have been found in a proportion of the brains of AD victims, but the findings are inconsistent (Assal and Cummings 2002).

Research that measures cerebral atrophy (indicated by a widening of the gyri, shrinkage of the sulci, and dilatation of the ventricles) in groups of AD and age-matched control subjects has demonstrated that atrophy is present in many but not all cases of dementia (Albert et al. 1984). Because some atrophy occurs with normal aging, it is often difficult to detect pathological atrophy in the individual demented patient from a gross inspection of CT scans, although MRI scans are more useful and thus increasingly used to assist with AD diagnosis. Atrophy appears to be more prevalent in cases of early-onset AD than in late-onset AD.

A phenomenon called Programmed Cell Death (PCD), or apoptosis, has also been shown to cause a cascade of nerve cell deaths in AD. However, it is not yet known whether this is a cause of AD or simply an immunological strategy whereby the brain is cleansed of damaged or dead nerve cells (Troy and Shelanski 2002).

Neurobehavioral and Psychosocial Deficits in AD

Usually the first symptom to emerge in AD and many other dementias is forgetfulness, which progresses until it becomes clear that it is not the mild memory disorder that commonly occurs as a consequence of normal aging but is pathological. As AD progresses, the patient finds it increasingly difficult to remember new information and forgets names, telephone numbers, routes once well known, conversations, and events of the day. If tasks are interrupted, they may be forgotten and left unfinished, and the simplest household chores may become a danger; for example, the stove may be left on or the bath left to overflow. Such all-encompassing memory problems lead to confusion and disorientation. In the late stages of dementia, memory loss for both past and recent events becomes profound, and the patient is unable to remember where she lives, who close family members are, what year it is, or even her own name.

Other cognitive functions usually become impaired after the memory problems become established. Speech and language are almost always affected to a lesser or greater degree, and speech content may become impoverished and concrete; the patient may find it difficult to stay on the topic being discussed. Speech is sometimes inarticulate and difficult to understand; as the dementia worsens, the patient may lose spontaneous speech and finally become mute. In the middle stages of AD, abstract thinking gradually becomes difficult, and the patient has trouble comprehending novel situations and subtle nuances of language and nonverbal expression. In the early and middle stages, the patient is aware of these difficulties and may avoid new situations to minimize embarrassment and failures.

A range of psychometric tools are used both in clinical practice and in research for measuring the progressive cognitive decline as well as functional decline in AD. The most common measure of global cognitive decline used is probably the Mini-Mental State Examination (MMSE; Folstein, Folstein, and McHugh 1975), although many more sophisticated measures have been developed, especially for research (Sarazin, Horne, and Dubois 2002). In general, these scales show a regular 6-monthly or annual decline in cognitive functioning, particularly in memory functioning, with a more rapid decline as the disease progresses. Whether this more rapid decline indicates a more rapidly progressing disease or a variable sensitivity of the tests to the various cognitive stages of the disease is not clear. Sarazin et al. (2002) and Walker and Salek (2002) provide summaries of studies using different psychometric tests to measure the rate of cognitive decline and functional decline, or "quality of life," respectively.

During the early and middle stages of AD, it is not uncommon for patients to become depressed as they realize what is happening. The depression usually takes the form of depressive symptomology, rather than major depressive episodes. One study found that 38% of their clinical population demonstrated symptoms of depression (Mega, Cummings, Fiorello, and Gornbein 1996). With progression of AD, the frontal lobes are increasingly affected, and patients gradually lose insight and in many cases become unconcerned about their behaviors and problems; thus, depression is alleviated. At this stage, poor judgment, poor impulse control, and disinhibited behaviors are common. The family must now cope with a relative who continually embarrasses them in social situations, wanders from home and cannot find her way back, is careless about personal cleanliness, and may be abusive toward family members and caregivers. Personality changes become predominant during this middle stage, and a previously energetic person can become apathetic, withdrawn, and unspontaneous, spending her days lying in bed or watching television with little comprehension of what she is watching. Rapid changes in emotion may also occur, and the patient may become irritable, angry, or euphoric for no apparent reason. Agitation is very common and was found in 60% of a clinical sample of AD patients (Mega et al. 1996). Occurrences of aggression and violence appear to be linked to agitation and signal the importance of finding ways to assist the patient to feel calm and avoid situations that increase agitation.

Psychotic symptoms in the form of delusions and hallucinations sometimes occur in the middle stages of dementia (Assal and Cummings 2002; McLean 1987b). One study found that delusions occur in 22% and hallucinations in 10% of AD patients (Mega et al. 1996). The delusions are often paranoid, and family members are often terribly upset by their relative's accusations that they steal her possessions, take her food, or are plotting to kill her. In recent years there has been an increasing awareness of the abuse of the elderly by caregivers, so in some cases the paranoia may be based on reality. Hallucinations, when they occur, tend to be visual rather than auditory, as in schizophrenia, although auditory and tactile hallucinations can also occur. In the final stages of AD, the patient exists in a vegetative state, mute, incontinent, and bedridden, with no awareness of the people around her and no memories of her past life.

Course and Management

Interventions   Many causes of dementia are potentially reversible, and in these cases treatment will depend on the etiology. In the case of AD, researchers are still some distance from finding a cure or a way to prevent AD. In the future perhaps the use of embryonic stem cells to replace dysfunctional acetylcholine-releasing nerve cells in AD, or to replace dead hippocampal neurons, will herald a more permanent "cure" for AD.

In the meantime, rapid pharmacological advances are being made that address the symptoms of AD. The most useful pharmacological interventions work on the cholinergic system. In AD, although numerous neurotransmitters seem to be deficient, the most convincing correlation with severity of AD is with a reduced choline acetyltransferase activity, resulting in reduced synthesis of acetylcholine. Drugs including acetylcholine precursors, cholinergic agonists, cholinesterase inhibitors, and enhancers of acetylcholine release have been trialed with the aim of increasing acetylcholine levels in the brain without producing unacceptable side effects. The acetylcholinesterase inhibitors (AchEIs) have proved the most promising drug treatment to date. Controlled clinical trials demonstrate that almost half of those patients who take AchEIs respond positively to them, with improvements on measures of cognitive, behavioral, and ADL (Activities of Daily Living) measures. Unfortunately, patients who do not respond to these drugs can not yet be predicted, and the cost of providing these drugs to AD sufferers is considerable. However, any drug that delays institutionalization for a number of months at least is likely to save money, as well as being welcomed by the patient (especially if in the early to middle stages of AD) and caregivers.

Experimentation is also in progress on monoamine oxidase (MAO) inhibitors (because of their antioxidant potential), Vitamin E, and memantine, and on extract of *Ginkgo biloba*. Anti-inflammatory drugs might prove useful in slowing the progression of AD, as inflammatory proteins are often present at AD lesion sites, and statins to reduce low-density lipoprotein (LDL) cholesterol in AD patients might also prove useful, as some studies have shown that there is a lower prevalence of AD in patients who take statins for cardiovascular problems (Richter and Richter 2002).

Some of the most useful treatments are those that alleviate coexisting medical conditions or treat the psychiatric symptoms of dementia. Antidepressants can be helpful in the early stages if the patient is severely depressed, and antipsychotic medications may reduce psychotic symptoms and decrease aggressive and agitated behaviors, and sleep disturbances can be treated with short-acting hypnotics. Drug therapies must be carefully monitored and introduced slowly to avoid overmedicating and to keep to a minimum unpleasant or even dangerous side effects.

Providing good nutrition, encouraging meaningful activities, and providing a familiar and calming environment will assist patients in the early and middle stages of AD to cope better and cause less stress to their caregivers. No longer is it wise to argue with a parent who now has AD and who once enjoyed nothing better than a good argument. No longer will new environments and new people stimulate, in a positive way, a mother who used to be the life and soul of the party, but who now has AD. Psychological interventions aimed at improving memory and decreasing confusion have been attempted, and these may certainly be helpful in the short-term; however, the cognitive decline continues unabated (Quayhagen and Quayhagen 1989) until the patient can no longer participate in sessions aimed at helping her to cope with everyday tasks.

Management in the early and middle stages of AD   In the early and middle stages of AD, the patient usually continues to be cared for at home, which is desirable because confusion and disorientation are minimized if the patient remains in a familiar environment. The caregivers, usually the family, need enormous support throughout this period, including sound information, respite care, home and nursing help, support from other families of AD sufferers, and psychological support and counseling. Knowledge about practical strategies that they can use to reduce the distress and antisocial behaviors of their AD relative can be both useful for the caregiver and empowering for the patient. For example, caregivers can practice ways to respond to their relative when she becomes agitated and abusive that do not involve arguing or correcting her or using logic to counteract her irrational complaints. Often "reflecting" the patient's comments in a calm and empathetic manner and, when possible, attempting to paraphrase, in simple language, the feelings that underlie the irrational or paranoid statements (perhaps of helplessness, fear, anger, or confusion) will calm the patient, and she usually quickly forgets what upset her. Confusion, forgetfulness, and paranoia can be reduced by keeping the patient's environment and routine as familiar as possible and by explaining in advance any changes in routine that are necessary.

In addition to using drugs such as AchEIs to reduce or delay the cognitive and behavioral symptoms of AD, a number of studies have demonstrated that in the early and middle stages of dementia, it is possible to assist patients, nonpharmacologically, in regaining some of the skills of daily living they have lost. Such programs include combinations of providing information, assisting with spatial orientation (e.g., learning to find their own way to the toilet), communication skills (e.g., learning to express their feelings of pleasure and displeasure), basic skills (such as feeding), and even more advanced skills like doing the laundry (Griffen and Mouheb 1987; McElvoy and Patterson 1986). Programs that target the caregivers can also help them to gain self-confidence in dealing with the patient and the symptoms of the disease as it progresses (Chiverton and Caine 1989).

Throughout the earlier stages of AD, care must be taken to monitor the patient's emotional state. The suicide risk must be assessed in all patients, especially those who are depressed, and the patient should be helped accordingly. Patients who are mildly or moderately depressed and who still have reasonable cognitive abilities can sometimes find a path out of their depression as a result of a process of "putting their house in order." This action could include discussing their future care with their family, making a will, planning the details of their funeral, and writing letters for their children and grandchildren to be read after the writer's death (e.g., on a grandchild's twenty-first birthday). Family photographs and mementoes from the past can be shared with family members and the patient encouraged to talk about the past (perhaps while being recorded) so that these memories can be passed on to younger and as-yet unborn family members. "Putting one's house in order" may involve the patient making peace with others and with herself, and it often paves the way to emotional acceptance that life is nearing completion. All these actions can be empowering for the patient and can form a positive part of the grieving process, both for the AD sufferer and the family.

Management in the later stages of AD   As the dementia worsens, the patient loses insight, becomes increasingly apathetic or disinhibited, is likely to wander without any idea of where she is going or how to find her way back, and requires considerable assistance with everyday activities, such as washing, dressing, eating, and using the toilet. At this stage, strategies that previously helped to calm the patient are no longer effective. This is the point at which families often must make the difficult decision to place their relative in a home, where she will die in the next few months or sometimes years. Understandably this is an intensely stressful time for families. They are physically and emotionally exhausted from years of caring for their loved one while she deteriorates into a person quite alien to the one they have known all their lives; in addition, they feel guilty because they feel they are abandoning the patient in her time of greatest need. If the patient is a parent or partner who has cared for the caregiver in past years, such abandonment cuts very deeply indeed.

Some family structures (particularly extended families and cultures that have great respect for their elderly) are able and willing to care for their relative until death, but for many families, continuing to care for someone in the last stages of dementia places an intolerable stress on the family or on particular family members. Psychological counseling may be helpful in assisting these families to understand that their relative can no longer appreciate them and, sadly, is unable to care whether she remains at home or is nursed in a hospital or hospice. The best that can be done for the patient at this stage is to make her as comfortable as possible and to ensure that she is not in pain, which often requires professional nursing and medical care.

Case Presentation

Background

Sophie was 51 when she was diagnosed with AD. Speaking at her funeral 5 years later, her daughter, Diane, gave her this eulogy. "Sophie was a strong, vital woman, a fine journalist, a radio talk-back host who kept everyone on their toes, my father's only love, and an irreplaceable Mum." Sophie was not the first member of Diane's family who had died of AD. Sophie's own mother was diagnosed with the disease at age 65 and was nursed by Sophie for several years before she died in a nursing home at the age of 70. This was a stressful period for the family, as they struggled with the tragedy of watching Sophie's mother become disinhibited, verbally abusive, and finally mute and incontinent. Diane was particularly upset, as she had enjoyed a close relationship with her grandmother, and she and Sophie gained some benefit from seeing a clinical psychologist over this period. When Sophie's mother was placed in a nursing home on the suggestion of the psychologist, Sophie assumed the task of researching and writing a series of articles for the local newspaper on AD and the problems this disease causes for families. This research helped her come to terms with her grief, and it also increased her knowledge about AD.

Thus, when by the age of 49 Sophie found herself forgetting the beginning of books before she reached the end, had to reread her own articles to remind herself what she had written only a few days previously, and forgot names and important dates, she became worried that she too had AD. As a journalist, she had prided herself on her excellent memory and often conducted an entire interview without taking notes. Her husband and friends told her this level of forgetfulness was normal for someone of her age and recounted instances when they forgot important dates and the names of their acquaintances. Sophie remained concerned and returned to the psychologist who had helped her previously.

The psychologist took her concerns seriously. Although she had only a basic training in neuropsychology, the psychologist gave Sophie a neuropsychological assessment that included the revised Wechsler Adult Intelligence Scale, the Wechsler Memory Scale, and the Rey Complex Figure (Rey 1941). She was pleased with the results: Sophie scored in the average range across all the tests except for the Rey Figure delayed recall, which fell two standard deviations (SD) below the average score for a woman Sophie's age. The psychologist attributed this low score to fatigue and anxiety and explained to Sophie that she was probably imagining her memory difficulties because her results on the formal memory tests were quite normal. Here lies a salient lesson for psychologists who are not fully trained in neuropsychology. Sophie's psychologist made the mistake of thinking that an *average* score is a normal score, whereas she should have compared the scores with an estimate of Sophie's premorbid abilities. Given Sophie's journalistic talents, it is extremely unlikely she would have scored in the average range on the Verbal subtests of the Wechsler Intelligence Scales, and the very simple WMS memory tests, had she been unimpaired. A different picture would probably have emerged had Sophie been given a more difficult verbal memory test. In retrospect, it was clear that Sophie's average and low-for-her scores on some of the Wechsler Verbal subtests were caused by word-finding difficulties, which were also already apparent in her normal conversation.

Sophie was nevertheless comforted for a time by these "good" results, but over the next 18 months, it became apparent even to her family that something was wrong. Sophie was retired from her radio talk-back show because she was frequently unable to find the words she wanted, a major disability for an interviewer known for her quick wit and fluent speech. In addition, Sophie would sometimes repeat questions she had asked only minutes before and forget the name of the person she was interviewing. Sophie was referred by her general practitioner to a geriatrician, and the assessment process began in earnest.

Assessment Process

Medical assessment   The doctor's aim is to assess whether there are sufficient symptoms of dementia to cause concern and, if so, to proceed with a range of medical investigations to rule out any causes that could be reversible or that require a particular treatment regimen. Sophie's doctor took note of the memory and word-finding problems observed by Sophie's husband, Peter, and the possibly relevant fact that Sophie's mother had died of AD. She then gave Sophie a screening test for dementia, the Mini-Mental State Examination (MMSE) (Folstein et al. 1975), and, on finding that Sophie's score on this fell in the moderately impaired range, she proceeded with exhaustive medical investigations and referred Sophie to a neuropsychologist.

Sophie had no history of hypertension, strokes, heart problems, metabolic imbalances, or endocrine disease that could account for her symptoms of memory impairment and speech difficulties. Sophie's work had never involved substances likely to cause neurotoxic or other physical effects, and she was not currently in an environment (such as living in a house that is being painted) that can cause transient problems such as headache, loss of concentration, and apparent memory problems for some people. She took no prescription medications and did not smoke or take recreational drugs, thus ruling out drug side effects, interactions, overdoses, or a gradual toxic buildup of medication. A thorough investigation of medications is particularly important in elderly patients because some patients may be taking several medications for various ailments. Sophie had no history of psychiatric disturbance, although she was currently feeling depressed and not sleeping or eating well. Sophie herself attributed these problems to anxiety about a probable diagnosis of AD.

Sophie's physical examination was normal and included an examination of her senses because deterioration of hearing or vision, again more common in an elderly population, can result in confusion, disorientation, apparent memory impairment, and paranoia and thus be misdiagnosed as dementia. Laboratory screening tests on Sophie's blood, urine, and cerebrospinal fluid ruled out any metabolic disorders that might account for the symptoms. A CT scan of Sophie's brain showed no areas of infarction (strokes) or any mass lesions. The lateral ventricles appeared slightly larger than normal for her age, however, and the possibility of some minor cortical atrophy could not be ruled out by the neuroradiologist.

The doctor's preliminary findings were that no clear cause could be found for Sophie's reported cognitive difficulties; in particular, she ruled out reversible causes of dementia. A patient who presents with an acute deterioration with an onset within the last 12 months, but who shows only mild dementia on a cognitive screening test, is more likely to have a reversible cause for her cognitive problems than a patient who has had a gradual deterioration over a period of 2 years or longer but demonstrates severe dementia on the cognitive screening test (Larson, Reifler, Canfield, and Cohen 1984). Sophie did not fall into the reversible dementia pattern, although she also was unable to be classified with certainty as having irreversible dementia at this point.

Unlike Sophie, in many cases of AD, the patient is clearly demented by the time of first assessment. Often the victim and family adapt to the gradual cognitive changes, excuse the changes on grounds of old age, and cover them by reducing the victim's participation in tasks she finds difficult. Such a "coverup" is particularly common for patients who have retired or who work in the home, where a cognitive decline may be less noticeable than in a job that requires a good memory and the ability to make decisions in novel situations. Obviously, a delay in diagnosis can be positive if indeed the patient is ultimately diagnosed with AD, as an early diagnosis may rather pointlessly precipitate the onset of the anguish the patient and family will surely suffer. The danger in delaying diagnosis lies in the possibility that there is another reversible or treatable cause for the cognitive decline and that in time the disorder may advance too far for optimal treatment.

The neuropsychological assessment   Sophie attended her initial session with me accompanied by her husband and her three children. My first impression of Sophie was of a tiny woman with dark hair and eyes and delicate facial features; she could have passed for 40 rather than 50. Her voice was strong and clear, and it quickly became apparent that she was had a vibrant personality, even in the face of her understandable anxiety. It was clear from the outset that her husband and children loved her dearly, and at first they were fiercely protective of her to the extent of minimizing many of her problems.

After spending some time explaining the neuropsychological assessment process, I first talked generally with the family, concentrating on the many positive aspects of their family life and Sophie's many achievements. When the family felt more at ease, I commenced a more structured approach by taking a careful history from each member of the family, including Sophie, regarding the onset of her cognitive symptoms. Important dates (e.g., each of Sophie's birthdays and Christmas day) were tagged and Sophie's behaviors and accomplishments at those times were explored to enable me to build a picture of a gradual decline of memory and word-finding abilities and a recent problem with finding her way around. This picture was consistent with a dementing process such as AD, but not with vascular dementia, which tends to have a more distinct onset and a stepwise progression. Likewise, if depression were the primary cause of Sophie's problems, the onset of memory and other cognitive difficulties would probably have been more abrupt. In addition, word-finding problems and difficulties finding one's way around are unlikely to be noticeable problems in cases of mild to moderate depression.

Sophie attended the following three sessions without her family and was assessed using a broad range of neuropsychological tests. The previous results of the Wechsler Intelligence and Memory Scales and the Rey Complex Figure were available, which made it possible to assess whether any deterioration had occurred over the past 18 months. In the previous assessment, in retrospect, Sophie had already been showing symptoms of verbal and visuospatial memory impairment and word-finding problems, despite having been told she had no problems, given her average scores. I gave Sophie a word pronunciation test, the National Adult Reading Test (NART) (Nelson and O'Connell 1978; Nelson and Willison 1991), which confirmed my hypothesis that, based on her past achievements, Sophie's estimated premorbid IQ should fall in the superior range at least. The NART is a test that enables an estimate of premorbid ability, at least in an English-speaking person who can read. It relies on the finding that the correct pronunciation of irregularly spelled English words does not deteriorate at the same rate as other cognitive abilities in dementia and has a high correlation with the WAIS IQ, presumably because both the NART and WAIS rely to some extent on formal education and level of reading ability as well as "intelligence."

The repeat of the Wechsler Intelligence Scale demonstrated that Sophie's scores on most of the subtests now fell 1 or 2 SD below average. Her lowest scores were on subtests involving visuospatial abilities (Block Design, Object Assembly, and Picture Arrangement) and on tests involving abstract concepts (Similarities and the questions asking for an explanation of proverbs in the Comprehension subtest). Sophie's responses were also slowed, which was very apparent on the Digit Symbol subtest. Her word-finding problem was very apparent, especially in the Vocabulary subtest, where she sometimes struggled to find the words to define a simple word that she was ultimately able to demonstrate she knew by describing it in a very roundabout way (called *circumlocution*).

To assess her visuospatial functions further, I gave Sophie the Rey Complex Figure, which she had been given 18 months earlier. Usually, I would give a parallel version of the Complex Figure, called the Taylor Figure (Taylor 1969) the second time, but considering Sophie's clear deterioration on other tests, I decided that any practice affect would be minimal over such a long time span, and repeating the identical test would allow any decline to be clearly evaluated. Her copies of the Rey Figure on the two occasions 18 months apart are shown in Figure 17-1. The deterioration on this difficult visuospatial task was dramatic, especially given Peter's comment that Sophie used to enjoy sketching and was very good at it. Sophie took considerable care and time with her copy of the Rey Figure and refused to stop even when it became apparent she was becoming upset by her performance. When she finally completed it after a 5-minute struggle, she was crying as she said, "How can I find that

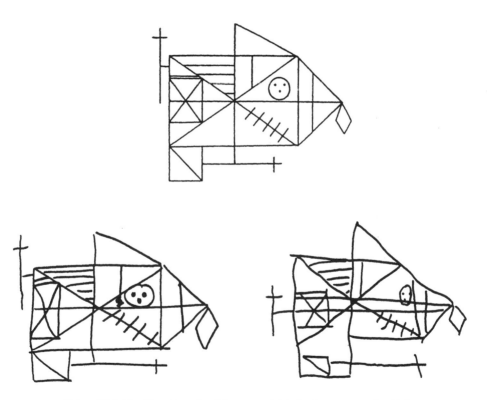

Figure 17-1 The Rey Complex Figure model is in the top row. Sophie's copy of it when she was in the early stages of dementia of Alzheimer's type is below this on the left, and her much deterioriated copy of it 18 months later is on the right.

so impossible? Look at it; it is dreadful, dreadful. A small child could do better than that."

Sophie was also given the Wisconsin Card Sorting Test (Heaton 1981) to assess her ability to make abstractions, given her lowered score on Similarities. This test requires the patient to sort cards according to categories, depending on the feedback they receive from the examiner after each card sort. Sophie seemed to grasp the first category after four card sorts; when, after 10 correct sorts, I changed the category without telling Sophie, she had difficulty changing to the new category despite being told that each card she sorted was incorrect. After eight incorrect sorts, she finally sorted to the correct category and was told it was correct, but then she immediately returned to the original category. Sophie became increasingly upset with each failure to sort correctly, and the test was terminated at this point. Sophie's performance suggested a number of things: First, she had difficulty making decisions involving abstract concepts; second, she had difficulty modifying her performance in response to verbal feedback; and third, she *perseverated* (returned to the original idea). Although poor performance on the WCST can occur after damage in cortical areas other than the frontal lobes (Anderson, Damasio, Jones, and Tranel 1991), in Sophie's case her difficulties were interpreted as indicative of frontal-lobe dysfunction, a finding consistent with the middle stages of AD.

In contrast, Sophie demonstrated insight into her difficulties by becoming upset by her poor performance, indicating that any frontal-lobe dysfunction was not yet advanced. Sophie's feelings of depression resulted from her still being able to understand what was happening to her, which had implications for her care and treatment. First, it could be helpful to treat Sophie's depression with antidepressants or with counseling; and second, Sophie still had the ability to think for herself and make decisions about her treatment and her future, and she should be given every assistance in doing this. This type of intervention would also allow Sophie to take some control over her current illness and future treatment, and that in itself should help to diminish feelings of depression, helplessness, and hopelessness.

On memory tests, including a repeat of some of the Wechsler Memory Scale subtests, Sophie's scores had also decreased significantly. On the Logical Memory passages, she could remember only four ideas from each story on immediate recall (an average score for her age was a recall of about eight ideas) and only two ideas from the first story and none from the second story after a delay of 10 minutes. On the Paired-Associates memory subtest, pairs of words that obviously go together (e.g., baby-cries) and pairs of words that are not usually associated (e.g., school-grocery) are learned over a number of trials. When Sophie was tested by being given the first word of each pair and asked for the word that went with it, she recalled all the obvious pairs by the second trial but none of the unusual pairs by the third trial. Her recall of the Rey Figure after a 45-minute delay consisted of a rectangle and nothing else.

Given her poor performance on the relatively simple Wechsler memory subtests, I considered it unnecessary to upset her further by giving her a more difficult, and therefore more sensitive, verbal memory test, such as the Oral Selective Reminding

Test (Bucshke and Fuld 1974). I did give her an easier memory test (the Recognition Memory Test; Warrington 1984), which relies on recognition rather than spontaneous recall, to see whether her memory had deteriorated to the extent that even this was impaired. On both word and face recognition, she scored 2 SD below average. She believed she had done quite well on this, as she was not given feedback, and her mood lifted a little.

Finally, Sophie was given some brief subtests from an aphasia battery to assess her language abilities. Comprehension was good, as were writing letters, numbers, and sentences to dictation. She could also repeat meaningful sentences accurately, but she had difficulty with some meaningless sentences (e.g., "The day, that the dream thought, jumped cheaply" from the Anomalous Sentences Repetition Test; Weeks 1988). This latter difficulty is considered a strong indicator of dementia. When asked to describe a picture, the content of her description was impoverished, consisting of a listing of objects with no indication of the actions depicted in the picture. This problem was clearly more than one of word-finding and indicated a marked decline from the previous fluent and rich content of her articles and interviews.

Sophie's memory for past events was informally assessed in the final session by inviting Peter in at the end, asking him to name events they had both attended, and then comparing Sophie's recollections with those of her husband. She was able spontaneously to recall some details of major events held in the past year, such as her own fiftieth birthday and her daughter's twenty-first birthday, both large social events, but she was unable to recall any details of a television series she and her husband had watched over a recent 6-week period. When Peter described it, she said she experienced a vague feeling of familiarity but could not add any details herself. She remembered that her last day at the radio studio had been celebrated but could recall no details. In fact, it was a formal dinner and presentation to Sophie of a painting and was attended by about 60 people. When Peter described the painting, she said she could now recall it and could see it in her mind's eye hanging over the fireplace, but her recall of the presentation of the painting remained vague. When asked to recall the names of her nieces and nephews (whom she knew quite well), she could not. She could, however, remember her own children's names, though was unable to recall the birth dates of her two sons and thought each was a year younger than he was.

The pattern of results from this assessment demonstrated a generalized cognitive decline compared with Sophie's previous assessment and a highly significant decline in relation to her estimated premorbid "superior" cognitive abilities. Sophie was clearly trying her best throughout the assessment and was distressed at times when she realized how poorly she was performing. These observations support other evidence (e.g., no history of depression and her current depressed mood appearing to be a direct result of her insight into her deteriorating cognitive abilities) that Sophie's poor performance was not a symptom of pseudodementia (i.e., depression). The assessment was spread over three sessions, and great care was taken to ensure that she was not tired; when she became upset, testing was terminated as soon as Sophie would allow. In an attempt to diminish her anxiety, whenever possible, difficult tests were followed by tests she was more likely to be able to accomplish. Despite these measures, her distress and anxiety probably had some negative influence on her performance, but these factors were by no means sufficient to explain her low scores.

Diagnosis

The neuropsychological assessment, coupled with the results from the medical investigations, was considered sufficient to enable the doctor to make a diagnosis of probable AD. Of particular importance was the fact that the cognitive deficits were progressive and included definite retrograde and anterograde memory impairments as well as deficits in language, abstract thinking, and visuospatial abilities that together made it impossible for Sophie to continue in her work or to socialize in the manner she had previously. Other causes for the dementia had been ruled out as carefully as possible, although a firm diagnosis of AD could not be made until her death and a postmortem on her brain.

Interventions and Management

The first intervention was the manner in which the diagnosis was revealed to Sophie. She and Peter were told together in a meeting with her doctor. Sophie, of course, was expecting bad news but nevertheless had continued to hold a small hope that her symptoms might have some other, less tragic cause. When this final ray of hope was dashed, her immediate reaction was to grimace and comment, "Well at least I'll have a good excuse for my crazy behavior now." She then fell silent, and her husband took her home after being given a firm appointment for as many members of the family who wished to meet with me in 2 days' time. It was made clear to them that they would have ongoing counseling and therapy available to them as well as other more practical help as they required it.

Peter and their three children attended the next session, which was taken up with listening to the grief and anger of each family member and answering their questions honestly. Sophie had remained almost mute for a day following her return home but had begun to cry when her 17-year-old son, Matthew, hugged her and told her he was going to make sure she was around for his twenty-first birthday. Since then Sophie continued to cry and sometimes fall asleep from exhaustion, and the family had decided to leave her in the care of a good friend from the Alzheimer's Support Group while they attended the counseling session.

The family decided to continue the same routine as long as possible but with a roster to ensure that at least one family member or one of Sophie's friends was in the house at all times to be available if Sophie should need them, want to talk, go out, or simply watch television with them. Peter had already decided to take partial leave from his law practice, which fortunately he was financially able to do, so that he could spend as much time with Sophie as possible before her dementia worsened to the point where she could not appreciate her family.

The possibility of suicide was discussed, and all her children said they would make their love and need of their mother so clear that she would not want to take her life. The importance of finding a nursing home or hospice where their mother could be cared for in her final months was also brought up by Diane, who had been the family member most involved in her grandmother's illness and care. It was agreed to put this on hold until Sophie felt ready to talk about it.

Within a week, Sophie felt able to see me for her first therapy session. Initially Sophie attended with her husband but then decided to continue weekly sessions alone. During these sessions, through me she wrote letters to her husband and to each of her children to be read after her death. She made a short audio tape recording for the entire family, made difficult by her word-finding problems, especially given her emotional state. With many stops and starts, however, she completed a very moving tape, which later became an important catalyst in the grieving and healing process for her family.

Once these tasks were completed, Sophie decided to have a session with her family to discuss her wish to be placed in a hospice when she needed full-time nursing care. She also talked with them about her wishes for her funeral and said she had written letters to be given to each of them after her death. This was a very positive session, after which the family members were able to talk at home with one another about many issues, both trivial and deep. Sophie did not ask for further therapy sessions, but on her request I visited her at home from time to time.

While Sophie was having her individual sessions with me, the other family members also attended sessions to talk about practical issues and concerns as well as to begin to work through their own grief. Diane found it particularly difficult because it brought back memories of her grandmother's dementia. All the children had concerns, at first unvoiced, that they too would end their days demented. This fear was discussed in terms of statistics (i.e., the many family members of AD patients who do not develop the disease); the massive research efforts going into finding the cause, a cure, and treatments for AD; the changing societal views and laws about euthanasia; and the many productive years the children had ahead of them before they need worry about the fairly unlikely possibility that they would also develop AD.

Sophie remained at home for 4 years. As she had requested in the early stages of her illness, she was placed in a hospice when she needed full-time nursing care. While at home she remained relatively easy to look after, and family members quickly learned ways to defuse potentially difficult situations. Sophie's depressed mood improved as her insight decreased, and within a year of diagnosis she no longer experienced periods of depression. She often made inappropriate or insensitive comments, frequently forgot or confused her children's names, and could not be left alone in the house for fear she would hurt herself or set fire to the house by leaving the stove on. The family continued to assist her to cook simple meals as long as she was able, as this gave her pleasure for a short time.

Sophie sometimes became agitated for no apparent reason, and she sometimes threw food or crockery if she did not like the food she was given. Her family members did not argue or correct her but simply removed the offending food, led her to her rocking chair, placed headphones over her ears, and played her favorite music. Matthew in particular spent many hours reading to her, playing simple card games of "snap" (and letting her win most of the time), and accompanying her on walks. Sophie retained his face and name in her memory longer than any others. After much soul-searching, Peter returned to his full-time law practice after 12 months, but he continued to keep most evenings free for Sophie. As he said, this work routine kept him "sane" and gave him the psychological strength to cope with Sophie.

Sophie deteriorated rapidly once in the hospice, and within 6 weeks she was mute and could recognize no one. Matthew had a small family gathering to celebrate his twenty-first birthday 3 months after Sophie entered the hospice, and Sophie came home for the occasion. To an onlooker she may have appeared unaware of what was going on, but Matthew insists that when he said to her, "See, Mum, I knew you would stick around for my twenty-first," she squeezed his hand and smiled at him. She died a month later, and a postmortem confirmed that she suffered from AD.

The family came to four therapy sessions following her death and were greatly helped and comforted by the audio tape and letters Sophie had left for them. Their grieving was already well advanced by the time Sophie died, and at the end her death came as a relief. Their support for one another was very strong, and they felt that as a family they had gained much of value as a consequence of the quality time they had been able to spend not only with Sophie but with each other. Matthew is now a hospice nurse.

Discussion

Dementia, whatever its cause, is a tragedy for the victim and for family and friends. It is also one of the most difficult areas for professionals, as they too must watch, helpless, as a person with a personality and intellect deteriorates into a "vegetable." It is perhaps this feeling of being unable to halt the inevitable decline that makes it so stressful to work or live with people with dementia. Therefore, any interventions, however small, that give the sufferer some control over her life (even if it is just controlling when she goes to bed) or that give the caregivers and family some means of improving the quality of the sufferer's daily existence will partially alleviate these feelings of helplessness and depression.

Families know the dementia sufferer best, and when given some encouragement, even small children can often come up with new and creative ways to ease the lives of the caregivers and bring some happiness into the patient's day. After the shock of the diagnosis has subsided and a routine of care has been established, it is important that all members of the family continue to live their own lives as well as sharing in the care of the patient if that is their wish. It is all too common for the bulk of the care to fall on the shoulders of one person, usually a woman relative; this situation should be avoided from the outset with the therapist encouraging the setting up of a roster system and using community services as well as family members.

Sophie was particularly fortunate in having a supportive family that was financially well off. Many elderly people who become demented have no family and are placed in a geriatric hospital early in their dementia, which often seems to precipitate their deterioration and death, perhaps because of a lack of stimulation or because they are still able to feel at some level that no one cares whether they live, and they simply give up.

Sophie's assessment and diagnosis were more straightforward than is often the case, primarily because of her own knowledge of the disease. In general, after the initial medical and neuropsychological assessment, a diagnosis would not be made until follow-up neuropsychological assessments demonstrated a progression of the cognitive deficits. A number of test batteries can be given over time to assess progressive dementia, and one of these could have been used instead of the Wechsler Scales. In Sophie's case, her earlier assessment with the Wechsler Scales acted as a useful baseline for the later assessment and made further longitudinal assessments unnecessary. In many cases, rating scales and questionnaires can be given to the caregivers at regular intervals to assess how well the patient is coping with everyday tasks and self-care. This practice provides another ongoing measure of the progress of the disease and also allows the professionals to organize appropriate nursing and home help and to suggest hospitalization at the appropriate time. Caregivers also need to have their coping abilities and stress levels monitored so that they can receive assistance and respite from their role before they collapse either physically or emotionally. Dementia is ultimately a tragedy for family and friends; their stress and grief continue for the duration of the disease and often long after the sufferer's death. For the dementia sufferer, the loss of insight that accompanies the middle and late stages of dementia spares them much emotional pain and embarrassment.

It is perhaps only when we watch a person who was once active, independent, intelligent, humorous, and loving gradually "losing her mind" that we begin to comprehend the magnificence and complexity of the human brain and want to discover more about what it can do, how it works, how it can overcome great adversity (including damage to itself), and how we may someday be able to fix it when it goes wrong. Part of the challenge for neuroscience researchers is to find answers to these questions. For the clinical neuropsychologist and other professionals working with neurologically impaired people, the human tragedy they see daily becomes one of the most salient reasons for persisting with this difficult but rewarding work.

18
■

SPLIT BRAIN, SPLIT MIND?
CASE L.B.

In 1981 Roger Sperry of the California Institute of Technology (Caltech) shared the Nobel Prize in Physiology and Medicine for his research on the behavior and neuropsychology of animals and people that had undergone an operation in which the *corpus callosum*, the large fiber tract connecting the two hemispheres of the brain, is split (Sperry 1982). Split-brain surgery (*commissurotomy*) was first performed in humans in the 1940s in an attempt to control epilepsy; a series of 26 adults and adolescents were operated on with mixed results (Akelaitis 1941; Escourolle, Hauw, Gray, and Henin 1975). It seems unlikely, however, that the corpus callosum was completely divided in most of these patients.

The first complete commissurotomies were performed by Professor P. J. Vogel and Dr. J.. Bogen of the Californian College of Medicine (Bogen and Vogel 1962). Beginning in 1961, they and their colleagues performed 10 commissurotomies, and many of the patients in this Californian series have been the subjects of neuropsychological research from the time of their operations to the present. The most prominent of the Californian patients are N.G., L.B., and A.A.; in addition to Roger Sperry, the most prominent researchers include Joseph Bogen, Michael Gazzaniga, Jay Myers, Eran and Dahlia Zaidel, and Jerre Levy.

Researchers from other parts of the United States and Canada have also contributed to the ever-increasing body of knowledge arising from studies of split-brain subjects. For example, numerous studies have been carried out by Professor Michael Gazzaniga and his colleagues, including among many others Donald Wilson, Joseph LeDoux, John Sidtis, and Jeff Holtzman. Gazzaniga first became involved in split-brain studies when he researched the Californian subjects for his doctoral thesis with Sperry as his advisor. Some of Gazzaniga's findings from later studies of split-brain subjects from

This chapter could not have been written without the kind permission and cooperation of L.B.; the encouragement and assistance of Professor Michael Corballis, who provided me with many personal anecdotes, interviewed L.B. for me, and critiqued drafts of this chapter; and Professor Joseph Bogen, who kindly gave me permission to write this chapter and critiqued it for me.

the eastern United States led to heated arguments between researchers from different laboratories (Gazzaniga 1983a, 1983b; Levy 1983; Zaidel 1983). Such controversy, when it arises from apparently incongruent research findings, is the stuff of good science if it leads to new and better interpretations of old data and the design of new experiments aimed at clarifying confusing results. Science that remains the realm of one laboratory is in danger of becoming entrenched within the mindset of that laboratory unless, of course, new students are given the freedom to explore their own fresh ideas, even when these do not fit the traditional mold. Sperry ran his Caltech laboratory in this open and stimulating way, as described by his ex-student Gazzaniga in a book he wrote many years later:

> One of the many things that made Sperry an excellent mentor was that he left you alone. He set a laboratory context for work, and he was always there working to make things better, to advise, to assist, and to guide. But he didn't order anyone around or tell anyone what to do. . . . We all freely interacted and talked all the time about everything. In the early years the work was being done primarily by Sperry, Bogen, and myself, but others were around too. (Gazzaniga 1985, p 37)

L.B., the man who is the focus of this chapter, is the most intensively studied of all the Californian split-brain subjects, perhaps because he is one of the most intelligent members of the group. Magnetic resonance imaging (MRI) studies by Bogen, Schultz, and Vogel (1988) confirmed that the operation performed on L.B. had successfully split all the fibers of the corpus callosum, making the results of studies of L.B. somewhat clearer to interpret than those of other people, in whom some fibers of the corpus callosum may have been (accidentally) left intact during the surgery.

L.B. is the only case in this book whom I have not had the privilege of meeting and assessing personally. Given the importance of the U.S. split-brain research to neuropsychology, it was clearly important to include a split-brain case in this book. Fortunately, my colleague Michael Corballis had assessed L.B. a number of times (Corballis and Ogden 1988; Corballis and Sergent 1988; Corballis and Trudel 1993) and was about to set off on another trip to California to test L.B. again. This time he was armed with various questions I wanted him to ask L.B., and he returned with an audio tape of a long conversation with L.B., who had readily agreed to my writing about him. Writing about someone about whom I have read and heard a great deal, but never met, increases the possibility that I will do L.B. an injustice in trying to convey the essence of his presence to the reader. By including some of L.B.'s own descriptions and obtaining feedback on early drafts of this chapter from people who know L.B. well, I hope I will not get it too wrong.

Why are split-brain patients so fascinating to neuroscientists and lay people alike? First, most people find the idea that we have two independently thinking and acting minds inside the same skull intriguing. Of course, in the normal state the two sides of our brain are connected, and to the owner of the brain as well as to the casual observer, they appear to act as one mind. It is only in the abnormal state when the two hemispheres are surgically separated that their potential for independence becomes apparent. Even then, it takes special equipment and clever experimentation to trick the brain into revealing its two independent minds; in everyday life split-brain subjects appear to think and behave exactly like everyone else. Second, the split-brain phenomenon has provided neuroscientists with a means of testing hypotheses about the specialist functions of the intact left and right hemispheres. For example, is language restricted to the left hemisphere, and can the right hemisphere perform visuospatial tasks better than the left? Third, hypotheses about the integration of functions across the two hemispheres can be tested. How important is the connection between the two sides of the brain given that split-brain subjects behave perfectly normally in nonexperimental situations? What can the connected brain do that the disconnected brain cannot? Can some information be transferred from one hemisphere to the other even when the brain is split? If so, what is the substance of this information, and how does it get from one side to the other?

One final and controversial area of inquiry involves consciousness and intelligence. The most dramatic difference between the disconnected hemispheres is that the left hemisphere can talk just as well as a normal person, but in most split-brain subjects, the right hemisphere is mute or at best has very limited speech and therefore cannot report orally what is happening in the right hemisphere. An extreme point of view would be that the right hemisphere is unintelligent as well as mute. Gazzaniga in particular has suggested that the disconnected, nonlinguistic right hemisphere is less intelligent than an ape. For example, in 1983 he wrote, "Indeed, it could well be argued that the cognitive skills of a normal disconnected right hemisphere without language are vastly inferior to the cognitive skills of a chimpanzee" (Gazzaniga 1983a, p. 536). Such an extreme stance is no longer held by most researchers in the field, and even Gazzaniga allows that the nonlinguistic right hemisphere is superior (over the left hemisphere and the apes) in its ability to perform some specialized, nonverbal visuospatial skills (Gazzaniga and Smylie 1983). The view that the right hemisphere is as intelligent as the speaking left hemisphere, but specialized for different functions, and that in addition it is equally self-aware and self-conscious, but at a nonverbal level, is certainly not universally held either (cf. Bogen 1993, 2000; Gazzaniga 1983a, 1983b; Levy 1983; Zaidel 1983).

Many answers to these questions have been found and even agreed on by most researchers in the field, but many remain unanswered, in part because of the variation in results among subjects. Split-brain subjects are like any other group of people: Although they have many similarities in terms of what their split brains can and cannot do, they also demonstrate individual differences. For example, the extent of their ability to comprehend language with the right hemisphere appears to vary considerably among subjects, leading to confusion for students struggling to understand the extensive research literature and stimulating controversy within the scientific community. As with all neuropsychological research, interpretations of old data must often be rethought and revised when new data that do not fit the original interpretation come to light. Thus, some of the interpretations of the data discussed in this chapter and throughout this book are likely to be obsolete in a few years. Nevertheless, if the data themselves are methodologically sound, they will remain valid and continue to serve as part of the data base for new hypotheses and new discoveries.

Theoretical Background

The Operation

In experimental animals, the corpus callosum connecting the two hemispheres is surgically cut along with the optic chiasm. Thus, with one eye covered, the animal receives visual input only in the hemisphere opposite the source of the visual stimulus. Behavioral responses to that visual information can then be interpreted as emanating from only one hemisphere. In the human, the corpus callosum is split for therapeutic purposes: The patient has intractable and debilitating epileptic seizures that cannot be satisfactorily controlled by anticonvulsant medication. The seizures are diffuse or of mixed types and cannot be localized to a defined area within the cortex. Therefore, it is not possible to cut out the epileptic focus surgically as in some cases of partial, focal seizures (see Chapter 4), and the two hemispheres (also called the forebrain) are disconnected in the hope of preventing the spread of the seizures from one hemisphere to the other. In many cases, the commissurotomy reduces seizure spread and frequency substantially, and in some cases it completely abolishes them. Some patients remain on anticonvulsant medication, but at much lower levels, whereas others may ultimately become seizure-free without medication.

A complete split or commissurotomy in humans usually includes not only the main fiber band, the corpus callosum, but also smaller commissures, including the anterior and hippocampal commissures. The Californian patients, including L.B., underwent a complete commissurotomy in one operation, but many of the East Coast patients had a staged commissurotomy in which only the corpus callosum was split (called a *callosotomy*), which division was often carried out in two stages over two operations. According to Wilson, Reeves, and Gazzaniga (1978), this approach seemed to be less debilitating and had a smaller risk of postoperative complications, usually with equally good therapeutic results. In humans, the optic chiasm is not split.

Acute Disconnection Syndrome

Acute Disconnection Syndrome occurs in most patients immediately after the commissurotomy and may last from a few days to several weeks. The patient is mute and can communicate only by using body language. The patients are often unable to perform purposeful movements with the left side of their body on verbal command (*left-sided apraxia*). Left-sided instability, incoordination, an unsteady wide-based gait, inattention to or neglect of stimuli on the left side, and apathy are also common. Sometimes competitive movements of the two hands may occur. For example, one hand may be unbuttoning the pajama jacket while the other buttons it up again. A partial or staged commissurotomy may reduce these symptoms considerably. Within days to weeks most of these symptoms resolve. Speech becomes normal, and the patient regains normal movement, although rapid, highly coordinated movements remain impaired.

Late Disconnection Syndrome

The most obviously bisected system of the commissurotomized brain is the visual system; all the visual information from the right visual field (i.e., to the right of the central visual fixation point) is projected to the left hemisphere, and vice versa. Tactile and auditory stimuli are projected predominantly to the opposite side of the brain, but weak ipsilateral connections (i.e., to the same side of the brain) are also present. In the split-brain subject, normal movements of the eyes and head readily compensate for the disconnection of the right and left visual systems, and hand movements and auditory cues also serve to distribute sensory information to both hemispheres. Therefore, to demonstrate the disconnection of the sensory systems, controlled testing procedures that ensure that the stimuli go only to one hemisphere are required. In this case, the sectioning of the corpus callosum prevents the crossing of information from one hemisphere to the other. If an object is placed in the unseen right hand of the split-brain subject, he will be able to say what it is; the tactile information travels directly to the left, speech hemisphere. If instead the subject is asked to write down the name of the object or pick it from a number of unseen objects with the left hand, he will not be able to do this because the information cannot be transmitted to the right hemisphere, which controls the left hand. Of course, if the left hemisphere first says the name of the object felt by the right hand, then the right hemisphere may be able to understand the simple noun and then pick the corresponding object from an array of objects with the left hand. This strategy is called *cross-cuing*, and experimenters must be on the alert for this and other cross-cuing strategies when assessing their subjects. As explained later, L.B. is a past master at subtle *cross-cuing*, which in the early days of experimentation probably resulted in a few otherwise inexplicable results!

When an object is placed, unseen, in the left hand, the subject cannot say what it is, nor can he pick it from an array with his right hand (controlled by the left hemisphere) because only the right, mute hemisphere has the information. If the subject is then shown an array of objects in free vision, however, he can point to the object with his left but not with his right hand. In these cases, the ipsilateral pathways from the hand to the brain are clearly inhibited by the more dominant contralateral pathways.

The visual disconnection is assessed by asking the subject to fixate on a point straight ahead and then briefly flashing a stimulus (a picture or a word) in one visual field or the other. As long as the stimulus is not exposed long enough to allow an eye saccade or movement toward it, it will be projected only to the visual cortex of the opposite hemisphere. Thus, when an object or word is flashed in the subject's right visual field, he will be able to tell the experimenter what it is; but when an object or word is flashed in the left visual field, he will deny having seen anything. If, however, he is shown an array of objects or printed words in free vision and asked to guess what was flashed in his left visual field, he will accurately point to the correct object or word with his left hand but will not be able to point to the correct object or word with his right hand. A most dramatic illustration of the split brain occurs when two different objects are flashed simultaneously, one image projecting to each hemisphere. If an apple is flashed in the left visual field, the left hand will pick up an apple from a bowl of fruit in open view. At the same time, an orange flashed in the right visual field will result in the right hand picking an orange from the fruit bowl. Asked what he saw, the subject will reply "an orange," because only the image of the orange was available to the speaking left hemisphere.

Other general findings following commissurotomy include normal writing with the right hand but poor or absent writing with the left hand and good drawing of cubes and other spatial, nonverbal pictures with the left hand and poor drawings with the right hand. The left hand is also better than the right at doing the Block Design subtest of the Wechsler Adult Intelligence Scale (WAIS). There is some evidence to suggest that these findings are not entirely an indication of right-hemispheric specialization for visuospatial perception but may also reflect a right-hemispheric specialization for manipulospatial skills. That is, a right-hemispheric superiority will be more apparent when a visuospatial task has a motor component. One study used a visuospatial task that did not require a motor component and found that the left hemisphere was as good as the right when asked to make discriminations or matches between patterns flashed into one visual field or the other (Le Doux, Wilson, and Gazzaniga 1978).

Still, the bulk of evidence supports the idea that the right hemisphere is specialized for the higher cognitive functions involved in tasks requiring a nonverbal, holistic, visuospatial approach, regardless of whether there is a motor component. Certainly some data are best able to be interpreted in this light. For example, using the visual modality, the right hemisphere is better at deciding what a three-dimensional object made by folding paper would look like if it was unfolded into the two-dimensional form (Levy-Agresti and Sperry 1968) and is better at recognizing faces (Gazzaniga and Smylie 1983; Levy, Trevarthen, and Sperry 1972).

Whereas the extent of the right hemisphere's role in visuospatial cognition is still controversial, the specialization of the left hemisphere for language is not in doubt and is clearly demonstrated by the normal ability of the disconnected left hemisphere to perform all language tasks. The extent of the language ability possessed by the right hemisphere is not so clear. Most of the right-handed split-brain subjects have a fairly good ability to comprehend single words that enter the right hemisphere via auditory, visual, or tactile routes. In addition, the disconnected right hemisphere can make lexical decisions (i.e., tell if a pronounceable letter string is a real word). This ability fits with the finding that patients undergoing a Wada test with the left hemisphere anesthetized before temporal lobe excision for epilepsy (see Chapter 4) can understand simple commands with their awake right hemisphere.

Understanding syntax and speaking and spontaneous writing with the right hemisphere are generally extremely poor or absent in most split-brain subjects who otherwise show good language comprehension. Most of the subjects' right hemispheres cannot use phonetic (sound) cues to assist comprehension. For example, they cannot tell whether words flashed to the right hemisphere rhyme or not (Levy and Trevarthen 1977). In the rare case where a right-handed split-brain subject appears to have more extensive language abilities in the right hemisphere (Gazzaniga and Le Doux 1978), this may be the result of early left-hemispheric damage and the consequent sharing of some language functions by the right hemisphere even before the commissurotomy was carried out. In some cases, subsequent sophisticated MRI has demonstrated that the corpus callosum was not completely split at the time of the operation, allowing information relayed to the right hemisphere to be transferred across to the left, speaking hemisphere.

Calculation abilities have also been shown to be a left-hemispheric ability. The method is as follows. The subject is shown a card in open view with numerals 1 to 8 printed on it. Then two blocks, each with one to four pegs inserted in it, are presented, one at a time, to the unseen left hand. The subject is then asked to point with the left hand to the sum of the two blocks. Most subjects could count the number of pegs on a single block but could sum two blocks only up to four and could not subtract one block from another or multiply. It is interesting to note that even in hemispherectomized patients in whom the isolated right hemisphere behaves more like a left hemisphere than a right one with respect to language functions, calculation beyond simple addition is still not possible (see Chapter 19). Further support for a left-hemispheric monopoly over calculation is found in cases of Gerstmann's syndrome, where a lesion in the posterior left hemisphere abolishes the ability to perform sums other than simple addition (see Chapter 6).

Case Presentation

Background

L.B. was delivered by caesarean section in May 1952. He was cyanotic and weighed 5 pounds at birth; he was placed in an incubator for 8 days. His early development was considered normal until he suffered his first epileptic seizure when he was 3.5 years old. Over the next 9 years, his seizures increased in severity. Nevertheless, he attended public school, although he did not do particularly well, often achieving grades of C or lower. When he was on light doses of anticonvulsant medication, he was a talkative, active, happy child and enjoyed physical activities, including swimming and skating. He particularly liked sketching and had an ambition to become a cartoonist. His seizures become particularly severe when he was about 12. Heavier doses of anticonvulsant medication did not help but simply put him to sleep in class (Bogen 1969; Bogen and Vogel 1975; Gazzaniga 1970; Levy, Nebes, and Sperry 1970).

Neurological examinations were unremarkable, and skull radiographs, a computed tomography (CT) brain scan, and a bilateral carotid angiogram were all normal. However, electroencephalographic (EEG) recordings did indicate diffuse abnormalities of his brain waves. It was decided that a complete commissurotomy would be the best treatment, and this was carried out by Dr. Bogen and Professor Vogel in April 1965 1 month before L.B.'s 13th birthday. At the time of his surgery, L.B. was in the seventh grade, he read normally for his age, and his Full-scale IQ on the Wechsler Intelligence Scale for Children was 115 (Verbal IQ 119, Performance IQ 108). He was right-handed but could also write less well with his left hand, and he was able to draw three-dimensional Necker cubes with either hand. As expected, before his corpus callosum was sectioned, he could easily identify objects placed in either hand and could read words flashed to either visual field.

The commissurotomy was uncomplicated, and the anterior and hippocampal commissures were cut as well as the corpus callosum. L.B. made a rapid recovery that was unusual in that he suffered only minimally the typical acute disconnection syndrome of mutism and poor left-sided motor control. The day after surgery, he was happy and talkative. He could hold up his left hand but could not hold up two fingers with his left hand on verbal command. He was unable to write with his left hand or copy figures with his right hand, but this defiency lasted for only a few weeks before he could once again copy figures and write with both hands (Bogen 1969; Bogen and Vogel 1975; Gazzaniga 1970; Levy et al. 1970).

Following surgery, his seizures were alleviated, although he continued on a reduced regime of anticonvulsant medication. He returned to school, and apart from having difficulty with mathematics, he continued to achieve at an average to low-average level in his other subjects. Three years after surgery, a number of left-sided focal motor seizures suggested he might have a right-sided abnormality, although no right-sided focus had been detected before surgery. Some minor right-sided damage may have occurred at the time of surgery when the right hemisphere was pulled back to allow the surgeon to access the corpus callosum (Zaidel 1988). According to L.B., his seizures now occur only about once every 6 months, usually in the early hours of the morning while he is asleep.

When Mike Corballis interviewed and assessed L.B. for me so that I could write this chapter, L.B. was 42 years old and had lived with a split brain for 29 years. He died a few years later, leaving as a legacy a large body of data that has contributed significantly to our understanding about the interrelationship of the two cerebral hemispheres and brainbehavior relations more generally. He was assessed numerous times, not only by the Caltech researchers but also by many other researchers from around the world. L.B. seemed to enjoy participating in the research projects and was a cooperative, cheerful subject. As he remarked to Mike Corballis in 1994, "I don't mind testing as long as they learn something. I like it; it's a game, sort of. I get a kick out of it." With reference to the many new researchers that arrive at Caltech to test him, he commented, "I'm a good person for someone starting out. I'll tell them if they're doing something wrong, or if I can see when I'm not meant to." (Personal communication from M. Corballis, 1994)

L.B. delighted in trying to trick and outwit the experienced researcher, and his skill at using peripheral cross-cuing has at times perplexed researchers and caused them to rethink their experimental setup to ensure that L.B. cannot cross-cue. Some of his tricks included using small movements of his nose, tongue, or lips to form a geometric shape flashed to his right hemisphere. This, he reported, allows his left hemisphere to see what the shape is so that he can name it. According to D. W. Zaidel (1988), this cross-cuing technique can be readily circumvented (Zaidel, Zaidel, and Bogen 1990).

When Mike Corballis asked L.B. to describe himself, L.B. replied, "I'm relatively kind. Semipolite. My feet always stay on the ground. I'm happy. No problems! I like simple food, a steak, a good hamburger. I hate cooking 'cause I know what went in it. I'm not a fashion plate. I like to be comfortable." L.B. said he had no friends, and most of the people he knew well were family members. He said he used to go out at night with friends but added, "I got tired of coming in at three or four in the morning because I was plastered. I decided, well, its time to straighten up here, get your act together." L.B. had been married and divorced and then until his death lived with his father and his father's wife.

Although L.B. was employed in various jobs from 1972 to 1989 (e.g., working in a tool shop), after that period he kept himself occupied at home, where he spent a lot of time writing, drawing, and playing cards and other games on his computer. He enjoyed listening to music from the 1920s to the 1980s, occasionally watched films on cable television, and read a little, although he stuck mostly to technical books on computers. Reading novels gave him a headache because he had difficulty with scanning from one line to the next. He did not follow any exercise program or participate in sports, but he did a lot of "speedy" walking. He conversed easily and fluently about current topics of interest and expressed firm and informed opinions about current and past political figures. When asked about religion, he replied, "God and I have a good understanding. I leave him alone and he leaves me alone. Don't bother me and I won't bother you."

Over the years of testing, L.B. obviously gained a good understanding of the split-brain phenomena, and every now and then reread all the articles written about him. This knowledge seemed to be purely "academic," however, as subjectively he felt the same as everyone else. Occasionally, he noticed that he was acting in a "split" manner: "I can be holding my keys in my left hand and my right hand will be looking for them in my pocket."

Neuropsychological Assessments

General intellectual abilities   Before surgery, L.B.'s general intellectual abilities fell easily within the average range or above and remained so after his surgery. At the age of 17, his Wechsler Adult Intelligence Scale (WAIS) Full-scale IQ was 106 (Verbal IQ 110, Performance IQ 100). His range of subtest scores was quite wide, however, with Digit Symbol (a test of visuospatial perception and psychomotor speed) falling below his age mean, as is fairly typical for people with brain damage of any kind. In contrast, on tests of verbal abstraction and conceptualization, he scored in the superior range. A further assessment on the WAIS in 1976 when L.B. was 23 demonstrated no significant change (Full-scale IQ 110, Verbal IQ 109, Performance IQ 110) (Campbell, Bogen, and Smith 1981; Levy et al. 1970).

L.B.'s reading ability was average, and his ability to draw spontaneously with both his right and left hands was good (see Figs. 18-1 and 18-2). He could also write with either hand. In rapidly reacquiring these abilities, he was unusual for a split-brain subject, as the hemispheric disconnection commonly produces a right-hand drawing impairment and a left-hand writing impairment (Bogen 1969). It seems likely that L.B. had acquired quite good ipsilateral control of his hands, which would explain his eventual lack of these disconnection problems.

His ability to copy the Rey Complex Figure with his right hand was not very good, however (see Fig. 18-3), and demonstrated considerable visuospatial impairment. His score of 17 of a possible 36 points fell well below the 10th percentile of 29. When asked to copy the Taylor Complex Figure with his left hand, his drawing was rather indistinct, with wobbly lines (probably because he was drawing with his left, nondominant hand), but the proportions of the figure were considerably more accurate than his previous right-handed copy (see Fig. 18-4). His score of 27.5 out of 36 (wobbly but otherwise correct lines were not penalized) still fell below the 10th percentile but was nevertheless considerably better than his score when he used his right hand. This result may indicate that each hand was controlled primarily by the opposite hemisphere while carrying out this novel visuospatial task and that ipsilateral

Figure 18-1 L.B.'s spontaneous drawings with his right hand. The "cartoon" on the right is a self-portrait of L.B. (With kind permission of L.B.)

Figure 18-2 L.B.'s spontaneous drawings with his left hand. (With kind permission of L.B.)

control was minimal, which would explain why his left-handed (right hemisphere) copy was better proportioned than his right-handed copy. An hour after copying each figure, L.B. was asked to draw the figures from memory using the same hand that he used to copy each figure. For both figures he recalled only the main details, and his recall scores fell well below the 10th percentile for both.

Receptive and expressive language   L.B.'s language functions were completely normal under everyday conditions. Likewise, under experimental conditions, his left hemisphere showed normal comprehension and expression of spoken and written language. His right hemisphere was able to comprehend nouns, adjectives, and verbs equally well when word-frequency factors were taken into account, but he could not carry out written commands lateralized to his right hemisphere (Gazzaniga 1970); that is, although he could comprehend verbs with his right hemisphere, he could not act on them.

Larry Johnson (1984) reported a study that suggested that L.B.'s right hemisphere could speak to some degree. Johnson found that L.B. could vocalize both stimuli presented simultaneously in his right and left visual fields, but he could not determine whether they were the same or different. This latter result appeared to suggest that there was no transfer of information between the hemispheres; thus, the left visual field stimulus must have been named by the right hemisphere.

Another interpretation for L.B.'s apparent ability to name stimuli with his right hemisphere was later suggested by Myers and Sperry (1985), who found that, in common with most split-brain subjects, L.B. was poor at processing language phonetically (by sound) in his right hemisphere. For example, he had difficulty recognizing that words rhymed when they were flashed to his right hemisphere. A study in which L.B. was able to respond with appropriate rhymes for single digits seen only by his right hemisphere was considered by Myers and Sperry (1985) to indicate that the left hemisphere had access to some information that gave a clue to the identity of the digit. Such information must be transferred subcortically, allowing the subject's left hemisphere to make an intelligent guess as to the identity of the digit seen only by the right hemisphere and then to provide a rhyming word. When doing these sorts of tasks, L.B. seemed to rehearse mentally all the possibilities until one "sticks out." Myers and Sperry likened this to the "tip of the tongue" phenomenon we all experi-

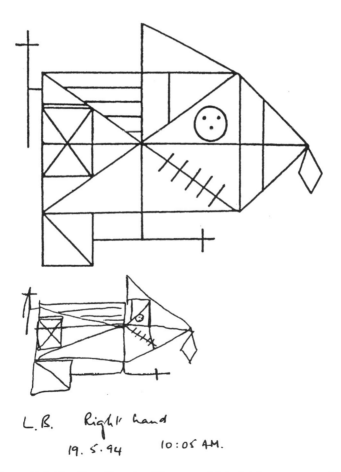

Figure 18-3 The Rey Complex Figure model is in the top row, with L.B.'s copy of it with his right hand below. (With kind permission of L.B.)

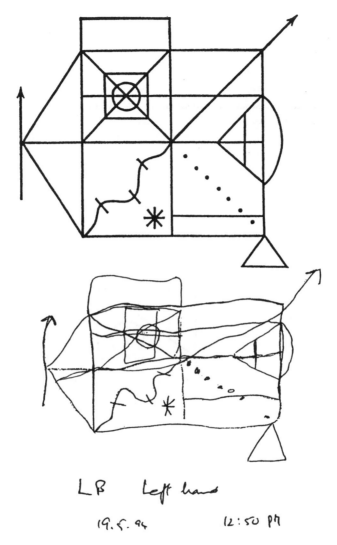

Figure 18-4 The Taylor Complex Figure model is in the top row, with L.B.'s copy of it with his left hand below. (With kind permission of L.B.)

ence at times. We know we know the elusive word and have some imprecise information about what it is. As soon as someone else says it, or we come across it while going through possible alternatives, we recognize it immediately.

Early on, the limitations of L.B.'s right hemisphere expressive language were explored by Levy et al. (1970) 4 years after his surgery. They found that L.B. could spell two- and three-letter words by ordering plastic letters with his unseen left hand, but when asked what word he had just correctly spelled he was unable to say. This finding demonstrated that there was no transfer from the right to left hemisphere and that his right hemisphere could not speak. He was then asked to run his left fingers over plastic letters already formed into words and either to write them with his left hand or to say them. He was able to write them but was never able to say them before writing them. He was able to say some words after writing them, which has been attributed to bilateral kinesthetic feedback allowing the left hemisphere to discriminate what the left hand has written. The left hemisphere then vocalizes the word.

L.B. was also asked to write with his left hand the names of objects placed in his unseen left hand. He would often clumsily write the first two letters of the name of the object, stop, hold the pencil more naturally, and then add some incorrect letters. For example, after holding a pipe, he slowly printed out *PI*, stopped, and then continued by changing the *I* into an *E* and adding *NCIL* to form *PENCIL*. He then scratched out the last four letters and said he did not know what the object was. Levy et al. (1970) believe these problems are the result of interference from the language-dominant hemisphere. The right hemisphere begins to write the simple word, but then the left hemisphere takes control of the left hand, presumably via ipsilateral pathways.

Dahlia Zaidel (1988) readministered some of these tests of expressive language 3 years later (i.e., 7 years postoperatively). She found a remarkable improvement in L.B.'s ability to vocalize words he had spelled out with plastic letters with his hidden left hand and already formed words he was asked to feel with his left hand. He could even vocalize irregularly spelled words (e.g., *walk* and *tight*) after feeling them with his left hand. Zaidel observed, however, that L.B. was far slower reading with the left hand than reading with the right hand, and he could take up to 45 seconds to read one left-hand word. In other tests, when L.B. was asked to write or name numbers, letters, objects, or shapes placed in his unseen left hand, his performance depended on how familiar the items were. If he had seen the range of objects before testing, he was more likely to be correct than if he had no idea what the objects might be. He was also better with one-digit numbers, where there are 10 possibilities (from 0 to 9), than on letters, where there are 26 possibilities (from A to Z). When manipulating the object to be named, he would take a long time, obviously feeling its weight, dimensions, and texture. It is possible that crude sensory information was transferred to the left hemisphere via ipsilateral sensory projection systems and that L.B.'s left hemisphere was then able to run through the various alternatives until he found one that matched the sensory properties of the object. Other tests, in which L.B. had to palpate an object with one hand and then pick it from an array with the other hand, showed some cross-transfer of tactual information from one hemisphere to the other.

Seven years postoperatively, L.B. was 73%–86% correct when asked to write with his left hand the names of short words, simple shapes, and pictures of familiar objects flashed in his left visual field. His verbal naming of these stimuli was much poorer, and he was correct only about 50% of the time. When single letters or numbers were flashed in his left visual field, he could name them correctly 92%–100% of the time (D. Zaidel 1988). As suggested by Myers and Sperry (1985), this good result may have been accomplished by the subcortical transfer of sufficient sensory information from the right to left hemisphere to enable L.B.'s left hemisphere to make a correct guess.

The right hemisphere's ability to express words in writing is much better than its ability to speak. L.B.'s left-hand-written responses tend to be in cursive script rather than printed, suggesting a development of linguistic maturity. D. Zaidel (1988) suggested that vocalization is not as easy a task for the right hemisphere to perform as writing because there is only a single speaking musculature, which is dominated by the left hemisphere.

Other split-brain functions   L.B.'s mathematical abilities were, as with most split-brain subjects, confined to the left hemisphere. With his right hemisphere, he was unable to do more than simple addition. As mentioned, his good ability to draw pictures and shapes spontaneously with his right hand as well as his left was unusual for a split-brain subject (see Figs. 18-1 and 18-2). This ability may not indicate that the left hemisphere is equal to the right for these abilities but, rather, that he had developed good ipsilateral control of his hands. That is, when he was drawing with his right hand, his hand movements may have been mediated by his right hemisphere. Objects that can be verbalized are readily recognized by both hemispheres in all split-brain subjects; like the other subjects, however, L.B. was faster at matching complex, relatively nonverbalizable patterns and unfamiliar faces with his right hemisphere. He was also better at copying complex figures (see Fig. 18-4), judging whole circle sizes from a small arc, making mental spatial transformations, and comprehending geometric principles with his right hemisphere (Sperry 1982).

Corballis and Sergent (1988), using mental rotation tasks, studied L.B.'s ability to generate images with each of his hemispheres. In these tasks, rotated letters or figures that face either forward or backward are flashed to one visual field (i.e., one hemisphere), and the subject must indicate whether the stimulus is forward or backward. It has been found that to do this, normal people turn the stimulus around in their mind until it reaches the upright position before they can decide whether it is forward or backward. Although it is an image they are rotating, the time they take to perform the task suggests that they proceed exactly as if the image were a real object. That is, when the letter is presented upside down, 180 degrees from upright, it takes longer to make a decision than when it is presented only 45 degrees from the upright. On these sorts of tasks, L.B. showed a strong left visual field (right hemispheric) advantage, and his right-hemisphere performance was just like that of normal subjects. His left hemisphere did improve with practice, but it was never able to reach the level of skill that the right hemisphere demonstrated.

Self-Awareness in the Right Hemisphere

Most researchers now agree that the right hemisphere possesses some degree of higher intellectual ability, albeit in the realm of visuospatial and nonverbal thought rather than in the logical and sequential thought processes exemplified by the sophisticated linguistic and mathematical skills of the left hemisphere. A separate question is whether each hemisphere contains an ability to be aware of itself and to be socially aware. Does each disconnected hemisphere have that sophisticated, reflective, self-conscious kind of inner awareness and a concern with the wider social world that most of us believe separates humans from other primates? (Bogen 2000; Zaidel, Jacoboni, Zaidel, and Bogen 2003). Obviously, in relation to the left hemisphere, this question is easily answered in the affirmative, as that hemisphere can speak for itself and express what it is doing, thinking, and feeling. It knows who it is and can reflect on itself. In the normal, connected brain, it may not be necessary for the right hemisphere to be self-aware, as the left hemisphere can be aware of and speak for both sides of the brain.

To test such complex questions required a means of ensuring that complex visual stimuli could be confined to only one side of the disconnected brain for longer periods than a split second. Sperry, Zaidel, and Zaidel (1979) used a specially designed optical system consisting of a special contact lens that when placed on the eye cut out one visual field while allowing the eyes to scan freely. If the other eye was covered, then the split-brain subject, using only one hemisphere, could visually scan an array of stimuli and think and respond to them while they were still in view. Using this procedure, L.B.'s right hemisphere was shown arrays of four to nine photographs, drawings, or printed material of neutral and emotionally laden photographs (e.g., faces, pets, and belongings, public and historical figures, etc.). He was asked to point with the left hand to items he recognized or liked or disliked. Sometimes he was asked to indicate with a "thumbs-up" or "thumbs-down" sign how he felt about particular items. L.B.'s facial expressions and exclamations were also noted. Follow-up oral questioning was directed to the speech hemisphere to ensure that the visual information seen by the right hemisphere had not crossed over to the left hemisphere.

The results were clear. Each hemisphere was equally good at recognizing photographs of L.B. as well as those of his relations, pets, belongings, familiar scenes, and well-known historical, political and entertainment figures. L.B.'s answers to follow-up questions after recognition by his right hemisphere demonstrated that he not only recognized that the person or item was familiar but knew the personal or social context of the item. When a photograph of L.B. was produced unexpectedly among unrelated items, in an inappropriate context, he demonstrated this by his emotional expression, or at some subcortical level the emotion he felt would cross to the left hemisphere, which might comment "What are they?" or "Was it me?" An actual example taken from Sperry et al. (1979) will best illustrate the social and self-awareness of L.B.'s right hemisphere: L.B.'s right hemisphere was shown an array of four pictures of people, singly and in groups. Three pictures contained unknown people, but the fourth contained Hitler in uniform standing with four other men. L.B. was asked to point to "any of these that you recognize." He examined the card for about 14 seconds and then pointed, with his left hand, to the face of Hitler. The following conversation and its interpretation by the researchers was reported by Sperry and colleagues in 1979.

> Examiner (Ex): Do you recognize that one? Is that the only one? (LB again inspected the full array but did not point to any others.)
>
> Ex: Well, on this: Is this one a "thumbs-up" or "thumbs-down" item for you?

LB: (Signaled "thumbs-down.")

Ex: That's another "thumbs-down"?

LB: Guess I'm antisocial. (Because this was his third consecutive "thumbs-down.")

Ex: Who is it?

LB: GI came to mind. I mean . . . (Subject at this point was seen to be tracing letters with the first finger of his left hand on the back of his right hand.)

Ex: You're writing with your left hand; let's keep the cues out.

LB: Sorry about that.

Ex: Is it someone you know personally, . . . or from entertainment, . . . or historical, or . . . ?

LB: (Interrupted and said) Historical.

Ex: Recent or . . . ?

LB: Past.

Ex: This country or another country?

LB: Uh-huh-okay.

Ex: You're not sure?

LB: Another country, I think.

Ex: Prime Minister, king, president, . . . any of them?

LB: Gee (and pondered with accompanying lip movements for several seconds).

Ex: (Giving further cues) Great Britain? . . . Germany?

LB: (Interrupted and said definitely) Germany (and then after a slight pause added) Hitler.

Interpretation: Right hemisphere readily identified the picture of Hitler and did not recognize any others. Left hemisphere cued by the mental aura which was generated by the picture and by the responses of the right hemisphere to examiner's questions guessed "government" and "historical," at the same time rejecting alternatives like a personal acquaintance or someone in entertainment. Subject's standard trick of trying to pass peripheral cues from the informed right hemisphere to the uniformed left was interrupted and did not help much. The continuing vagueness of the speaking hemisphere's orientation is illustrated in the hesitancy and comments like "Another country, I think." The accurate identification in the mute hemisphere is indicated in the negative responses to the series of false vocal cues and the immediate, firm positive response to "Germany" followed shortly by vocal confirmation of the correct identification of Hitler (Sperry et al. 1979, pp. 159–160).[1]

L.B.'s right hemisphere also gave the "thumbs-down" sign to pictures of Castro, a war scene, and overweight women in swim suits, whereas the "thumbs-up" sign was given for Churchill, Johnny Carson, and pretty girls. When he was shown a picture of himself, he gave a "thumbs-down" sign, but this was accompanied by a broad, sheepish grin. When asked whose picture it was, after a short hesitation he replied "myself."

1. Reprinted from *Neuropsychologia* vol. 17 (1979), R. W. Sperry, E. Zaidel, and D. Zaidel, "Self-Recognition and Social Awareness in the Deconnected Minor Hemisphere," pp. 159–160, with kind permission from Elsevier Science Ltd., Kidlington, UK.

Emotional Expression, Interpersonal Relationships, Fantasy, and Dreaming

In common with most of the split-brain subjects, L.B. appeared to demonstrate some degree of *alexithymia*, which refers to a poor ability to express feelings verbally, impoverished reports of fantasies, and interpersonal relationships that were over-conforming and lacking in intense emotion (Hoppe 1977; Hoppe and Bogen 1977; TenHouten, Hoppe, Bogen, and Walter 1986). Hoppe and Bogen (1977) compared their impressions of the Californian split-brain subjects on various aspects, including whether the subjects described endless details rather than feelings, whether they used appropriate words to describe emotions, and whether they had rich fantasy lives. Their independent impressions matched quite well, and by quantifying their results and comparing the mean scores of the split-brain group with the mean scores of psycho-somatic patients considered to demonstrate alexithymic tendencies, they concluded that the split-brain subjects had an even greater tendency toward alexithymia than the psychosomatic patients. A taped conversation between L.B. and Mike Corballis provides some support for this. When asked about friends, L.B. said he had none by choice, and that all the people he knew quite well were family members and their children. For example, he only knew his next-door neighbor by sight. He remarked, "I'm generally an isolationist, someone who sticks to themselves a lot. Basically my slogan is "Why worry?" When the conversation was steered around to personal relationships, he replied in a very matter-of-fact, nonemotive manner. When asked if he had dreams, he replied, "If I do, I don't remember. I've tried to keep a dream diary many times. A couple of times I've had a dream, nothing significant. I've had a sense of falling. I've dreamed about running. I've dreamed I'm a businessman locked in an office—couldn't get out." A cynic might suggest that this last dream was a reflection of the many hours L.B. spent shut up in a laboratory performing computerized cognitive tasks for psychologists.

Although emotions are perceived and represented at some level by both hemispheres, it has been postulated that the right hemisphere plays a special role in the perception of emotions (Tucker, Watson, and Heilman 1977; Heilman and Satz 1983). Hoppe and colleagues suggested that the alexithymia demonstrated by split-brain subjects results from the disconnection of the two hemispheres. That is, the cognitive representations of emotions perceived by the right hemisphere are unable to cross over to the left hemisphere for verbalization (Hoppe 1977; TenHouten et al. 1986).

Personal and Social Consequences

Without doubt, L.B.'s life was greatly improved by his split-brain surgery; as a consequence of the procedure, his epilepsy was brought under control with much lower doses of anticonvulsant medication. His good level of premorbid intelligence, the early age at which he had his surgery, and the apparent lack of significant brain damage he sustained before, during, or after surgery probably contributed to his excellent short- and long-term outcome.

Although L.B. had not been steadily employed throughout his adult life, he enjoyed his involvement with the researchers and visiting scientists to the Caltech laboratory. His cross-cuing tricks were well known, although when asked to do so, he always tried to control his own tendency to use one side of his brain to let the other side know what the other half was doing. Nevertheless, he was not above trying out new ways of cross-cuing, which kept the experimenters on their toes. Because of his intelligence and personal dedication to split-brain research, he proved to be the most important split-brain subject in the Californian series. Professor Sperry's studies on him and others in the Caltech series resulted in Sperry being awarded the Nobel Prize in Physiology and Medicine in 1981. This in itself is an honor few neuropsychological "subjects" could claim. Indeed, as a result of participating in many PhD projects, L.B. claimed that he himself had earned lots of PhD degrees!

L.B.'s social life was, by choice, very restricted. He clearly did not seek out friendships and preferred his own company and that of his computer to the company of people outside his close family circle. Although L.B. did not seek company, he did not appear to be shy or awkward when with others. He conversed in a relaxed manner with researchers, who knew him as a happy person who enjoyed telling jokes and delighted in beating them at their own sophisticated games. How closely L.B.'s "isolationist" lifestyle was tied to his commissurotomy is impossible to say; in any case, he seemed content with his lifestyle.

Discussion

Split-brain subjects have been the focus of numerous clever studies aimed at enlightening us further about the specialist functions of each hemisphere and the intricate ways the two sides of the brain communicate with each other both when split and compared with normal brains when connected. Many issues have been clarified, but many controversies remain. In part, such controversies are the result of the variation across the split-brain population. One answer may be to accept the truism that there are subtle individual differences in the functioning of the right and left hemispheres. Nevertheless, in general terms, the findings of unilateral lesion studies are confirmed in that the left hemisphere is dominant for language, especially speech functions, as well as other logical, sequential functions such as mathematics; the right hemisphere tends to be better at performing many visuospatial and nonverbal functions. Both hemispheres are self-aware and socially aware, and both appear to feel emotions, although there is some evidence that the verbal left hemisphere is not very good at expressing some emotions.

In many situations, it appears that some types of nonspecific information can be transferred subcortically to the opposite hemisphere, providing cues to aid that hemisphere to "guess" more accurately what has been received by the other hemisphere. How much this occurs in the normal connected hemisphere is not known. Possibly with time and practice the split-brain subject develops the functioning of these subcortical pathways.

Perhaps the most important message to come out of the split-brain research is the fact that in everyday life these people seem relatively unaffected by their split. Only when neuroscientists trick them using clever techniques is the disconnection detected. However, Zaidel et al. (2003) have argued that the subjective feelings of conflict that healthy people without split brains sometimes experience may imply that the two hemispheres can conduct partially separate parallel processing (Bogen 2000). In support of this, Iacoboni, Rayman, and Zaidel (1996) found that some normal people responded like split-brain subjects in lateralized tests, suggesting some sort of functional disconnection. Nevertheless, in most non-brain-damaged people, the two sides of the brain generally seem to work together, at least at a conscious level. The suggestions of the popular press that we can readily consciously train one hemisphere to perform certain specialized tasks independent of the other thus seem unlikely.

19
■

A WHOLE LIFE WITH HALF A BRAIN

KATE'S STORY

If I were asked to describe Kate's most obvious characteristics, I would say she is assertive, witty, and verbally "quick." She is also a middle-aged woman who works full-time in a large city library, has been married and divorced, and enjoys an active social life. Kate, however, is different in one important way from the innumerable other women who would fit a similar description: She has only half a brain.

Hemispherectomy, the removal of one cerebral hemisphere of the brain, must surely be the most drastic of all neurosurgical operations. Most people would probably find it difficult to believe that a person left with half a brain could survive, let alone cope independently in the world. There are, however, a number of cases of hemispherectomy that demonstrate beyond doubt that under certain circumstances humans can live full lives following the removal of either the right or left cerebral hemisphere. Kate, whose story is told in this chapter, is one of these remarkable cases.

Her story and the story of others like her is not simply a curiosity or a tale of courage and determination but adds to our knowledge about the ability of the human brain to adapt and "make do" with far fewer neurons and cerebral structures than are found in the normal brain. A careful examination of the spared abilities and impairments found following hemispherectomy can provide us with clues about which functions can be taken over by other parts of the brain or by other functional systems in the brain, and which functions cannot. Although these people may indeed cope extremely well, careful assessment reveals some areas of impairment, both in the simple sensory and motor domains and in areas of higher cognitive functioning. Nevertheless, the overriding impression for everyone who meets, talks with, and assesses Kate is one of amazement. Typical comments are, "I don't believe it! She can't really have only one hemisphere! That can't be a computed tomography (CT) scan of her brain!"

There are of course many people who have had hemispherectomies and who are

Kate, under the initials K.O.F, has been featured in a number of scientific papers, including Cavazutti and Erba (1976), Corballis and Ogden (1988), and Ogden (1988a, 1989, 1996). Detailed descriptions of her abilities and impairments and those of hemispherectomized people like her can be found in these papers.

severely impaired. Usually these people were mentally retarded before the hemispherectomy, possibly because they had extensive damage or abnormal brain structures in both hemispheres of the brain. It is generally thought that damage to one hemisphere of the brain must occur in infancy if removal of that hemisphere is to improve the person's chance of a normal life. People who have normally functioning brains in their childhoods and who in adulthood have one hemisphere extensively damaged or removed because of a tumor are left with severe impairments that relate specifically to the hemisphere that was removed or damaged. Recovery of these deficits (e.g., usually language impairments following the removal of a left hemisphere and visuospatial deficits following the removal of a right hemisphere) tends not to occur.

The usual reason for performing a hemispherectomy is to remove a severely diseased, damaged, or atrophied hemisphere that is already substantially nonfunctional. The damaged hemisphere often causes frequent and severe epileptic seizures such that the other, "good" hemisphere is unable to function well either. In many cases, removal of the nonfunctional hemisphere results in a marked reduction or complete elimination of the seizures. This frees the individual to use the remaining hemisphere without constant interruption from the effect of the electrical activity of the seizures on the brain and the depressive effect of anticonvulsant medication. Disruption to the person's family, social, and educational activities caused by the seizures also lessens.

People who undergo hemispherectomy who are not severely retarded are frequently used as experimental subjects to test hypotheses about the ability of one hemisphere to take over the specialist functions usually mediated predominantly by the other hemisphere. Some of the studies that have been undertaken in an attempt to answer these questions are summarized in the next section, and the case of Kate provides some more detailed examples of experimental assessments that can result in furthering our understanding of brain–behavior relations in a more general sense.

Theoretical Background

Hemispheric Specialization

In approximately 96% of right-handers and 70% of left-handers, the left hemisphere is dominant for language functions (Milner 1975), including verbal memory (Blakemore and Falconer 1967), and the right hemisphere is dominant for visuospatial functions (Franco and Sperry 1977), including nonverbal memory (Milner 1965, 1968b; Milner and Taylor 1972) and emotional expression (Bryden and Ley 1983; Heilman, Scholes, and Watson 1975; Ross 1981; Tucker, Watson, and Heilman 1977). The specialization of the right hemisphere for visuospatial functions and emotional expression is by no means as clear as the specialization of the left hemisphere for language. Nevertheless, there is no doubt that posterior right-hemispheric lesions give rise to a greater range and severity of visuospatial deficits than do posterior left-hemispheric lesions (Benton 1959; Benton and Hecaen 1970; Carmon and Bechtoldt 1969; Heilman, Watson, and Valenstein 1993; Milner 1965), and this is supported by

data from subjects with complete forebrain commissurotomies (i.e., split-brain subjects; see Chapter 18). In these subjects the isolated right hemisphere can perform
visuospatial tasks better than the left hemisphere can (Franco and Sperry 1977; Puccetti 1981).

Equipotentiality and Plasticity

Recovery of specialized language and visuospatial abilities after massive damage to
one or the other hemisphere raises questions about the equipotentiality and plasticity
of different brain areas and systems with respect to their ability to mediate and take
over a range of functions. There is ample evidence that the younger the person is
when the brain damage occurs, the more likely he is to recover the functions usually
mediated by the damaged brain systems; this is particularly true for language. Children
who sustain extensive damage to the left "speech" hemisphere early in life commonly
demonstrate recovery or continued development of language functions (Basser 1962;
Ogden 1989, 1996), but older children and adults who sustain damage to the language
areas of their left hemisphere are unlikely to regain full language. One reason may be
that it takes many years for the undamaged parts of the brain to take over the functions
previously mediated by the damaged brain areas. The long-term survival rate of adult
subjects who sustain massive brain damage is poor; thus, their failure to recover specialized functions may simply reflect the fact that their brains have not had time to
restore complex functions (St. James-Roberts 1981).

In patients who have had left hemispherectomies (removal of the left cerebral
hemisphere of the brain), language functions must be mediated entirely by the right
hemisphere. Detailed studies of these cases allow us to assess how similar and how
different the two hemispheres are at mediating different aspects of language. For example, Dennis (1980), Dennis and Kohn (1975), and Dennis and Whitaker (1976) all
claim that when the right hemisphere takes over language in infancy, it does so in a
degraded form, which suggests that hemispheric specialization is already fixed in
infancy so that the isolated right hemisphere performs language tasks in a qualitatively
different way from the left hemisphere. In support of this finding, they also found that
left-hemispherectomized subjects had difficulty understanding passive-negative sentences (e.g., "the girl is not pushed by the boy"). Bishop (1983) questioned the significance of these findings, however, and argued that adolescents with a low mental
age perform at chance on this test and that even some older teenagers of average
intelligence make frequent errors on these sentences. Ogden's (1988a, 1996) studies
on Kate and other left hemispherectomized people supported this, as these individuals
were able to improve their performances on passive-negative sentences if they were
permitted to read rather than hear the sentences and were given unlimited time to
decide on the correct answer.

These contradictory research findings underline the importance of taking careful
note of the methodologies used in different studies when evaluating them. In the
examples above, it is important to understand that participants may make errors on

tasks for many different reasons, and teasing apart the various reasons for their poor performance is essential if a correct interpretation of brain–behavior relations is to be made. In studies of the comprehension of passive-negative sentences, it is clear that if brain-damaged participants can attain near perfect scores if given sufficient time, but make numerous errors if given only a brief time to respond, then their ability to understand this complex sentence structure is intact, but their ability to process information at a normal speed is not. It is well established that brain damage generally results in a slowing of information processing, and that this can occur even after mild closed head injury (see Chapter 11). Thus, it is hardly surprising that slowed information processing should be a significant problem for people who have had an entire hemisphere removed, and this must be factored into any study examining other aspects of cognition in these individuals.

The ability of one hemisphere to mediate memory efficiently is an interesting issue, especially given the finding that subjects whose two hemispheres have been disconnected from each other (commissurotomy or split-brain subjects) have poor recent memories (Milner and Taylor 1972; Sperry, Gazzaniga, and Bogen 1969). This has been attributed to the fact that the two hemispheres cannot communicate (Zaidel and Sperry 1974) and might suggest that subjects with only one hemisphere may also have impaired memories for recent material.

Another interesting area of inquiry posed by these unusual cases is that of the fate of functions normally mediated predominantly by the right hemisphere (Ogden 1989). At one extreme is the possibility that the solitary right hemisphere continues to mediate visuospatial and other "right-hemispheric" functions as well as language; at the other extreme is the possibility that the traditional right-hemispheric functions are lost or severely degraded as a consequence of the right hemisphere's involvement in language. An intermediate hypothesis is that some right-hemispheric functions are impaired and others remain substantially normal.

A number of studies have examined speech, reading, and spelling functions of subjects following left hemispherectomy (Dennis 1980; Dennis and Kohn 1975; Dennis and Whitaker 1976; Gott 1973a; Ogden 1988a, 1996; Smith 1966; St. James-Roberts 1981), but studies of memory abilities following hemispherectomy are rare (Gott 1973b; Ogden 1988a), as are detailed studies of visuospatial functions in left-hemispherectomized subjects (Gott 1973b; Ogden 1989).

Case Presentation

Background

I first met Kate in Boston, when she was 45 years old. In the past she had been the subject of various experimental investigations both at the Boston Children's Hospital and at Massachusetts Institute of Technology (MIT). I contacted her and asked if she would be willing to participate again in various experiments. She was amenable and agreed to come to the MIT Clinical Research Center for 2 full days of testing. Although I had read her medical file before meeting her, it did not provide a clear picture of Kate as a "person" but, rather, concentrated on her very extensive medical history. I had also seen her CT brain scan (see Fig. 19-1) taken a year previously and was thus prepared to meet a woman with significant physical impairments, perhaps with at least some speech difficulties and possibly displaying some unusual behaviors. The only clue that the woman who confidently and fluently greeted me was the "owner" of the CT scan was her right arm, which she held in a flexed position. My initial impression of total normality has not changed over a 7-year period. Even when she had difficulty with some of the neuropsychological tests, she continued to communicate and react in a perfectly appropriate fashion. Her behavior had not always been so normal, however, as seen from her childhood history.

Kate had an uncomplicated birth and a normal development until the age of 10 months, when she fell from her cot, hitting the left side of her head. This fall resulted in a right hemiplegia, and as a consequence she is left-handed. Because her grandparents, parents, and five siblings are all right-handed, Kate's left-handedness is almost certainly a result of her early left-hemispheric damage. She had another fall, again hitting her head, when she was 5 years old, and an electroencephalogram (EEG) at this time showed some seizure activity in the left occipital area. Kate began to have generalized seizures when she was 9 years old, and at this time a radiographic test called a pneumoencephalogram demonstrated an enlarged left lateral ventricle and extensive subarachnoid air over the left hemisphere. The interpretation of this finding was that the left hemisphere had almost totally atrophied. By the time she was 15 years old, Kate was having 25 seizures a day. Many anticonvulsant medications were

Figure 19-1 A computed tomography scan of Kate's brain taken when she was 44 years old. The left side of the scan (on the left of the figure) shows the fluid-filled space where most of the left hemisphere was removed. All that remains is the medial surface of the occipital pole. The remaining right ventricle is dilated. (Reprinted from Ogden 1988a, p. 649, with kind permission from Elsevier Science Ltd., Kidlington, UK.)

tried but with little success. Physically, she managed quite well and was able to walk with a leg brace. She attended a special school for 8 years, completing the eighth grade, and her level of ability was reported to be within the "dull normal to borderline" IQ range up until the age of 14. Her spoken language was quite good.

Kate displayed a number of behavioral and emotional problems that worsened in adolescence. She was difficult to manage at school and at home and was frequently aggressive, rude, and inappropriate. As a result, her social development was stunted, and she had no friends.

When Kate reached adolescence, a difficult decision was made to remove the atrophied left hemisphere surgically in the hope of reducing her debilitating seizures. Three brain operations were performed when she was between the ages of 15 and 17 years, resulting in virtually all the left hemisphere being removed, including the wall of the lateral ventricle, its choroid plexus, parts of the corpus callosum, the basal ganglia, and the left hippocampus, leaving only the medial surface of the occipital lobe. A CT scan of her brain carried out many years later when she was 44 years old demonstrates the dramatic consequences of her hemispherectomy (see Fig. 19-1).

Following the operations, Kate was left with a dense right homonymous hemianopia (the loss of her right visual field), which has remained ever since. Her language abilities remained unchanged, and her behavior improved markedly. Kate has been completely free of seizures since her final operation, and she has not taken anticonvulsant medication since she was 21 years old. At the time of most of the assessments reported here, when Kate was 45, she had held a steady job in charge of a library photocopying machine for 22 years. She retired from that job at the age of 50, not because she could no longer perform well but because she wanted time to spend on other leisure activities. She lives independently, having been married and divorced, and is outgoing and sociable. She walks without aid and with a slight limp, but her right arm is wasted and she holds it in the flexed position.

Kate was given an extensive neuropsychological assessment to determine how well her right hemisphere had taken over language functions and the effect this might have had on the visuospatial functions usually mediated predominantly by the right hemisphere. She clearly enjoyed doing the neuropsychological tests, and she remained motivated and cooperative throughout, even after 2 full days of testing. She was a pleasure to test because of her delightful sense of humor and down-to-earth, assertive manner. She had strong opinions on a number of topics and readily expressed these opinions in conversation during breaks. Her long medical history had made her somewhat skeptical about the medical profession and its fund of knowledge (or lack of it) about the brain, in part because of her own ability to perform many tasks that she had been told she would never be able to do.

Neuropsychological Assessment

Overall verbal and visuospatial abilities   Kate's IQ scores on the Wechsler Intelligence Scales from 1958 (before her hemispherectomy) until 1986 are given in Table 19-1.

Table 19-1 Kate's WAIS-R and WMS results from 1958 until 1986

Year	Age (years)	Test	Verbal	Perform	Full-Scale	WMS Quotient
				IQ		
1958	16	W-B*	69	67	64	—
1974	33	W-B*	97	87	92	97
1977	36	WAIS	94	91	92	—
1979	38	WAIS	100	89	95	—
1981	41	WAIS-R	82	78	80	103
1986	45	WAIS-R	93	82	87	118

The "average" age-adjusted score for all the Wechsler IQs and the WMS Memory Quotient are 100 with a standard deviation of 15. Kate's operations were in 1957 (age 15) and 1959 (age 17).

W-B, Wechsler-Bellevue Intelligence Scale for Adults and Adolescents; WAIS, Wechsler Adult Intelligence Scale; WAIS-R, revised WAIS.

Given that the revised Wechsler Adult Intelligence Scales WAIS-R (Wechsler 1981) results in lower IQ scores (7–8 IQ points) than the WAIS, Kate's IQ has remained in the low-average to average range since 1974. Her Verbal IQ is 11 points higher than her Performance IQ. Her average scores on tests of Vocabulary and Comprehension are the best indicators that she is of average verbal ability, and it is her markedly low score on Arithmetic that pulls her Verbal IQ down. When given simple addition, subtraction, multiplication, and division sums to do either mentally or on paper, Kate could do only simple addition, demonstrating a severe impairment of calculation. Kate's scores on the visuospatial subtests were generally lower than her scores on the verbal tests; therefore, her visuospatial abilities were examined in more detail (described later).

Language abilities   Kate demonstrated normal and fluent expressive language and comprehension. For example, if asked to "Pick up the pencil and draw a circle on the paper, and then put it down and pick up the dime and give it to me," she could perform without hesitation or error. Even on the comprehension of passive-negative sentences (e.g., "the truck is not pulled by the car"), she gained a perfect score when she read the sentences for herself rather than having them read to her (Ogden 1988a). This finding contradicts the finding of Dennis (1980), Dennis and Kohn (1975), and Dennis and Whitaker (1976), that left-hemispherectomized subjects are unable to do this difficult language task. Her spoken language was entirely normal, and her language was both rich and expressive. She could write spontaneously, copy, and write to dictation. She could also read fluently but slowly, and on an extensive test requiring her to read lists of regular, irregular, and nonwords, she performed normally. She did, however, have some difficulty spelling irregular words (Ogden 1996). On a word fluency test, she was asked to give as many words as possible in 1 minute, starting with a particular letter; on this test she performed at about a 10-year-old level (Ogden 1988a).

Further tests of visuospatial functions   *Constructional apraxia*: Kate was severely impaired on copying a Necker cube and a five-pointed star (Fig. 19-2). On the copy of the Rey Complex Figure (Rey 1941), a test of visuospatial perception, planning, and construction, Kate was also severely impaired (Fig. 19-3). Her copy of the Taylor Complex Figure (Taylor 1969) was much better, although still below the 25th percentile for normal adults (Lezak 1983). Because she recalled copying the Taylor Complex Figure 12 years earlier, there may have been a practice effect.

Mental rotation and spatial relations: On the 10 two-dimensional mental rotation problems taken from the Luria-Nebraska Neuropsychological Battery (Golden, Hammeke, and Purisch 1980), a simple task requiring the subject mentally to turn an object around in two-dimensional space, Kate scored at chance (4 of 10). Normal adults make no errors on this test.

The Spatial Relations test comprised 10 examples taken from the Spatial Relations of the Differential Aptitude Tests (Bennett, Seashore, and Wesman 1962). The subject views a two-dimensional drawing of a shape that, if folded along the lines indicated on the drawing, will form a three-dimensional structure. The subject must choose the correct three-dimensional structure from four drawings. This test is a difficult one

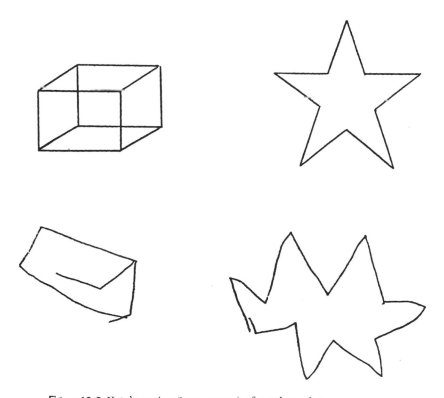

Figure 19-2 Kate's copies (bottom row) of a cube and star.

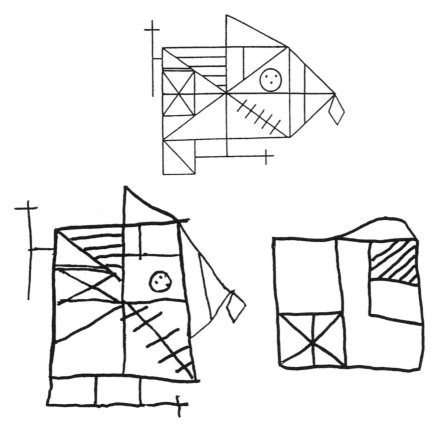

Figure 19-3 The Rey Complex Figure. The model for the copy is at the top, Kate's copy is on the left, and her recall is on the right.

involving mental manipulation of a visuospatial image. Kate scored at chance on this (3 of 10). Normal adults score between 7 and 10 on these examples.

Unilateral neglect: On a test of neglect designed by Mesulam (1985) in which the subject is asked to circle every *A* inserted randomly among other letters arranged in rows on a page, Kate missed 5 of 30 on the right and none on the left, which may indicate a mild form of hemineglect (see Chapter 7). On all other tasks, including reading, writing, visually bisecting lines, crossing out lines scattered randomly over a page (Albert 1973), and copying a line drawing of a simple scene shown to be sensitive to neglect (Ogden 1985a), she performed normally. The fact that Kate is unaware of her right visual-field defect may also be a consequence of neglect.

Face recognition: Kate demonstrates normal recognition of familiar faces, and in everyday life she appears to experience no difficulty in recognizing recently seen faces. On Benton's test of Face Recognition (Benton, Hamsher, Varney, and Spreen 1983), faces photographed in various degrees of shadow are matched with a number of different faces with the aim of recognizing the same face under different lighting conditions. On this test Kate obtained a normal score of 46 of 50. On Mooney's Closure Faces test (Mooney 1957), the subject is required to sort transformed drawings of human faces with the shadows rendered in black and the highlights in white into categories of *man, woman, old man, old woman, girl, boy*, and *left over*; Kate scored 50% correct. According to Lansdell (1968), patients with right temporal resections are impaired on this test relative to patients with left temporal resections. The mean percentage correct for the left temporal resection group is 83.5%, (with a standard deviation [SD] of 8.2), and for the right temporal resection group it is 71.8% (SD 15.5). Therefore, Kate scored well below the impaired right temporal resection group.

Tests of orientation: On Benton's Judgment of Line Orientation test (Benton et al. 1983), a simple perceptual task, Kate's score of 23 was in the average range. On the Body Scheme test (Semmes, Weinstein, Ghent, and Teuber 1963), a test of personal orientation, she gained perfect scores. In this test, the subject points to parts of her own body on verbal command and then she names the body parts, when indicated, on herself with eyes open and closed; she also touches on command body parts on the tester and touches body parts on herself that the tester touches on herself and body parts indicated by numbers on a drawing of a person facing forward and backward. Kate was also correct on right-left discriminations, even when a transposition was required before matching her own body parts onto another body facing the opposite way.

On Money's Road Map test (Money 1965), a test of directional sense, Kate's score of 29/32 was at the 17-year-old level. On Locomotor Mazes (Rudel and Teuber 1971; Semmes et al. 1963), a test of extrapersonal orientation, she was severely impaired. On this test the subject is required to walk a path between nine circular markers according to a visual map indicating the path to be followed, with north marked on one side of the markers and on the map. Kate was correct on only one of the five maps and correctly walked only 23 of the total of 44 paths (from one marker to the next).

Memory abilities   On the Wechsler Memory Scale (WMS) (Wechsler 1945), in 1986 Kate's Memory Quotient (MQ) was 118. As the MQ is scaled so that it approximately parallels the Wechsler Full-scale IQ, Kate performed at a much higher level than would be predicted by her average IQ. The WMS is primarily a test of simple verbal memory, and the visuospatial nonverbal memory component is small. Kate's scores on the verbal learning and memory subtests (Paired-Associates and Logical Memory) were particularly impressive. However, when I reassessed Kate on the WMS 6 years later, when she was aged 51 years, her MQ had decreased to 94, with her Logical Memory Score dropping from 11 in 1986 to 7 in 1992, and her Paired Associates score dropping from 17.5 to 9 (Ogden 1996). Her MQ and Logical Memory score were still, however, within the normal range. Other left-hemispherectomized individuals with a normal Verbal IQ have also demonstrated normal scores on the relatively simple verbal memory tests of the WMS, but on a more challenging list learning test, the California

Verbal Learning Test (Delis, Kramer, Kaplan, and Ober 1987), they have demonstrated severe verbal memory impairments (Abbott 1995).

The delayed recall of the Rey (see Fig. 19-3) and Taylor Complex Figures were given as tests of nonverbal, visuospatial memory. The Taylor Figure had been given previously in 1974, and the Rey was given in 1986 when she was age 45, and again in 1992. On all occasions her recall scores fell below the 10th percentile for normal adults. In fact, her recall scores have worsened significantly over the years since her hemispherectomy. In contrast, her scores on the verbal memory subtests of the WMS improved over the first 30 years after her hemispherectomy. In 1974 when Kate was 32, 15 years posthemispherectomy, Kate's WMS MQ was 97, and she recalled 55% of her copy of the Taylor Complex Figure. Twelve years later, in 1986, her WMS MQ had increased to 118, and she recalled only 25% of her copy of the Taylor Figure. Her increased MQ was primarily a result of an increase on the Verbal Memory subtests, as her Digit Span score and her scores on the simple WMS visual memory test remained stable (Ogden 1988a).

That Kate's Memory Quotient showed a significant decrease of 24 points from her assessment when aged 45 years to her assessment when aged 51 years shows that Kate is experiencing a more rapid decline in verbal memory as she ages than is seen in the normal population. As most people in their fifties can attest, an increasing difficulty with new verbal learning and memory (such as remembering names) is common (Baddeley 1999) and gets worse as we get older, but is not as precipitous as Kate's memory decline.

Tests of prosody   Emotional tone in speech (prosody) is thought to be a right hemispheric ability (Ross 1981), so it was of interest to assess Kate on this. She was asked to identify the tone of voice when hearing the sentence "I am going to the movies" recorded on tape by the voices of a man, woman, and child. Each voice said the sentence in six different tones—happy, angry, disinterested, sad, surprised, and tearful—recorded in different orders for each voice. Kate was also asked to repeat the sentence in the same tone of each of the voices and to say the sentence with the six different intonations on command. In addition, she had to identify visually the facial expressions intended to convey the same six emotions made by the tester, copy these expressions, and make the facial expressions on command. Kate performed perfectly on all these tasks of prosody. In addition, throughout the days of testing, which also included extensive interviews about her life, she expressed a range of emotions appropriate to the situation.

Personal and Social Consequences

As a young child and teenager, Kate's life was ruled by frequent severe seizures. She performed poorly at school, and her behavior was disturbed. Much of her time was spent in hospitals. Following her hemispherectomy, an immediate and almost miraculous change in her behavior was apparent to the doctors and nurses who knew her and to her family. Her seizures stopped, and she was gradually weaned off her anti-epileptic medication, which would have had the effect of increasing her level of cortical arousal, enabling her more readily to attend to important information and learn from it. Fifteen years after her final hemispherectomy operation, an assessment of her IQ demonstrated that it had improved from a preoperative assessment of "borderline" IQ to an "average" IQ. In concert with these intellectual improvements, Kate also developed a normal ability to form and retain friendships, to marry, and to hold a job. These new-found life skills probably relied on her increased intellectual abilities as well as on her release from the ever-present seizures.

Few other hemispherectomized people demonstrate intellectual abilities as remarkable as those demonstrated by Kate. It is therefore likely that Kate would have been of superior intelligence had she not suffered damage to her left hemisphere as an infant. Although her ability on several higher cognitive tasks remains compromised, Kate's life does not seem to be affected by this, perhaps because she never had the ability to perform these tasks.

Kate's attitude toward health, hospitals, and researchers has been influenced by her experiences; she has a healthy if rather cynical approach to medicine and science, and she avoids doctors as much as possible. When she does attend a doctor, she is assertive about her needs and her right to information. She enjoys assisting in research projects if it fits with her social schedule: The research is fully explained to her, and she is provided with the results and any articles arising from the studies in which she has been involved. She is rightly proud of her achievements, and she delights in the enthusiastic, often incredulous comments of researchers about her abilities.

Discussion

When subjects who have had infantile hemispherectomies or extensive unilateral damage are assessed on the WAIS-R, there is generally only a small and insignificant difference between the Verbal and Performance IQs, with the Verbal IQ being slightly higher no matter which hemisphere has been damaged (Smith 1978; St. James-Roberts 1981). The Performance tests of the WAIS-R do not assess right-hemispheric functions in depth, however; to obtain a true picture of the ability of the solitary right hemisphere to mediate visuospatial and other nonverbal functions, a more detailed assessment is required.

Many years following a left hemispherectomy, Kate displayed remarkably intact language and verbal memory abilities, possibly as a consequence of long recovery times (Ogden 1988a, 1996; St. James-Roberts 1981). Her verbal memory did begin to deteriorate once she reached her fifties, suggesting accelerated aging affects (Ogden 1996).

Kate did, however, demonstrate constructional apraxia, possible mild right visuospatial neglect, and moderate to severe impairment on tasks of spatial relations, face perception, mental rotation, and nonverbal memory. Deficits on all these tasks are usually associated with right-hemispheric lesions (De Renzi 1982). In contrast, prosody, considered a "right-hemispheric" function (Heilman et al. 1975; Ross 1981), remained normal.

On tests of left-right discrimination (Money's Road Map test) and personal orientation (Body Scheme test), she performed normally. Kohn and Dennis (1974) also found three of their four left hemidecorticates unimpaired on these tests. There is evidence that both these functions are mediated by the left hemisphere in normally lateralized adults. Lesions of the left parietal lobe can result in an inability to discriminate left from right (Benton 1959; Ogden 1985c), and left-hemispheric lesions also result in impairments of personal orientation (Semmes et al. 1963). The rare disorder of autotopagnosia (Ogden 1985c) is always associated with a left parietal lesion, and this disorder also involves a disturbance of the body schema.

On a simple perceptual task involving the judgment of line orientation, Kate was also normal. On Locomotor Mazes, however, a task of extrapersonal orientation involving mental rotation and spatial relations in addition to the judgment of line orientation, she was severely impaired, which is in contrast to three of the four left-hemidecorticate subjects assessed by Kohn and Dennis (1974). On the same test, their subjects were unimpaired. These subjects, whose onset of hemiplegia was before the age of 2 years and who underwent hemidecortication at age 14–18 years, were tested at age 18–25 years, 4–7 years following the surgery; thus, they had had much shorter recovery periods than Kate. Length of recovery time, therefore, cannot be positively correlated with this ability (cf. Ogden 1988a, 1989; St. James-Roberts 1981). One hypothesis that might explain these results and Kate's normal ability to comprehend syntactically complex sentences (Ogden 1988a, 1996) is that when all functions are mediated by the right hemisphere, aging factors interact with recovery period such that increasing recovery time is associated with improving verbal functions, and aging is associated with further impairment of nonverbal functions and, at a later age, new verbal learning and memory. Thus, Kate's solitary right hemisphere, although continuing to improve on complex language skills (e.g., passive-negative sentences) as recovery time lengthens, over the same time span becomes increasingly impaired on visuospatial functions, nonverbal memory, and extrapersonal orientation. That is, the aging right hemisphere first loses those functions that have always had the most tenuous "foothold" in hemispherectomized subjects.

An alternative hypothesis is that removal of the cortex only, as in the subject of Kohn and Dennis (1974), may allow the deeper structures of the decorticate hemisphere to continue to function to some degree. If this were the case, the visuospatial functions of these subjects might still be mediated in part by the decorticate hemisphere.

This study on Kate makes no statement about the ability of the left hemisphere to take over nonverbal functions after early right hemispherectomy. Kohn and Dennis's four right-hemidecorticate subjects are significantly more impaired than their left-hemidecorticate subjects on Money's Road Map test and on the test of extrapersonal orientation, but they are unimpaired on tests of personal orientation. The severity of their impairment on the test of extrapersonal orientation equals that of Kate. Other studies of subjects who have sustained massive damage to one hemisphere early in life suggest that the intact hemisphere will take over both verbal and spatial abilities; regardless of which hemisphere remains intact, spatial skills are likely to be more impaired than verbal abilities (Bigler and Naugle 1985; Franzen, Tishelman, Seine, and Friedman 1986).

Overall, studies of people who sustain the removal or damage of one hemisphere in infancy suggest that at birth the two hemispheres are equipotential for language and that language functions take priority over specialized visuospatial and other nonverbal functions. Corballis and Morgan (1978) have hypothesized a biological left-right maturational gradient that favors earlier development on the left than on the right. Thus, the right hemisphere becomes "ready" to develop language later than the left hemisphere. In the normal brain, once language is established in the left hemisphere, it inhibits the right hemisphere from developing these functions, freeing it to develop fully nonverbal functions.

Early extensive damage to one hemisphere results in the remaining hemisphere developing language functions first and the lower priority nonverbal functions second. If the left hemisphere is the intact one, language skills develop at a normal rate, and nonverbal skills are disadvantaged. If the right hemisphere is the intact one, language abilities again develop first, but the more subtle and complex aspects of language develop more slowly, as the right hemisphere does not attain the maturational stage necessary for the development of these skills until later in life (Ogden 1988a, 1996). Some nonverbal skills do not develop or are degraded as a result of the right-hemisphere's involvement in language (Ogden 1989). Because these nonverbal skills are so poorly developed, they may be the first to suffer from the effects of aging.

One right-hemispheric function, prosody, does not seem to be disadvantaged by the development of language in the right hemisphere, perhaps because prosody is so intimately tied in with speech. Ross (1981) has postulated that right-hemispheric lesions may disrupt prosody in terms of comprehension, repetition, and production in the same manner that left-hemispheric lesions disrupt propositional speech and that the corresponding affective aspects of speech are mediated by the homologous cortical areas and pathways in the right hemisphere. Therefore, following hemispherectomy, perhaps the cortical areas normally involved in the different aspects of propositional or affective speech can develop both types of speech in concert. This makes evolutionary sense, given that both aspects of speech are necessary for clear communication.

Under the rare circumstances of hemispherectomy, it is evident that in some cases it is possible for the remaining hemisphere to develop a range of skills sufficient for independent survival. The independent and normal life led by Kate provides testimony to this possibility.

REFERENCES

Abbott, S. D. 1995. *Living With Half a Brain: Outcome, Equipotentiality and Blindsight Following Hemispherectomy*. Unpublished master's thesis, Auckland, New Zealand, University of Auckland.

Af Bjorksen, G., and V. Halonen. 1965. Incidence of intracranial vascular lesions in patients with subarachnoid haemorrhage investigated by 4-vessel angiography. *Journal of Neurosurgery* 23:29–32.

Aimola Davies, A. 2004. Disorders of spatial orientation and awareness: Unilateral neglect. In: J. Ponsford, ed., *Cognitive and Behavioral Rehabilitation: From Neurobiology to Clinical Practice* (pp. 175–224). New York: Guilford Press.

Akelaitis, A. J. 1941. Studies on the corpus callosum; higher visual functions in each homonymous field following complete section of corpus callosum. *Archives of Neurology and Psychiatry (Chicago)* 45:788.

Albert, M. L. 1973. A simple test of visual neglect. *Neurology* 23:658–664.

Albert, M. S., M. A. Naeser, H. L. Levine, and J. Garvey. 1984. Ventricular size in patients with presenile dementia of the Alzheimer's type. *Archives of Neurology* 41:1258–1263.

Albert, M. S., R. W. Sparks, and N. A. Helm. 1973. Melodic intonation therapy for aphasia. *Archives of Neurology* 29:130–131.

American Psychiatric Association. 1994. *Diagnostic and Statistical Manual of Mental Disorders, 4th Edition* (DSM-IV). Washington, DC: American Psychiatric Association.

Anderson, S. W., H. Damasio, R. D. Jones, and D. Tranel. 1991. Wisconsin Card Sorting Test performance as a measure of frontal lobe damage. *Journal of Clinical and Experimental Neuropsychology* 13:909–922.

Anderson, S. W., J. Hathaway-Nepple, D. Tranel, and H. Damasio. 2000. Impairments of strategy application following focal prefrontal lesions. *Journal of the International Neuropsychological Society* 6:205.

Anderson, V. 2001. *Developmental Neuropsychology: A Clinical Approach*. Philadelphia: Psychology Press.

Andrew, S. E., Y. P. Goldberg, and M. R. Hayden. 1997. Rethinking genotype and phenotype correlations in polyglutamine expansion disorders. *Human Molecular Genetics*, 6:2005–2010.

Archer, J., R. S. Briellmann, D. Abbott, A. Syngeniotis, and G. D. Jackson. 2001. Spike triggered fMRI: a technique for understanding the aetiology of epileptiform activity. *NeuroImage* 13:S768.

Ardila, A., M. Rosseli, and F. Ostrosky. 1992. Sociocultural factors in neuropsychological assessment. In: A. E. Puente and R. J. McCaffrey, eds., *Psychobiological Factors in Clinical Neuropsychological Assessment* (pp. 181–192). New York: Plenum Press.

Ardila, A., M. Rosseli, and P. Rosas. 1989. Neuropsychological assessment in illiterates: visuospatial and memory abilities. *Brain and Cognition* 11:147–166.

Arlien-Soberg, P. 1985. Chronic effects of organic solvents on the central nervous system and diagnostic criteria. In: *Chronic Effects of Organic Solvents on the Central Nervous System and Diagnostic Criteria* (pp. 197–218). Copenhagen: World Health Organization.

Arlien-Soberg, P., P. Bruhn, C. Gyldensted, and B. Melgaard. 1979. Chronic painters' syndrome: toxic encephalopathy in house painters. *Acta Neurologica Scandinavica* 60:149–156.

Assal, F., and J. Cummings. 2002. Neuropathological; changes underlying neuropsychiatric symptoms in Alzheimer's disease. In: S. Gauthier and J. L. Cummings, eds., *Alzheimer's Disease and Related Disorders Annual 2002* (pp. 199–215). London: Martin Dunitz.

Baddeley, A. 1999. *Essentials of Human Memory*. Hove: Psychology Press.

Baddeley, A., and B. A. Wilson. 1994. When implicit learning fails: amnesia and the problem of error elimination. *Neuropsychologia* 32:53–68.

Baddeley, A., S. Bressi, S. Della Sala, R. Logie, and H. Spinnler. 1991. The decline of working memory in Alzheimer's disease. *Brain* 114:2521–2542.

Baker, E. L., and A. M. Seppalainen. 1986. Session 3: Human aspects of solvent neurobehavioural effects. Report of the workshop on clinical and epidemiological topics. *Neurotoxicology* 7:43–56.

Barlow, D. H., and M. Hersen. 1984. *Single case experimental designs: strategies for studying behavior change, 2nd Edition*. New York: Pergamon Press.

Barona, A., and R. L. Chastain. 1986. An improved estimate of premorbid IQ for blacks and whites on the WAIS-R. *International Journal of Clinical Neuropsychology* 8:169–173.

Barona, A., C. R. Reynolds, and R. L. Chastain. 1984. A demographically-based index of premorbid intelligence for the WAIS-R. *Journal of Consulting and Clinical Psychology* 52: 885–887.

Basser, L. S. 1962. Hemiplegia with early onset and the faculty of speech with special reference to the effects of hemispherectomy. *Brain* 85:427–460.

Bauer, R. M., and J. A. Demery. 2003. Agnosia. In: K. M. Heilman and E. Valenstein, eds., *Clinical Neuropsychology, 4th Edition* (pp. 236–295). New York: Oxford University Press.

Bauer, R. M., L. Grande, and E. Valenstein. 2003. Amnesic disorders. In: K. M. Heilman and E. Valenstein, eds., *Clinical Neuropsychology, 4th Edition* (pp. 495–573). New York: Oxford University PressBeck, A. T., G. Emery, and R. L. Greenberg. 1985. *Anxiety Disorders and Phobias: A Cognitive Perspective* (p 167). New York: Basic Books.

Beck, A. T., R. A. Steer, and G. K. Brown. 1996. *Beck Depression Inventory (2nd Edition) Manual*. New York: The Psychological Corporation.

Bell, B. A., and L. Symon. 1979. Smoking and subarachnoid haemorrhage. *British Medical Journal* 1:577–578.

Bennett, G. K., H. G. Seashore, and A. G. Wesman. 1962. *Differential Aptitude Tests: Space Relations*. New York: The Psychological Corporation.

Bentin, S., R. Silverberg, and H. W. Gordon. 1981. Asymmetrical cognitive deterioration in demented and Parkinson patients. *Cortex* 17:533–534.

Benton, A. L. 1959. *Right-Left Discrimination and Finger Localization*. New York: Hoeber-Harper.

Benton, A. L., and K. de S. Hamsher 1976. *Multilingual Aphasia Examination*. Iowa City: University of Iowa.

Benton, A. L., and H. Hecaen. 1970. Stereoscopic vision in patients with unilateral cerebral disease. *Neurology* 20:1084–1088.

Benton, A. L., and D. Tranel. 1993. Visuoperceptual, visuospatial, and visuoconstructive disorders. In: K. M. Heilman and E. Valenstein, eds., *Clinical Neuropsychology, 3rd Edition* (Chapter 8, pp. 165–213). New York: Oxford University Press.

Benton, A. L., K. de S. Hamsher, N. R. Varney, and O. Spreen. 1983. *Contributions to Neuropsychological Assessment. A Clinical Manual* (pp. 30–54). New York: Oxford University Press.

Ben-Yishay, Y. 1978. Working approaches to remediation of cognitive deficits in brain damaged persons. *Rehabilitation Monograph 59.* New York: New York University Medical Center.

Berg, L. 1988. The aging brain. In: R. Strong, W. G. Woods, and W. Burke, eds., *Central Nervous System Disorders of Aging* (pp. 1–16). New York: Raven Press.

Berkowitz, H. L. 1981. House officers knowledgeability of organic brain syndromes. *General Hospital Psychiatry* 3:231–234.

Bigler, E. D., and R. I. Naugle. 1985. Case studies in cerebral plasticity. *International Journal of Clinical Neuropsychology* 1:12–23.

Binder, J. R., S. J. Swanson, T. A. Hammeke, G. L. Morris, W. M. Mueller, M. Fischer, S. Benbadis, J. A. Frost, S. M. Rao, and V. M. Haugton. 1996. Determination of language dominance using functional MRI: a comparison with the Wada test. *Neurology* 46:978–984.

Bishop, D.V.M. 1983. Linguistic impairment after left hemidecortication for infantile hemiplegia? A reappraisal. *Quarterly Journal of Experimental Psychology* 35A:199–207.

Bisiach, E., and C. Luzzatti. 1978. Unilateral neglect of representational space. *Cortex* 14:129–133.

Bisiach, E., C. Luzzatti, and D. Perani. 1979. Unilateral neglect, representational schema and consciousness. *Brain* 102:609–618.

Blakemore, C. B., and M. A. Falconer. 1967. Long term effects of anterior temporal lobectomy on certain cognitive functions. *Journal of Neurology, Neurosurgery, and Psychiatry* 30:364–367.

Blessed, G., B. E. Tomlinson, and M. Roth. 1968. The association between quantitative measures of dementia and senile change in the cerebral gray matter of elderly subjects. *British Journal of Psychiatry* 114:797–811.

Bogen, J. E. 1969. The other side of the brain I: dysgraphia and dyscopia following cerebral commissurotomy. *Bulletin of the Los Angeles Neurological Society* 31:73–105.

Bogen, J. E. 1993. The callosal syndromes. In: K. M. Heilman, and E. Valenstein, eds., *Clinical Neuropsychology, 3rd Edition* (pp. 337–406). New York: Oxford University Press.

Bogen, J. E. 2000. Split-brain basics: relevance for the concept of one's other mind. *Journal of the American Academy of Psychoanalysis* 28:341–369.

Bogen, J. E., and P. J. Vogel. 1962. Cerebral commissurotomy in man. *Bulletin of the Los Angeles Neurological Society* 27:169–172.

Bogen, J. E., and P. J. Vogel. 1975. Neurologic status in the long term following complete cerebral commissurotomy. In: F. Michel and B. Schott, eds., *Les Syndromes de Disconnexion Calleuse Chez L'Homme.* Lyon: Hopital Neurologique.

Bogen, J. E., D. H. Schultz, and P. J. Vogel. 1988. Completeness of callosotomy shown by magnetic resonance imaging in the long term. *Archives of Neurology* 45:1203–1205.

Bogen, J. E., R. W. Sperry, and P. J. Vogel. 1969. Addendum: Commissural section and propagation of seizures. In: H. H. Hasper, A. A. Ward, and A. Pope, eds., *Basic Mechanisms of the Epilepsies* (pp 439–440). Boston: Little, BrownBohnen, N., A. Twijnstra, and J. Jolles 1993. Persistence of postconcussional symptoms in uncomplicated, mildly head-injured patients: a prospective cohort study. *Neuropsychiatry, Neuropsychology, and Behavioral Neurology* 6:193–200.

Bond, M. R. 1975. Assessment of the psychosocial outcome after severe head injury. In: *Ciba Foundation Symposium, no. 34 (new series), Outcome of Severe Damage to the Central Nervous System* (pp. 141–157). Amsterdam: Elsevier-Excerpta Medica.

Bonita, R. 1986. Cigarette smoking, hypertension and the risk of subarachnoid haemorrhage: a population-based case-control study. *Stroke* 17:831–835.

Bonita, R., and S. Thomson. 1985. Subarachnoid hemorrhage: epidemiology, diagnosis, management, and outcome. *Stroke* 16:591–594.

Bonita, R., R. Beaglehole, and J.D.K. North. 1983. Subarachnoid haemorrhage in New Zealand: an epidemiological study. *Stroke* 14:342–347.

Borkowski, J. G., A. L. Benton, and O. Spreen, 1967. Word fluency and brain damage. *Neuropsychologia* 5:135–140.

Bornstein, R. A., B.K.A. Weir, K. C. Petruk, and L. B. Disney. 1987. Neuropsychological function in patients after subarachnoid haemorrhage. *Neurosurgery* 21:651–654.

Brain, W. R. 1941. Visual disorientation with special reference to lesions of the right cerebral hemisphere. *Brain* 64:244–272.

Brandstadter, D., and W. H. Oertel. 2003. Depression in Parkinson's disease. In: A. Gordin, S. Kaakkola, and H. Teravainen, eds., *Advances in Neurology, Vol 91, Parkinson's Disease* (pp. 1–8). Philadelphia: Lippincott Williams and Wilkins.

Brinkman, R. R., M. M. Mezei, J. Theilmann, E. Almqvist, and M. R. Hayden. 1997. The likelihood of being affected with Huntington's disease by a particular age, for a specific CAG size. *American Journal of Human Genetics* 60:1202–1210.

Broca, P. 1861. Remarques sur le siege de la faculte du langage articule suivie d'une observation d'aphemie. *Bulletin de la Societe Anatomique de Paris* 6:330. (Translated in Herrnstein, R., and E. G. Boring. 1965. *A Source Book in the History of Psychology*. Cambridge, MA: Harvard University Press.)

Brookmeyer, R., S. Gray, and C. Kawas. 1998. Projections of Alzheimer's disease in the United States and the public health impact of delaying disease onset. *American Journal of Public Health* 88:1337–1342.

Brooks, D. N., and W. McKinlay. 1983. Personality and behavioral change after severe blunt head injury—a relative's view. *Journal of Neurology, Neurosurgery, and Psychiatry* 46:336–344.

Brooks, N. 1984. Head injury and the family. In: N. Brooks, ed., *Closed Head Injury: Psychological, Social, and Family Consequences* (pp. 123–147). Oxford: Oxford University Press.

Brown, R. G., and C. D. Marsden. 1988. "Subcortical dementia": The neuropsychological evidence. *Neuroscience* 25:363–387.

Brown, R. G., and C. D. Marsden. 1990. Cognitive function in Parkinson's disease: from description to theory. *Trends in Neuroscience* 13:21–29.

Bruhn, P., and O. A. Parsons. 1977. Reaction time variability in epileptic and brain-damaged patients. *Cortex* 13:373–384.

Bruhn, P., P. Arlien-Soberg, C. Gyldensted, and E. L. Christensen. 1981. Prognosis in chronic toxic encephalopathy. *Acta Neurological Scandinavica* 64:259–272.

Bryden, M. P., and R. G. Ley. 1983. Right-hemispheric involvement in the perception and expression of emotion in normal humans. In: K. M. Heilman and P. Satz, eds., *Neuropsychology of Human Emotion* (pp. 6–44). New York: Guilford Press.

Buschke, H., and K. Fuld. 1974. Evaluating storage, retention, and retrieval in disordered memory and learning. *Neurology* 11:1019–1025.

Calne, D. B. 2003. Parkinson's disease over the last 100 years. In: A. Gordin, S. Kaakkola, and

H. Teravainen, eds., *Advances in Neurology, Vol 91, Parkinson's Disease* (pp. 1–8). Philadelphia: Lippincott Williams and Wilkins.

Campbell, A. L. Jr., J. E. Bogen and A. Smith. 1981. Disorganization and reorganization of cognitive and sensorimotor functions in cerebral commissurotomy: compensatory roles of the forebrain commissures and cerebral hemispheres in man. *Brain* 104:493–511.

Caplan, D. 2003. Aphasic syndromes. In: K. M. Heilman and E. Valenstein, eds., *Clinical Neuropsychology, 4th Edition* (pp. 14–34). New York: Oxford University Press.

Carmon, A., and H. P. Bechtoldt. 1969. Dominance of the right cerebral hemisphere for steriopsis. *Neuropsychologia* 7:29–39.

Carramazza, A., and M. McCloskey. 1988. The case for single-patient studies. *Cognitive Neuropsychology* 5:517–528.

Cassitio, M. G. 1992. Current behavioural techniques. In: R. Gilioli, M. G. Cassitto, and V. Foa, eds., *Neurobehavioural Methods in Occupational Health* (pp. 27–38). Oxford: Pergamon Press.

Cavanaugh, J. B. 1985. Mechanisms of organic solvent toxicity: morphological changes. In: *Chronic Effects of Organic Solvents on the Central Nervous System and Diagnostic Criteria* (pp. 110–135). Copenhagen: World Health Organization.

Cavazutti, V., and G. Erba. 1976. Deficit mnestici dopo emisferectomia totale sinistra in pazienti con emiplegia spastica infantile. *Rivista Sperimentale di Freniatria* 20:585–612.

Cermak, L. S., N. Talbot, K. Chandler, and L. R. Wolbarst. 1985. The perceptual priming phenomenon in amnesia. *Neuropsychologia* 23:615–622.

Chandra, V., E. Kokmen, B. S. Schoenberg, and C. M. Beard. 1989. Head trauma with loss of consciousness as a risk factor for Alzheimer's disease. *Neurology* 39:1576–1578.

Charcot, J. M. 1883. Un cas de suppression brusque et isolee de la vision mentale des signes et des objects (formes et coleurs). *Progress Medicale* 11:568–571.

Chiverton, P., and E. D. Caine. 1989. Education to assist spouses in coping with Alzheimer's disease. A controlled trial. *Journal of the American Geriatrics Society* 37:593–598.

Christensen, A.-L. 1979. *Luria's Neuropsychological Investigation. Text, 2nd Edition.* Copenhagen: Munksgaard.

Chui, H. C., J. A. Mortimer, U. Slager, C. Zarow, W. Bondareff, and D. D. Webster. 1986. Pathological correlates of dementia in Parkinson's disease. *Archives of Neurology* 43: 991–995.

Cohen, N. J. 1984. Preserved learning capacity in amnesia: Evidence for multiple memory systems. In: L. Squire and M. Butters, eds., *Neuropsychology of Memory* (pp. 83–103). New York: Guilford PressCohen, N. J., and S. Corkin. 1981. The amnesic patient H.M.: Learning and retention of a cognitive skill. *Society for Neuroscience Abstracts* 7:517–518.

Cohen, N. J., and L. Squire. 1980. Preserved learning and retention of pattern-analyzing skill in amnesia: dissociation of knowing how and knowing that. *Science* 210:207–210.

Cools, A. R., J.H.L. Van den Bercken, M.W.I. Horstink, K.P.M. Van Spaendonck, and H.J.C. Berger. 1984. Cognitive and motor shifting aptitude disorder in Parkinson's disease. *Journal of Neurology, Neurosurgery, and Psychiatry*, 47, 443–453.

Corballis, M. C., and J. A. Ogden, 1988. Dichotic listening in commissurotomized and hemispherectomized subjects. *Neuropsychologia* 26:565–573.

Corballis, M. C., and M. J. Morgan, 1978. On the biological basis of human laterality. I. Evidence for a maturational left-right gradient. *Behavioral and Brain Sciences* 1:261–269.

Corballis, M. C., and J. Sergent. 1988. Imagery in a commissurotomised patient. *Neuropsychologia* 26:13–26.

Corballis, M. C., and C. I. Trudel. 1993. Role of forebrain commissures in interhemispheric integration. *Neuropsychology* 7:306–324.

Corkin, S. 1965. Tactually guided maze learning in man: effects of unilateral cortical excisions and bilateral hippocampal lesions. *Neuropsychologia* 3:339–351.

Corkin, S. 1968. Acquisition of motor skill after bilateral medial temporal-lobe excision. *Neuropsychologia* 6:255–265.

Corkin, S. 1981. Brain acetylcholine, aging and Alzheimer's disease: implications for treatment. *Trends in Neuroscience* 4:287–290.

Corkin, S. 1982. Some relationships between global amnesia and the memory impairments in Alzheimer's disease. In: S. Corkin, K. L. Davis, J. H. Growdon, E. Usdin, and R. J. Wurtman, eds., *Alzheimer's Disease: A Report of Progress in Research* (pp. 149–164). New York: Raven Press.

Corkin, S. 1984. Lasting consequences of bilateral medial temporal lobectomy: clinical course and experimental findings in H.M. *Seminars in Neurology* 4:249–259.

Corkin, S., D. G. Amaral, R. G. Gonzalez, K. A. Johnson, and B. T. Hyman. 1997. H.M.'s medial temporal lobe lesion: Findings from magnetic resonance imaging. *The Journal of Neuroscience* 17:3964–3979.

Corkin, S., Cohen, N. J., and H. J. Sagar. 1983. Memory for remote personal and public events after bilateral medial temporal lobectomy. *Society for Neuroscience Abstracts* 9:28.

Coslett, H. B. 2003. Acquired dyslexia. In: K. M. Heilman and E. Valenstein, eds., *Clinical Neuropsychology, 4th Edition* (pp. 108–125). New York: Oxford University Press.

Crease, R. 1993. Biomedicine in the age of imaging. *Science* 261:554–561.

Critchley, M. 1953. *The Parietal Lobes*. London: Edward Arnold and Co.

Critchley, M. 1966. The enigma of the Gerstmann's syndrome. *Brain* 89:183–198.

Crompton, M. 1964. The pathogenesis of cerebral infarction following the rupture of cerebral berry aneurysms. *Brain* 87:491–510.

Cummings, J. L., and D. F. Benson, 1986. Dementia of the Alzheimer's Type. An inventory of diagnostic clinical features. *Journal of the American Geriatrics Society* 34:12–19.

Dalrymple-Alford, J. C., A. S. Kalders, R. D. Jones, and R. W. Watson. 1994. A central executive deficit in patients with Parkinson's disease. *Journal of Neurology, Neurosurgery, and Psychiatry* 57:360–367.

Damasio, A. R., and S. W. Anderson. 2003. The frontal lobes. In: K. M. Heilman and E. Valenstein, eds., *Clinical Neuropsychology, 4th Edition* (pp. 404–446). New York: Oxford University Press.

Damasio, A. R., H. Damasio, and C. Chang Chui. 1980. Neglect following damage to frontal lobe and basal ganglia. *Neuropsychologia* 18:123–132.

Damasio, A., H. Damasio, and G. W. Van Hoesen. 1982. Prosopagnosia: Anatomic basis and behavioral mechanisms. *Neurology* 32:331–341.

Damasio, A. R., P. A., Lima, and H. Damasio. 1975. Nervous function after right hemispherectomy. *Neurology* 24:89–93.

Dpp. e Renzi, E. 1982. *Disorders of Space Exploration and Cognition*. Chichester: John Wiley & Sons.

De Renzi, E., and P. Faglioni. 1963. L'autotopoagnosia. *Archivio di Psicologia, Neurologia, e Psichiatria* 24:288–322.

De Renzi, E., and P. Faglioni. 1978. Normative data and screening power of a shortened version of the Token Test. *Cortex* 14:41–49.

De Renzi, E., P. Faglioni, and G. Scotti. 1970. Hemispheric contribution to exploration of space through the visual and tactile modality. *Cortex* 6:191–203.

De Renzi, E., A., Pieczuro, and L. Vignolo. 1966. Oral apraxia and aphasia. *Cortex* 2:50–73.

De Renzi, E., A., Pieczuro, and L. Vignolo. 1968. Ideational apraxia: a quantitative study. *Neuropsychologia* 6:41–52.

De Renzi, E., and G. Scotti, 1970. Autotopagnosia; fiction or reality? Report of a case. *Archives of Neurology* 23:221–227.

De Santis, A., M. Laiacona, R. Barbarotto, A. Basso, R. Villani, D. Spagnoli, and E. Capitani. 1989. Neuropsychological outcome of patients operated upon for intracranial aneurysm: analysis of general prognostic factors and of the effects of the location of the aneurysm. *Journal of Neurology, Neurosurgery, and Psychiatry* 52:1135–1140.

De Vreese, L. P. 1991. Two systems for colour-naming deficits: verbal disconnection vs colour imagery disorder. *Neuropsychologia* 29:1–18.

Delaney, R. C., A. J. Rosen, R. H. Mattson, and R. A. Novelly. 1980. Memory function in focal epilepsy: a comparison of non-surgically unilateral temporal lobe and frontal lobe samples. *Cortex* 16:103–117.

Delis, D., E. Kaplan, and J. Kramer. 2001. *Delis-Kaplan Executive Function System (D-KEFS)*. New York: The Psychological Corporation.

Delis, D. C., J. H. Kramer, E. Kaplan, and B. A. Ober. 1987. *CVLT California Verbal Learning Test, Adult Version Manual, USA*. San Antonio: The Psychological Corporation, Harcourt Brace Jovanovich.

Demaree, H. A., J. DeLuca, E. A. Gaudino, and B. J. Diamond. 1999. Speed of information processing as a key deficit in multiple sclerosis: implications for rehabilitation. *Journal of Neurology, Neurosurgery, and Psychiatry*, 67:661–663.

Denburg, N. L., and D. Tranel. 2003. Acalculia and disturbances of the body schema. In: K. M. Heilman and E. Valenstein, eds., *Clinical Neuropsychology, 4th Edition* (pp. 161–184). New York: Oxford University Press.

Dennerll, R. D. 1964. Cognitive deficits and lateral brain dysfunction. *Epilepsia* 5:177–191.

Dennis, M. 1976. Dissociated naming and locating of body parts after left anterior temporal lobe resection: an experimental case study. *Brain and Language* 3:147–163.

Dennis, M. 1980. Capacity and strategy for syntactic comprehension after left and right hemidecortication. *Brain and Language* 10:287–317.

Dennis, M., and B. Kohn. 1975. Comprehension of syntax in infantile hemiplegics after cerebral hemidecortication: left hemisphere superiority. *Brain and Language* 2:472–482.

Dennis, M., and H. A. Whitaker. 1976. Language acquisition following hemidecortication: Linguistic superiority of the left over the right hemisphere. *Brain and Language* 3:404–433.

Dikmen, S. S., N. Temkin, and G. Armsden. 1989. Neuropsychological recovery: relationship to psychosocial functioning and postconcussional complaints. In: H. S. Levin, H. M. Eisenberg, and A. L. Benton, eds., *Mild Head Injury* (pp. 229–241). New York: Oxford University Press.

Diller, L. 1976. A model for cognitive retraining in rehabilitation. *The Clinical Psychologist* 29:13–15.

Diller, L., and Y. Ben-Yishay. 1987. Outcomes and evidence in neuropsychological rehabilitation in closed head injury. In: H. S. Levin, J. Grafman, and H. M. Eisenberg, eds., *Neurobehavioral Recovery from Head Injury* (pp. 146–165). New York: Oxford University Press.

Dodrill, C. B. 1982. Neuropsychology. In: J. Laidlaw and A. Richens, eds., *A Textbook of Epilepsy* (pp. 282–291). Edinburgh: Churchill Livingstone.

Drachman, D. A., and J. Arbit. 1966. Memory and the hippocampal complex. *Archives of Neurology* 15:52–61.

Dryson, E., and J. A. Ogden. 1998. Chronic solvent neurotoxicity in New Zealand: notified cases between 1993 and 1997. *New Zealand Medical Journal* 111:425–427.

Dryson, E., and J. A. Ogden. 2000. Organic solvent induced chronic toxic encephalopathy:

Extent of recovery. And associated factors, following cessation of exposure. *Neuro-Toxicology* 21:659–666.

Dubois, P. H. 1939. A test standardised on Pueblo Indian children. *Psychological Bulletin* 36: 523–545.

Durie, M. H. 1977. Maori attitudes to sickness, doctors and hospitals. *New Zealand Medical Journal* 86:483–485.

Durie, M. H. 1984. Te taha hinengaro: an integrated approach to mental health. *Community Mental Health in New Zealand* 1:4–11.

Dustman, R. E., R. Y. Emmerson, L. A. Steinhaus, D. E. Shearer, and T. J. Dustman. 1992. The effects of videogame playing on neuropsychological performance of elderly individuals. *Journal of Gerontology* 47:168–171.

Dustman, R. E., R. O. Ruhling, E. M. Russell, D. E. Shearer, H. W. Bonekat, J. W. Shigeoka, J. S. Wood, and D. C. Bradford. 1984. Aerobic exercise training and improved neuro-psychological function of older individuals. *Neurobiology of Aging* 5:35–42.

Edling, C., K. Ekberg, G. Ahlborg, R. Alexandersson, L. Barregard, L. Ekenvall, L. Nilsson, and B. G. Svensson. 1990. Long term follow-up of workers exposed to solvents. *British Journal of Industrial Medicine* 47:75–82.

Eriksson, P. S., E. Perfilieva, T. Björk-Eriksson, A-M. Alborn, C. Nordborg, D. A. Peterson, and F. H. Gage. 1998. Neurogenesis in adult human hippocampus. *Nature Medicine* 4: 1313–1317.

Escourolle, R., J. J. Hauw, F. Gray, and D. Henin. 1975. Aspects neuropathologiques des lesions due corps calleux. In: F. Michel and B. Schott, eds., *Les Syndromes de Disconnexion Calleuse Chez l'Homme* (pp. 41–51). Lyon: Hopital Neurologique.

Fabrigoule, C., I. Rouch, A. Taberly, L. Letenneur, D. Commenges, J. M. Mazaux, J. M. Or-gogozo, and J. F. Dartigues. 1998. Cognitive process in preclinical phase of dementia. *Brain* 121:135–141.

Facca, G., and W. C. Koller. 2003. Differential diagnosis of parkinsonism. In: A. Gordin, S. Kaakkola, and H. Teravainen, eds., *Advances in Neurology, Vol 91, Parkinson's Disease* (pp. 383–396). Philadelphia: Lippincott Williams and Wilkins.

Farah, M. 1984. The neurological basis of mental imagery: a componential analysis. *Cognition* 18:241–269.

Farah, M. 1989. The neuropsychology of mental imagery. In: A. Damasio, ed., *Handbook of Neuropsychology: Disorders of Visual Processing, vol II* (pp. 395–413). Amsterdam: El-sevier Science.

Farah, M. 1990. *Visual Agnosia: Disorders of Object Recognition and What They Tell Us About Normal Vision.* Cambridge, MA: MIT Press.

Farah, M. 1991. Patterns of co-occurence among the associative agnosias: implications for visual object representation. *Cognitive Neuropsychology* 8:1–19.

Fedio, P., and A. F. Mirsky 1969. Selective intellectual deficits in children with temporal lobe or centrecephalic epilepsy. *Neuropsychologia* 7:287–300.

Flowers, K. A., and C. Robertson. 1985. The effect of Parkinson's disease on the ability to maintain a mental set. *Journal of Neurology, Neurosurgery, and Psychiatry* 48:517–429.

Flowers, K. A., I. Pearce, and J.M.S. Pearce. 1984. Recognition memory in Parkinson's disease. *Journal of Neurology, Neurosurgery, and Psychiatry* 47:1174–1181.

Fogelholm, R., and K. Murros. 1987. Cigarette smoking and subarachnoid hemorrhage: a population-based case-control study. Journal of *Neurology, Neurosurgery, and Psychiatry* 50:78–80.

Folstein, M. F., S. E. Folstein, and P. R. McHugh. 1975. "Mini-Mental State": a practical method for grading the mental state of patients for the clinician. *Journal of Psychiatric Research* 12:189–198.

Folstein, S. E. 1989. *Huntington's Disease.* Baltimore, MD: John Hopkins University Press.

Folstein, S. E., G. A. Chase, W. E. Wahl, A. M. McDonnell, and M. F. Folstein. 1987. Huntington's disease in Maryland: clinical aspects of racial variation. *American Journal of Human Genetics* 41:168–179.

Fornazzari, L., D. A. Wilkinson, B. M. Kapur, and P. L. Carlen. 1983. Cerebellar, cortical and functional impairment in toluene abusers. *Acta Neurologica Scandinavica* 67:319–329.

Franco, L., and R. W. Sperry, 1977. Hemisphere lateralization for cognitive processing of geometry. *Neuropsychologia* 15:107–111.

Franzen, J. 2001. *The Corrections.* London: 4th Estate.

Franzen, M. D., A. C. Tishelman, R. J. Seine, and A. Friedman. 1986. Case study: neuropsychological evaluation of an individual with congenital left-hemisphere porencephaly. *International Journal of Clinical Neuropsychology* 8:156–163.

Frassinetti, F., V. Angeli, F. Meneghello, S. Avanzi, and E. Làdavas. 2002. Long-lasting amelioration of visuospatial neglect by prism adaptation. *Brain* 125:608–623.

Freeman, W., and J. W. Watts. 1942. *Psychosurgery.* Springfield, IL: Thomas.

Funkenstein, H. H. 1988. Cerebrovascular disorders. In: M. S. Albert and M. B. Moss, eds., *Geriatric Neuropsychology* (pp. 179–207). New York: Guilford Press.

Gabrieli, J.D.E. 1986. *Memory systems of the human brain: Dissociations among learning capacities in amnesia.* Unpublished doctoral dissertation, Cambridge, MA, Massachusetts Institute of Technology.

Gabrieli, J.D.E., N. J., Cohen, and S. Corkin, 1988. The impaired learning of semantic knowledge following bilateral medial temporal-lobe resection. *Brain and Cognition* 7:157–177.

Gainotti, G. 1972. Emotional behavior and the hemispheric side of the lesion. *Cortex* 8:41–54.

Gainotti, G. 1984. Some methodological problems in the study of the relationships between emotions and cerebral dominance. *Journal of Clinical Neuropsychology* 6:111–121.

Gainotti, G., P. Messerli, and R. Tissot. 1972. Qualitative analysis of unilateral spatial neglect in relation to laterality of cerebral lesions. *Journal of Neurology, Neurosurgery, and Psychiatry* 35:545–550.

Gazzaniga, M. S. 1970. *The Bisected Brain.* New York: Meredith Corporation.

Gazzaniga, M. S. 1983a. Right hemisphere language following brain bisection. *American Psychologist* May 1983:525–537.

Gazzaniga, M. S. 1983b. Reply to Levy and Zaidel. *American Psychologist* May 1983:547–549.

Gazzaniga, M. S. 1985. *The Social Brain.* New York: Basic Books.

Gazzaniga, M. S., and J. E. Le Doux, 1978. The Integrated *Mind.* New York: Plenum Press.

Gazzaniga, M. S., and C. S. Smylie. 1983. Facial recognition and brain asymmetries: Clues to underlying mechanisms. *Annals of Neurology* 13:536–540.

Gershon, E. S., and R. O. Rieder. 1992. Major disorders of mind and brain. *Scientific American*, September:127–133.

Gerstmann, J. 1927. Fingeragnosie und isolierte Agraphie: ein neues Syndrom. *Zeitschrift fur Neurologie und Psychiatrie* 108:153–177.

Gerstmann, J. 1930. Zur Symptomatologie der Hirnlasionen im Uebergangsgebiet der unteren parietal-und mittleren. Occipitalwindung. *Nervenarzt* 3:691–695.

Geshwind, N. 1965. Disconnection syndromes in animals and man. *Brain* 88:237–294.

Gianutsos, R. 1992. The computer in cognitive rehabilitation: it's not just a tool any more. *Journal of Head Trauma Rehabilitation* 7:26–35.

Goetz, C. G. 1999. Hallucinations in Parkinson's disease: The clinical syndrome. In: G. M.

Stern, ed., *Advances in Neurology, Vol 80, Parkinson's disease* (pp. 419–423). Philadelphia: Lippincott Williams and Wilkins.

Gold, G., P. Giannakopoulos, and C. Bouras. 1998. Reevaluating the role of vascular changes in the differential diagnosis of Alzheimer's disease and Vascular dementia. *European Neurology* 40:121–129.

Golden, C. J., T. A. Hammeke, and A. D. Purisch. 1980. *The Luria-Nebraska Neuropsychological Battery Manual*. Los Angeles: Western Psychological Services.

Goodglass, H., and E. Kaplan. 1983. *Boston Diagnostic Aphasia Examination (BDAE)*. Philadelphia: Lea and Febiger. (Distributed by Psychological Assessment Resources, Odessa, FL.)

Gott, P. S. 1973a. Language after dominant hemispherectomy. Journal of Neurology, *Neurosurgery and Psychiatry* 36:1082–1088.

Gott, P. S. 1973b. Cognitive abilities following right and left hemispherectomy. *Cortex* 9:266–274.

Gould, E., A. Beylin, P. Tanapat, A. Reeves, and T. J. Shors. 1999. Learning enhances adult neurogenesis in the hippocampal formation. *Nature Neuroscience* 2:260–265.

Grafman, J., and S. Salazar. 1987. Methodological considerations relevant to the comparison of recovery from penetrating and closed head injuries. In: H. S. Levin, J. Grafman, and H. M. Eisenberg, eds., *Neurobehavioral Recovery from Head Injury*. New York: Oxford University Press.

Grafman, J., B. Jonas, and A. Salazar. 1990. Wisconsin Card Sorting Test performance based on location and size of neuroanatomical lesions in Vietnam veterans with penetrating head injury. *Perceptual and Motor Skills* 71:1120–1122.

Grant, D. A., and E. A. Berg. 1981. *Wisconsin Card Sorting Test*, Odessa, Florida: Psychological Assessment Resources, Inc.

Grant, I., and W. Alves. 1987. Psychiatric and psychosocial disturbances in head injury. In: H. S. Levin, J. Grafman, and H. M. Eisenberg, eds., *Neurobehavioral Recovery from Head Injury* (pp. 232–261). New York: Oxford University Press.

Graves, A. B., E. White, T. D. Koepsell, B. V. Reifler, G. van Belle, E. B. Larson, and M. Raskind. 1990. The association between head trauma and Alzheimer's disease. *American Journal of Epidemiology* 131:491–501.

Green, J. B., and L. G. Hartlage. 1971. Comparative performance of epileptic and non-epileptic children and adolescents. *Disorders of the Nervous System* 32:418–421.

Griffen, R. M., and F. Mouheb. 1987. Work therapy as a treatment modality for the elderly patient with dementia. *Physical and Occupational Therapy in Geriatrics* 5:67–72.

Gronwall, D. 1977. Paced Auditory Serial Addition Task: A measure of recovery from concussion. *Perceptual and Motor Skills*, 44:367–373.

Gronwall, D., and P. Wrightson. 1975. Cumulative effect of concussion. *Lancet* 2:995–997.

Gronwall, D., P. Wrightson, and P. Waddell. 1998. *Head Injury. The Facts, 2nd Edition*. Oxford: Oxford University Press.

Grote, E., and W. Hassler. 1988. The critical first minutes after subarachnoid hemorrhage. *Neurosurgery* 22:654–661.

Gusella, J. F., N. S. Wexler, P. M. Conneally, S. L. Naylor, M. A. Anderson, R. E. Tanzi, P. C. Watkins, K. Ottina, M. R. Wallace, A. Y. Sakaguchi, A. B. Young, I. Shoulson, E. Bonilla, and J. B.Martin.1983. A polymorphic DNA marker genetically linked to Huntington's Disease. *Nature* 306:234–238.

Hackett, M. L., and C. S. Anderson. 2000. Health outcomes 1 year after subarachnoid hemorrhage: an international population-based study. *Neurology* 55:658–662.

Hagen, C. 1982. Language cognitive disorganisation, following closed head injury: a conceptualization. In: L. E. Trexler ed., *Cognitive Rehabilitation: Conceptualization and Intervention* (pp. 131–151). New York: Plenum Press.

Halligan, P. W., and J. C. Marshall. 1994. Toward a principled explanation of unilateral neglect. *Cognitive Neuropsychology* 11:167–206.

Halstead, W. C. 1947. *Brain and Intelligence.* Chicago: University of Chicago Press.

Hanninen, H. 1982. Psychological test batteries: new trends and developments. In: R. Gilioli, M. G. Cassitto, and V. Foa, eds., *Neurobehavioural Methods in Occupational Health* (pp. 123–129). Oxford: Pergamon Press.

Harlow, J. M. 1868. Recovery from the passage of an iron bar through the head. *Publications of the Massachusetts Medical Society (Boston)* 2:327–346.

Harper, P. 1996. The epidemiology of Huntington's Disease. In: P. S. Harper, ed., *Huntington's Disease, 2nd Edition* (pp. 201–239). London, W.B. Saunders.

Harper, P., G. Houlihan, and A. Tyler. 1996. Genetic counselling in Huntington's Disease. In: P. S. Harper, ed., *Huntington's Disease, 4th Edition* (pp. 359–393). London, W.B. Saunders.

Harper, P., and M. Morris. 1996. Introduction: A historical background to Huntington's Disease. In: P. S. Harper, ed., *Huntington's Disease, 2nd Edition* (pp. 1–29). London, W.B. Saunders.

Harper, P., J. Soldan, and A. Tyler. 1996. Predictive tests in Huntington's Disease. In: P. S. Harper, ed., *Huntington's Disease, 2nd Edition* (pp. 395–424). London, W.B. Saunders.

Hartman, D. E. 1995. *Neuropsychological Toxicology. Identification and Assessment of Human Neurotoxic Syndromes, 2nd Edition* (Chapter 4). New York: Pergamon Press.

Heaton, R. K. 1981. *A Manual for the Wisconsin Card Sorting Test.* Odessa, Florida: Psychological Assessment Resources.

Heilman, K. M. 1982. Right hemisphere dominance for attention. In: S. Katsuki, T. Tsubaki, and Y. Toyokura, eds., *Neurology. Proceedings of the 12th World Congress of Neurology, Kyoto, Japan* (pp. 20–26). Amsterdam: Excerpta Medica,

Heilman, K. M., and E. Valenstein. 1972. Frontal lobe neglect in man. *Neurology* 22:660–664.

Heilman, K. M., and P. Satz. 1983. *Neuropsychology of Human Emotion.* New York: Guilford Press.

Heilman, K. M., R. Scholes, and T. R. Watson. 1975. Auditory affective agnosia: Disturbed comprehension of affective speech. *Journal of Neurology, Neurosurgery, and Psychiatry* 38:69–72.

Heilman, K. M., R. T. Watson, and D. Bowers. 1983. Affective disorders associated with hemispheric disease. In: K. M. Heilman and P. Satz, eds., *Neuropsychology of Human Emotion* (pp. 45–64). New York: Guilford Press.

Heilman, K. M., R. T. Watson, and E. Valenstein. 1993. Neglect and related disorders. In: K. M. Heilman and E. Valenstein, eds., *Clinical Neuropsychology, 3rd Edition* (pp. 279–336). New York: Oxford University Press.

Heilman, K. M., R. T. Watson, and E. Valenstein. 2003. Neglect and related disorders. In: K. M. Heilman and E. Valenstein, eds., *Clinical Neuropsychology, 4th Edition* (pp. 296–346). New York: Oxford University Press.

Hendrie, H. C. 1998. Epidemiology of dementia and Alzheimer's disease. *American Journal of Geriatric Psychiatry* 6:S3–18.

Hoehn, M. M., and M. D. Yahr. 1967. Parkinsonism: onset, progression, and mortality. *Neurology* 17:427–442.

Holland, A. 1980. *The Communicative Abilities in Daily Living: Manual.* Austin, TX: Pro-Ed.

Holland, A. 1984. *Language Disorders in Adults: Recent Advances.* San Diego, CA: College Hill Press.

Hop, J. W., G.J.E. Rinkel, A. Algra, and J. van Gijn. 1998. Quality of life in patients and partners after aneurysmal subarachnoid haemorrhage. *Stroke* 29:798–804.

Hoppe, K. D. 1977. Split brains and psychoanalysis. *Psychoanalytic Quarterly* 46:220–244.

Hoppe, K. D., and J. E. Bogen. 1977. Alexithymia in twelve commissurotomized patients. *Psychotherapy and Psychosomatics* 28:148–155.

Humphreys, G. W., and M. J. Riddoch. 1987. *To See But Not To See. A Case Study of Visual Agnosia.* London: Lawrence Erlbaum Associates.

Huntington, G. 1872. On Chorea. *Medical and Surgical Reporter* 26:320–321.

Huntington's Disease Collaborative Research Group. 1993. A novel gene containing a trinucleotide repeat that is expanded and unstable on Huntington's disease chromosomes. *Cell* 72:971–983.

Huntington Study Group. 1996. Unified Huntington's disease rating scale: reliability and consistency. *Movement Disorders* 11:136–142.

Iacoboni, M., J. Rayman, and E. Zaidel. 1996. Left brain says yes, right brain says no: normative duality in the split brain. In: S. R. Hameroff, A. W Kasniak, and A. C. Scott, eds., *Toward a Scientific Basis of Consciousness* (pp. 197–202). Cambridge, MA: MIT Press.

Inagawa, T., and A. Hirano. 1990. Autopsy study of unruptured incidental intracranial aneurysms. *Surgical Neurology* 34:361–365.

International Huntington Association and World Federation of Neurology. 1994. Guidelines for the Molecular Genetics Predictive Test in Huntington's Disease. *Neurology* 44:1533–1536.

International Subarachnoid Aneurysm Trial Collaborative Group. 2002. International subarachnoid aneursym trial (ISAT) of neurosurgical versus endovascular coiling in 2143 patients with ruptured intracranial aneurysms: a randomised trial. *The Lancet* 360:1267–1274.

International Study of Unruptured Intracranial Aneurysm Investigators. 1998. Unruptured intracranial aneurysms—risk of rupture and risks of surgical intervention. *The New England Journal of Medicine* 339:1725–1733

Jackson, G. D., A. Connelly, J. H. Cross, I. Gordon, and D. G. Gadian. 1994. Functional magnetic resonance imaging of focal seizures. *Neurology* 44:850–856.

Jackson, H. 1876. Case of large cerebral tumour without optic neuritis and with left hemiplegia and imperception. In: J. Taylor, ed., Selected *Writings of John Hughlings Jackson* (pp. 146–152). London: Hodden and Stoughton.

Jackson, J. 1878. Remarks on non-protrusion of the tongue in some cases of aphasia. *Lancet* 1:716; *Brain* 38:104 (1915 reprint).

Jacobs, D. H., J. Shuren, and K. M. Heilman. 1995. Impaired perception of facial identity and facial affect in Huntington's disease. *Neurology*, 45:1217–1218.

Jelinek, G. 2001. *Taking Control of Multiple Sclerosis. Natural and Medical Therapies to Prevent its Progression.* Melbourne, Australia: Hyland House Publishing.

Jellinger, K. 1979. Pathology and aetiology of intracranial aneurysms. In: H. W. Pia, C. Langmaid, and J. Zierski, eds., *Cerebral Aneurysms. Advances in Diagnosis and Therapy* (pp. 5–19). New York: Springer.

Jennett, B., and Bond, M. 1975. Assessment of outcome after severe brain damage. *Lancet* 1: 480–484.

Jennett, B., G. Teasdale, R. Braakman, J. Minderhoud, and R. Knill-Jones. 1976. Predicting outcome in individual patients after severe head injury. *Lancet* 1:1031–1035.

Johnson, L. D., J. G. Bachman, and P. M. O'Malley. 1979. *Drugs and the Nation's High School*

Students: Five Year Trends, 1979 Highlights. Rockville, MD: National Institute on Drug Abuse.

Johnson, L. E. 1984. Bilateral visual cross-integration by human forebrain commissurotomy subjects. *Neuropsychologia* 22:167–175.

Jones, M. K. 1974. Imagery as a mnemonic aid after left temporal lobectomy: contrast between material-specific and generalized memory disorders. *Neuropsychologia* 12:21–30.

Jones-Gotman, M. 1987. Commentary: Psychological evaluation-testing hippocampal function. In: J. Engel Jr., ed., *Surgical Treatments of the Epilepsies* (pp. 203–211). New York: Raven Press.

Jones-Gotman, M., and B. Milner. 1977. Design fluency: the invention of nonsense drawings after focal cortical lesions. *Neuropsychologia* 15:653–674.

Jordan, B. D., N. R. Relkin, L. D. Ravdin, A. R. Jacobs, A. Bennett, and S. Gandy, 1997. Apolipoprotein E epsilon4 associated with chronic traumatic brain injury in boxing. *Journal of the American Medical Association* 278:136–140.

Juntunen, J. 1983. Neurological examination and assessment of the syndromes caused by exposure to neurotoxic agents. In: R. Gilioli, M. G. Cassitto and V. Foa, eds., *Neurobehavioral Methods in Occupational Health* (pp. 3–10). Oxford: Pergamon Press.

Juvela, S., M. Porras, and K. Poussa. 2000. Natural history of unruptured intracranial aneurysms: probability of and risk factors for aneurysm rupture. *Journal of Neurosurgery* 93: 379–387.

Kaplan, E. 1988. A process approach to neuropsychological assessment. In: T. Boll and B. K. Bryant, eds., *Clinical Neuropsychology and Brain Function: Research, Measurement and Practice* (pp. 129–167). Washington, DC: American Psychological Association.

Kaplan, E., D. Fein, R. Morris, and D. Delis. 1991. *WAIS-R NI Manual.* San Antonio, TX: The Psychological Corporation.

Kapur, N., ed. 1997. *Injured brains of medical minds. Views from within.* Oxford: Oxford University Press.

Karnath, H.-O., S. Ferber, and M. Himmelbach. 2001. Spatial awareness is a function of the temporal not the parietal lobe. *Nature* 411:950–953.

Karnath, H-O., M. Himmelbach, and C. Rorden. 2002. The subcortical anatomy of human spatial neglect: Putamen, caudate nucleus and pulvinar. *Brain* 125:350–60.

Kay, J., R. Lesser, and M. Coltheart. 1992. *PALPA. Psycholinguistic Assessments of Language Processing in Aphasia.* East Sussex: Lawrence Erlbaum Associates.

Keane, M. M., J.D.E. Gabrieli, and S. Corkin. 1987. Multiple relations between fact learning and priming in global amnesia. *Society for Neuroscience Abstracts* 13:1454.

Keller, A. Z. 1970. Hypertension, age, and residence in the survival of people with subarachnoid haemorrhage. *American Journal of Epidemiology* 91:139–147.

Kendall, P. C., and S. D., Hollon, eds. 1979. *Cognitive-Behavioral Interventions: Theory, Research and Procedures.* New York: Academic Press.

Kendall, P. C., and S. D. Hollon, eds. 1981. *Assessment Strategies for Cognitive-Behavioral Interventions.* New York: Academic Press.

Khan-Bourne, N., and R. G. Brown. 2003. Cognitive behaviour therapy for the treatment of depression in individuals with brain injury. *Neuropsychological Rehabilitation* 13:89–107.

Kimura, D. 1964. Cognitive deficit related to seizure patterns in centrecephalic epilepsy. *Journal of Neurology, Neurosurgery, and Psychiatry* 27:291–295.

Kinsbourne, M. 1977. Hemi-neglect and hemisphere rivalry. In: E. A. Weinstein and R. P. Friedland, eds., *Advances in Neurology, vol 18.* New York: Raven Press.

Kinsbourne, M. 1993. Orientational bias model of unilateral neglect: Evidence from attentional gradients within hemispace. In: I. H. Robertson and J. C. Marshall, eds., *Unilateral Neglect: Clinical and Experimental Studies* (pp. 63–86). East Sussex: Lawrence Erlbaum Associates, Ltd.

Kinsbourne, M. 1994. Mechanisms of neglect: Implications for rehabilitation. *Neuropsychological Rehabilitation* 4:151–154.

Kinsbourne, M., and D. B. Rosenfield. 1974. Agraphia selective for written spelling. *Brain and Language* 1:215–226.

Kishimoto, K., N. Nakamura, and Y. Sotokawa. 1957. Population genetics study—Huntington's chorea in Japan. *Annual Report, Research Institute of Environmental Medicine* 9:195–211.

Knopman, D., and O. Selnes. 2003. Neuropsychology of dementia. In: E. M. Heilman, and E. Valenstein, eds., *Clinical Neuropsychology, 4th Edition* (pp. 574–616). New York: Oxford University Press.

Kogeorges, J., and D. F. Scoot. 1981. Biofeedback and its clinical applications. *British Journal of Hospital Medicine* 25:601–603.

Kohn, B., and Dennis, M. 1974. Selective impairments of visuospatial abilities in infantile hemiplegics after right cerebral hemidecortication. *Neuropsychologia* 12:505–512.

Kokmen, E., J. P. Whisnant, W. M. O'Fallon, C. P. Chu, and C. M. Beard. 1996. Dementia after ischemic stroke: A population-based study in Rochester, Minnesota (1960–1984). *Neurology* 46:154–159.

Kopelman, M., B. Wilson, and A. Baddeley. 1990. *The Autobiographical Memory Interview*. Bury St. Edmunds: Thames Valley Test Company.

Kossyln, S. M. 1981. The medium and message in mental imagery. *Psychological Review* 88:46–66.

Kossyln, S. M. 1983. *Image and Mind*. Cambridge, MA: Harvard University Press.

Kurtzke, K. F. 1983. Epidemiology of MS. In: J. F. Hallpike, C.W.M. Adams, and W. W. Tourtellotte, eds., *Multiple Sclerosis* (pp. 49–95). Baltimore, MD: Williams and Wilkins.

Lakke, P.W.F. 1981. Classification of extrapyramidal disorders. Proposal for an international classification and glossary of terms. *Journal of the Neurological Sciences* 51:313–327.

Lang, A. E., A. Lozana, E. B. Montgomery, R. R. Tasker, and W. D. Hutchison. 1999. Posteroventral medial pallidotomy in advanced Parkinson's disease. In: G. M. Stern, ed., *Advances in Neurology. Volume 80. Parkinson's Disease* (pp. 575–583). Philadelphia: Lippincott Williams and Wilkins.

Lang, A.E.T., and S. Fahn. 1989. Assessment of Parkinson's disease. In: T. L. Munsat, ed., *Quantification of Neurologic Deficit* (pp. 285–389). Stoneham, MA: Butterworths.

Langston, J. W., P. Ballard, and J. Irwin. 1983. Chronic parkinsonism in humans due to a product meperidine-analog synthesis. *Science* 219:979–980.

Lansdell, H. 1968. Effect of extent of temporal lobe ablations on two lateralised deficits. *Physiology and Behaviour* 3:271–273.

Larsen, J. P. 2003. Sleep disorders in Parkinson's disease. In: A. Gordin, S. Kaakkola, and H. Teravainen, eds., *Advances in Neurology, Vol 91, Parkinson's Disease* (pp. 329–334). Philadelphia: Lippincott Williams and Wilkins.

Larson, E. B., B. V. Reifler, C. Canfield, and G. D. Cohen. 1984. Evaluating elderly outpatients with symptoms of dementia. *Hospital and Community Psychiatry* 35:425–428.

Lawrence, A. D., B. J. Sahakian, J. R. Hodges, A. E. Rosser, K. W. Lange, and T. W. Robbins. 1996. Executive and mnemonic functions in early Huntington's disease. *Brain* 119:1633–1645.

Le Doux, J. E., D. H. Wilson, and M. S. Gazzaniga. 1978. Block Design performance following callosal sectioning: observations on functional recovery. *Archives of Neurology* 35:506–508.

Levin, H. S. 1995. Outcome from mild head injury. In: R. Narayan, J. Wilberger, and J. Povlishock, eds., *Neurotrauma* (pp. 749–754). New York: McGraw-Hilll.

Levin, H. S., H. E. Gary, W. M. High, S. Mattis, R. M. Ruff, H. M. Eisenberg, L. F. Marshall, and K. Tabbador. 1987a. Minor head injury and the postconcussional syndrome: methodological issues in outcome studies. In: H. S. Levin, J. Grafman, and H. M. Eisenberg, eds., *Neurobehavioral Recovery From Head Injury* (pp. 262–275). New York: Oxford University Press.

Levin, H. S., S. Mattis, R. M. Ruff, H. M. Eisenberg, L. F. Marshall, and K. Tabbador. 1987b. Neurobehavioral outcome of minor head injury: a three center study. *Journal of Neurosurgery* 66:234–243.

Levin, H. S., V. M. O'Donnell, and R. G. Grossman. 1979. The Galveston Orientation and Amnesia Test: a practical scale to assess cognition after head injury. *Journal of Nervous and Mental Disorders* 167:675–684.

Levine, D. N., and E. Sweet. 1983. Localization of lesions in Broca's motor aphasia. In: A. Kertesz, ed., *Localization in Neuropsychology* (pp. 185–208). New York: Academic Press.

Levine, S. 1997. *A Year to Live: How to live this year as if it were your last.* New York: Bell Tower.

Levy, J. 1983. Language, cognition, and the right hemisphere. A response to Gazzaniga. *American Psychologist* May 1983:538–541.

Levy, J., R. D. Nebes, and R. W. Sperry. 1970. Expressive language in the surgically separated minor hemisphere. *Cortex* 7:49–58.

Levy, J., and C. Trevarthen. 1977. Perceptual, semantic and phonetic aspects of elementary language processes in split-brain patients. *Brain* 100:105–118.

Levy, J., C. Trevarthen, and R. W. Sperry. 1972. Perception of bilateral chimeric figures following hemispheric deconnection. *Brain* 95:61–78.

Levy-Agresti, J., and R. W. Sperry. 1968. Differential processing capacities in major and minor hemispheres. *Proceedings of the National Academy of Science U.S.A.* 61:1158.

Lezak, M. D. 1983. *Neuropsychological Assessment, 2nd Edition.* New York: Oxford University Press.

Lezak, M. D. 1995. *Neuropsychological Assessment, 3rd Edition.* New York: Oxford University Press.

Lieberman. A. 1996. Adolf Hitler had post-encephalitic Parkinsonism. *Parkinsonism and Related Disorders* 2:95–103.

Liepmann, H. 1900. *Das Krankheitsbild der Apraxie ('motorischen Asymbolie').* Berlin: Karger.

Liepmann, H. 1905. Der weitere Krankheitsverlauf bei dem einseitig Apraktischen und der Gehirnbefund auf Grund von Serienschnitten. *Monatsschrift fur Psychiatrie und Neurologie* 17:283–311.

Lindvall, O. 1999. Neural transplantation: Can we improve the symptomatic relief? In: G. M. Stern, ed., *Advances in Neurology, vol 80, Parkinson's disease* (pp. 635–640). Philadelphia: Lippincott Williams and Wilkins.

Lipchik, E. 1988. Interviewing with a constructive ear. *Dulwich Centre Newsletter* Winter:3–5.

Lipchik, E., and S. de Shazer. 1986. The purposeful interview. *Journal of Strategic and Systemic Therapies* 5:88–99.

Lissauer, H. 1890. Ein fall von seelenblindheit nebst einem beitrage zur theorie derselben. *Archiv fur Psychiatrie und Nervenkrankheiten* 21:222–270.

Ljunggren, B., B. S. Sonesson, H. Saveland, and L. Brandt, 1985. Cognitive impairment and adjustment in patients without neurological deficits after aneurysmal SAH and early operation. *Journal of Neurosurgery* 62:673–679.

Loiseau, P., E. Stube, D. Broustet, S. Battelliochi, C. Gomeni, and P. D. Morselli. 1980. Evaluation of memory function in a population of epileptic patients and matched control. *Acta Neurologica Scandinavica* 62:80, 58–61.

Long, C. G., and J. R. Moore. 1979. Parental expectations for their epileptic children. *Journal of Child Psychology and Psychiatry* 20:313–324.

Loranger, A. W., H. Goodell, F. H. McDowell, J. E. Lee, and R. D. Sweet. 1972. Intellectual impairment in Parkinson's syndrome. *Brain* 95:405–412.

Luria, A. R. 1966. *Higher Cortical Functions in Man* (B. Haigh, translator). New York: Basic Books.

Luria, A. R. 1970. The functional organization of the brain. *Scientific American* 222:2–9.

Luria, A. R. 1971. Memory disturbances in local brain lesions. *Neuropsychologia* 9:367–376.

Luria, A. R. 1973. *The Working Brain*. London: Penguin Press.

Maguire, A. M. 2000. Reducing neglect by introducing ipsilesional global cues. *Brain and Cognition* 43:328–332.

Maguire, A. M., and J. A. Ogden. 2002. MRI brain scan analyses and neuropsychological profiles of nine patients with persisting unilateral neglect. *Neuropsychologia* 40:879–887.

Manly, T., K. Hawkins, J. Evans, K. Woldt, and I. H. Robertson. 2002. Rehabilitation of executive function: facilitation of effective goal management on complex tasks using auditory alerts. *Neuropsychologia* 40:271–281.

Marsel-Wilson, W. D., and H.-L. Teuber. 1975. Memory for remote events in anterograde amnesia: recognition of public figures from news photographs. *Neuropsychologia* 13:353–364.

Marshall, J. C., and P. W. Halligan. 1994a. Left in the dark: The neglect of theory. *Neuropsychological Rehabilitation* 4:161–168.

Martin, R., and H. F. McFarland. 1993. Role of genetic factors for the autoimmune pathogenesis of multiple sclerosis. In: U. Halbreich, ed., *Multiple Sclerosis: A Neuropsychiatric Disorder* (pp. 73–96). Washington, DC: American Psychiatric Press.

Martin, W. E., R. B. Loewenson, J. A. Resch, and A. B. Baker. 1973. Parkinson's disease: clinical analysis of 100 patients. *Neurology* 23:783–790.

Matarazzo, J. D., and A. Prifitera. 1989. Subtest scatter and premorbid intelligence: lessons from the WAIS-R standardization sample. *Psychological Assessment* 1:186–191.

Mattingley, J. B. 2002. Visuomotor adaptation to optical prisms: a new cure for spatial neglect? *Cortex* 38:277–283.

Mattis, S. 1976. Mental status examination for organic mental syndrome in the elderly patient. In: L. Bellak and T. B. Karasu, eds., *Geriatric Psychiatry* (pp. 77–122) New York: Grune and Stratton.

Mattis, S., and R. Kovner. 1978. Different patterns of mnemonic deficits in two organic amnestic syndromes. *Brain and Language* 6:179–191.

Mayeux, R., and Y. Stern. 1983. Intellectual dysfunction and dyslexia in Parkinson's disease. In: R. F. Mayeux and W. G. Rosen, eds., *The Dementias* (pp. 211–227). New York: Raven Press.

Mayeux, R., Y. Stern, L. Cote, and J.B.W. Williams. 1984. Altered serotonin metabolism in depressed patients with Parkinson's disease. *Neurology* 34:642–646.

Mayeux, R., and Y. Stern, R. Rosenstein et al. 1988. An estimate of the prevalence of dementia in idiopathic Parkinson's disease. *Archives of Neurology* 45:260–262.

Mayeux, R., Y. Stern, J. Rosen, and J. Leventhal. 1981. Depression, intellectual impairment, and Parkinson's disease. *Neurology* 31:645–650.

McCarthy, R. A., and E. K. Warrington. 1990. *Cognitive Neuropsychology. A Clinical Introduction.* San Diego, CA: Academic Press.

McCormick, W. F., and Schmalstieg, E. J. 1977. The relationship of arterial hypertension to intracranial aneurysms. *Archives of Neurology* 34:285–287.

McElvoy, C. L., and R. L. Patterson. 1986. Behavioral treatment of deficit skills in dementia patients. *Gerontologist* 26:475–478.

McKenna, P., and E. K. Warrington. 1978. Category specific naming preservation: a single case study. *Journal of Neurology, Neurosurgery, and Psychiatry* 41:571–574.

McKenna, P., J. R. Willison, D. Lowe, and G. Neil-Dwyer. 1989. Cognitive outcome and quality of life one year after subarachnoid haemorrhage. *Neurosurgery* 24:361–367.

McKenzie, K. G., and G. Kaczanowski. 1964. Prefrontal leucotomy. A five year controlled study. *Canadian Medical Journal* 91:1193–1196.

McKhann, G., D. Drachman, M. Folstein, R. Katzman, D. Price, and E. M. Stadlan. 1984. Clinical diagnosis of Alzheimer's disease: report of the NINCDS-ADRDA Work Group under the auspices of Department of Health and Human Services Task Force on Alzheimer's Disease. *Neurology* 34:939–944.

McLean, A., S. Dikmen, N. Temkin, A. R. Wyler and J. L. Gale. 1984. Psychosocial functioning at one month after head injury. *Neurosurgery* 14:393–399.

McLean, S. 1987a. Assessing dementia. Part 1: difficulties, definitions and differential diagnosis. *Australian and New Zealand Journal of Psychiatry* 21:142–174.

McLean, S. 1987b. Assessing dementia. Part 2: clinical, functional, neuropsychological and social issues. *Australian and New Zealand Journal of Psychiatry* 21:284–304.

Mega, M. S., J. L. Cummings, T. Fiorello, and J. Gornbein. 1996. The spectrum of behavioral changes in Alzheimer's disease. *Neurology* 46:130–135.

Messerli, P., X. Seron, and P. Tissot. 1979. Quelques aspects de la programmation dans le syndrome frontal. *Archives Suisses de Neurologie, Neurochirurgie, et de Psychiatrie* 125: 23–35.

Mesulam, M.-M. 1981. A cortical network for directed attention and unilateral neglect. *Annals of Neurology* 10:309–325.

Mesulam, M.-M. 1983. The functional anatomy and hemispheric specialization for directed attention. *Trends in Neurosciences* 6:384–387.

Mesulam, M.-M. 1985. *Principles of Behavioral Neurology* (pp. 86–90). Philadelphia: F. A. Davis.

Meyer, V., and H. J. Yates. 1955. Intellectual changes following temporal lobectomy for psychomotor epilepsy. *Journal of Neurology, Neurosurgery, and Psychiatry* 18:44–52.

Meyers, J. E., and K. R. Meyers. 1995. *The Meyers Scoring System for the Rey Complex Figure Test and Recognition Trial: Professional Manual.* Odessa, FL: Psychological Assessment Resources.

Mickel, S. F., J.D.E. Gabrieli, T. J. Rosen, S. Corkin and J. H. Growdon. 1986. Mirror tracing: preserved learning in patients with global amnesia and some patients with Alzheimer's disease. *Society for Neuroscience Abstracts* 12:20.

Milner, B. 1954. Intellectual function of the temporal lobes. *Psychological Bulletin* 51:42–62.

Milner, B. 1963. Effects of different brain lesions on card sorting. *Archives of Neurology* 9:90–100.

Milner, B. 1965. Visually guided maze learning in man: effects of bilateral hippocampal, bilateral frontal, and unilateral cerebral lesions. *Neuropsychologia* 3:317–338.

Milner, B. 1966. Amnesia following operation on the temporal lobes. In: C.W.L. Whitty and O. L. Zangwill, eds., *Amnesia* (pp. 109–133). London: Butterworths.

Milner, B. 1968a. Disorders of memory after brain lesions in man. *Neuropsychologia* 6:175–179.

Milner, B. 1968b. Visual recognition and recall after right temporal-lobe excision in man. *Neuropsychologia* 6:191–208.

Milner, B. 1975. Psychological aspects of focal epilepsy and its neurosurgical management. In: D. P. Purpura, J. K. Penry, and R. D. Walters, eds., *Advances in Neurology, vol 8* (pp. 299–320). New York: Raven Press.

Milner, B., and Taylor, L. 1972. Right hemisphere superiority in tactile pattern-recognition after cerebral commissurotomy: evidence for nonverbal memory. *Neuropsychologia* 10:1–15.

Milner, B., S. Corkin, and H.-L. Teuber. 1968. Further analysis of the hippocampal amnesic syndrome: 14-year follow-up study of H.M. *Neuropsychologia* 6:215–234.

Mirsky, A. F., D. W. Primac, C. A. Marsan, H. E. Rosvold, and J. R. Stevens. 1960. A comparison of the psychological test performance of patients with focal and non-focal epilepsy. *Experimental Neurology* 2:75–89.

Mohr, E., J. Juncos, C. Cox, I. Litvan, P. Fedio, and T. N. Chase. 1990. Selective deficits in cognition and memory in high-functioning parkinsonian patients. *Journal of Neurology, Neurosurgery, and Psychiatry* 53:603–606.

Mistry, R. 2002. *Family Matters*. London: Faber & Faber.

Money, J. 1965. *A Standardized Road-Map Test of Direction Sense*. Baltimore, MD: John Hopkins University Press.

Moniz, E. 1954. How I succeeded in performing the prefrontal leucotomy. *Journal of Clinical and Experimental Psychopathology* 15:373–379.

Mooney, C. M. 1957. Age in the development of closure ability in children. *Canadian Journal of Psychology* 11:219–226.

Morris, M. 1991. Psychiatric aspects of Huntington's disease. In: P. S. Harper, ed., *Huntington's Disease* (pp. 81–126). London: W.B. Saunders.

Morris, M., and J. Scourfield. 1996. Psychiatric aspects of Huntington's Disease. In: P. S. Harper, ed., *Huntington's Disease, 2nd Edition* (pp. 73–121). London: W.B. Saunders.

Mort, D. J., P. Malhotra, S. K. Mannan, C. Rorden, A. Pambakian, C. Kennard, and M. Husain. 2003. The anatomy of visual neglect. *Brain* 126:1986–1997.

Mortimer, J. A. 1983. Alzheimer's disease and senile dementia; prevalence and incidence. In: B. Reisberg, ed., *Alzheimer's Disease* (pp. 141–148). New York: The Free Press.

Mortimer, J. A., L. R. French, J. T. Hutton, and L. M. Schuman. 1985. Head injury as a risk factor for Alzheimer's disease. *Neurology* 35:264–266.

Mortimer, J. A., and A. B. Graves. 1993. Education and other socio-economic determinants of dementia and Alzheimer's disease. *Neurology* 43:S39–S44.

Mortimer, J. A., and F. J. Pirozzolo. 1985. Remote effects of head trauma. *Developmental Neuropsychology* 1:215–229.

Mortimer, J. A., C. M. van Duijn, V. Chandra, L. Fratiglioni, A. B. Graves, A. Heyman et al. 1991. Head trauma as a risk factor for Alzheimer's disease: a collaborative re-analysis of case-control studies. EURODERM Risk Factors Research Group. *International Journal of Epidemiology 20 Suppl* 2:S28–S35.

Mortimer, J. A., F. J. Pirozzola, E. C. Hansch, and D. D. Webster. 1982. Relationship of motor symptoms to intellectual deficits in Parkinson's disease. *Neurology* 32:133–137.

Myers, J. J., and R. W. Sperry. 1985. Interhemispheric communication after section of the forebrain commissures. *Cortex* 21:249–260.

Nelson, H. E. 1976. A modified card sorting test sensitive to frontal lobe defects. *Cortex* 12: 313–324.

Nelson, H. E., and A. O'Connell. 1978. Dementia: the estimation of premorbid intelligence levels using the New Adult Reading Test. *Cortex* 14:234–244.

Nelson, H. E., and J. Willison. 1991. *National Adult Reading Test (NART), 2nd Edition.* Windsor, UK: NFER-Nelson.

Neugebauer, R., and M. Susser. 1979. Some epidemiological aspects of epilepsy. *Psychological Medicine* 9:207–215.

Newcombe, F. 1969. *Missile Wounds of the Brain.* Oxford: Oxford University Press.

NIOSH 1987. *Current Intelligence Bulletin 48, Organic Solvent Neurotoxicity.* Ohio: U.S. Department of Health and Human Services.

Nissen, M. J., N. J. Cohen, and S. Corkin. 1981. The amnesic patient H. M.: learning and retention of perceptual skills. *Society for Neuroscience Abstracts* 7:517.

Nutt, J. G. 1989. Excitatory amino acids and Huntington's disease. *Genetics Northwest* 6:4–5.

Oddy, M, M. Humphrey, and D. Uttley. 1978. Subjective impairment and social recovery after closed head injury. *Journal of Neurology, Neurosurgery, and Psychiatry* 41:611–616.

Ogden, J. A. 1983. *Out of Mind, Out of Sight: Unilateral Spatial Disorders in Brain-Damaged Patients.* Unpublished doctoral thesis, Auckland, New Zealand, University of Auckland.

Ogden, J. A. 1984. Dyslexia in a right-handed patient with a posterior lesion of the right cerebral hemisphere. *Neuropsychologia* 22:265–280.

Ogden, J. A. 1985a. Anterior-posterior interhemispheric differences in the loci of lesions producing visual hemineglect. *Brain and Cognition* 4:59–75.

Ogden, J. A. 1985b. Contralesional neglect of constructed visual images in right and left brain-damaged patients. *Neuropsychologia* 23:273–277.

Ogden, J. A. 1985c. Autotopagnosia: occurrence in a patient without nominal aphasia and with an intact ability to point to parts of animals and objects. *Brain* 108:1009–1022.

Ogden, J. A. 1987a. The "neglected" left hemisphere and its contribution to visuospatial neglect. In: M. Jeannerod, ed., *Neuropsychological and Physiological Aspects of Spatial Neglect* (pp. 215–233). Amsterdam: Elsevier Science Publishers.

Ogden, J. A. 1987b. The recovery of spatial deficits in a young man with a fronto-parietal infarct of the right hemisphere. *New Zealand Journal of Psychology* 16:72–78.

Ogden, J. A. 1988a. Language and memory functions after long recovery periods in left-hemispherectomized subjects. *Neuropsychologia* 26:645–659.

Ogden, J. A. 1988b. Onset of motor neglect following a right parietal infarct and its recovery consequent on the removal of a right frontal meningioma. *New Zealand Journal of Psychology* 17:24–31.

Ogden, J. A. 1989. Visuospatial and other "right-hemispheric" functions after long recovery periods in left-hemispherectomized subjects. *Neuropsychologia* 27:765–776.

Ogden, J. A. 1993a. Visual object agnosia, prosopagnosia, achromatopsia, loss of visual imagery, and autobiographical amnesia following recovery from cortical blindness: case M.H. *Neuropsychologia* 31:571–589.

Ogden, J. A. 1993b. The psychological and neuropsychological assessment of chronic occupational solvent neurotoxicity: a case series. *New Zealand Journal of Psychology* 23:83–94.

Ogden, J. A. 1996. Phonological dyslexia and phonological dysgraphia following left and right hemispherectomy. *Neuropsychologia* 34:905–918.

Ogden, J. A. 2001a. First do no harm. Culturally appropriate neuropsychological assessment for indigenous people: a position paper. *Brain Impairment* 2:1–10.

Ogden, J. A. 2001b. Cognitive and psychosocial outcome of chronic occupational solvent neurotoxicity. In: G. Wypych, ed., *Handbook of Solvents* (pp. 1326–1333). Ontario: ChemTec Publishing.

Ogden, J. A. 2002. Daisy, daisy, Give me your answer do! Case studies of left visual neglect in patients with acute cerebral lesions. *Brain Impairment* 3:54–63.

Ogden, J. A., and K. Barker. 2001. Imagery used in autobiographical recall in early and late blind adults. *Journal of Mental Imagery* 25:153–176.

Ogden, J. A., E. Cooper, and M. Dudley. 2003. Adapting neuropsychological assessments for minority groups: a study comparing white and Maori New Zealanders. *Brain Impairment* 4:122–134.

Ogden, J. A., and S. Corkin. 1991. Memories of H. M. In: W. C. Abraham, M. C. Corballis, and K. G. White, eds., *Memory Mechanisms: A Tribute to G. V. Goddard* (pp. 195–215). Hillsdale, NJ: Lawrence Erlbaum.

Ogden, J. A., J. H. Growdon and S. Corkin. 1990. Deficits on visuospatial tests involving forward planning in high-functioning Parkinsonians. *Neuropsychiatry, Neuropsychology, and Behavioral Neurology* 3:125–139.

Ogden, J. A., P. L. Levin, and E. W. Mee. 1990. Long-term neuropsychological and psychosocial effects of subarachnoid hemorrhage. *Neuropsychiatry, Neuropsychology, and Behavioral Neurology* 3:260–274.

Ogden, J. A., and G. McFarlane-Nathan. 1997. Cultural bias in neuropsychological assessment of young Maori men. *New Zealand Journal of Psychology*, 26:2–12.

Ogden, J. A., E. W. Mee, and M. Henning. 1993a. A prospective study of impairment of cognition and memory and recovery after subarachnoid hemorrhage. *Neurosurgery* 33:572–587.

Ogden, J. A., E. W. Mee, and M. Henning. 1993b. Life-events stress: a significant precursor to subarachnoid hemorrhage. *Neuropsychiatry, Neuropsychology, and Behavioral Neurology* 6:219–228.

Ogden, J. A., E. W. Mee, and M. Henning. 1994. A prospective study of psychosocial adaptation following subarachnoid haemorrhage. *Neuropsychological Rehabilitation* 4:7–30.

Ogden, J. A., E. W. Mee, and T. Utley. 1998. Too little, too late: Does Tirilazad Mesylate reduce fatigue following SAH? *Neurosurgery* 43:782–787.

Ogden, J. A., T. Utley, and E. W. Mee. 1997. Neurological and psychosocial outcome 4 to 7 years after subarachnoid hemorrhage. *Neurosurgery* 41:25–34.

Ohm, T., H. Muller., H. Braak, and J. Bohl. 1995. Close-meshed prevalence rates of different stages as a tool to uncover the rate of Alzheimer's disease-related neurofibrillary changes. *Neuroscience* 64:209–217.

Ojemann, G. 1979. Individual variability in cortical localization of language. *Journal of Neurosurgery* 50:164–169.

Ojemann, G. 1980. Brain mechanisms for language: observations during neurosurgery. In: J. Lockhard and A. A. Ward, eds., *Epilepsy: A Window to Brain Mechanisms* (pp. 243–260). New York: Raven Press.

Osterrieth, P. A. 1944. Le test de copie d'une figure complexe. *Archives de Psychologie* 30: 206–356.

Owen, A. M., A. C. Roberts, J. R. Hodges, B. A. Summers, C. E. Polkey, and T. W. Robbins. 1993. Contrasting mechanisms of impaired attentional set-shifting in patients with frontal-lobe damage or Parkinson's disease. *Brain* 116:1159–1175.

Parkarinen S. 1967. Incidence, aetiology, and prognosis of primary subarachnoid haemorrhage:

a study based on 589 cases diagnosed in a defined urban population during a defined period. *Acta Neurologica Scandinavia* 29(Suppl.):1–128.

Parkinson, J. 1817. *An essay on the Shaking Palsy.* London: Sherwood, Nesly, and Jones.

Parsonson, B., and J. F. Smith. 1986. Seizures. In: N. J. King and A. Remenyi, eds., *Health Care, A Behavioural Approach* (pp. 125–132). New South Wales: Grune and Stratton.

Paulsen, J. S., R. E. Ready, J. M. Hamilton, M. S. Mega, and J. L. Cummings. 2001. Neuropsychiatric aspects of Huntington's disease. *Journal of Neurology, Neurosurgery, and Psychiatry,* 71:310–314.

Penfield, W., and B. Milner. 1958. Memory deficits produced by bilateral lesions in the hippocampal zone. *Archives of Neurology and Psychiatry* 79:475–497.

Penfield, W., and L. Roberts. 1959. *Speech and Brain Mechanisms.* Princeton, NJ: Princeton University Press.

Peretz, I., R. Kolinsky, M. Tramo, R. Labrecque, C. Hublet, G. Demeurisse, and S. Belleville, S. 1994. Functional dissociations following bilateral lesions of auditory cortex. *Brain* 117(Pt 6):1283–1301.

Perkin, G. D., and J. S. Wolinsky. 2000. *Multiple Sclerosis.* Oxford, Health Press Ltd.

Perlesz, A., M. Furlong, and D. McLachlan. 1992. Family work and acquired brain damage. *Australia New Zealand Journal of Family Therapy* 13:145–153.

Perret, E. 1974. The left frontal lobe of man and the suppression of habitual responses inverbal categorical behaviour. *Neuropsychologia* 12:323–330.

Peterson, R. C., G. E. Smith, R. J. Ivnik, E. G. Tangalos, D. J. Schaid, S. N. Thibodeau, E. Kokmen, S. C. Waring, and L. T. Kurland.. 1995. Apolipoprotein E status as a predictor of the development of Alzheimer's disease in memory-impaired individuals. *Journal of the American Medical Association* 273:1274–1278.

Piccirilli, M., T. Sciarma, and S. Luzzi. 2000. Modularity of music: evidence from a case of pure amusia. *Journal of Neurology, Neurosurgery, and Psychiatry*69:541–545.

Pick, A. 1922. Storung der Orientierung am eigenen Korper. Beitrag zur Lehre vom Bewusstsein des eigenen Korpers. *Psychologische Forschung* 1:303–318.

Pirozzolo, F. J., E. C. Hansch, J. A. Mortimer, D. D. Webster, and M. A. Kuskowski. 1982. Dementia in Parkinson's disease: a neuropsychological analysis. *Brain and Cognition* 1: 71–83.

Poirier, J. 2002. Cholesterol transport and synthesis are compromised in the brain in sporadic Alzheimer's disease: from risk factors to therapeutic targets. In: S. Gauthier and J. L. Cummings, eds., *Alzheimer's Disease and Related Disorders Annual 2002* (pp. 1–21). London: Martin Dunitz Ltd.

Ponsford, J. 1995. Mechanisms, recovery and sequelae of traumatic brain injury: A foundation for the REAL approach. In: J. Ponsford, S. Sloan, and P. Snow, eds., *Traumatic Brain Injury: Rehabilitation for Everyday Living* (pp. 1–31). Hove: Lawrence Erlbaum Associates.

Ponsford, J., S. Sloan, and P. Snow. 1995. *Traumatic Brain Injury: Rehabilitation for Everyday Living.* Hove: Lawrence Erlbaum Associates.

Porteus, S. D. 1931. *The Psychology of a Primitive People.* New York: Longmans, Green.

Posner, M. I., Y. Cohen, and R. D. Rafal. 1982. Neural systems control of spatial orienting. *Philosophical Transactions of the Royal Society of London Series B* 298:60–70.

Posner, M. I., J. Walker, F. J. Friedrich, and R. D. Rafal. 1984. Effects of parietal lobe injury on covert orienting of visual attention. *Journal of Neuroscience* 4:163–187.

Postle, B. R., J. S. Berger, and M. D'Esposito. 1999. Functional neuroanatomical double dissociation of mnemonic and executive control processes contributing to working memory performance. *Proceedings of the National Academy of Science U.S.A.* 96:12959–12964.

Prigatano, G. P. 1991. Disturbances of self-awareness of deficit after traumatic brain injury. In: G. P. Prigatano and D. L. Schacter, eds., *Awareness of Deficit after Brain Injury* (pp. 111–126). New York: Oxford University Press.

Prigatano, G. P. 1994. Individuality, lesion location, and psychotherapy after brain injury. In: A.-L. Christianson and B. P. Uzzell, eds., *Brain Injury and Neuropsychological Rehabilitation* (pp. 173–186). Hillsdale, NJ: Lawrence Erlbaum Associates.

Prisko, L. 1963. *Short-term memory in focal cerebral damage.* Unpublished doctoral dissertation, Montreal, McGill University.

Puccetti, R. 1981. The alleged manipulospatiality explanation of right hemisphere visuospatial superiority. *Behavioural and Brain Sciences* 4:75–76.

Quayhagen, M. P., and M. Quayhagen. 1989. Differential effects of family-based strategies on Alzheimer's disease. *The Gerontologist* 29:150–155.

Raaymakers, T. W. 2000. Functional outcome and quality of life after angiography and operation for unruptured intracranial aneurysms. *Journal of Neurology, Neurosurgery, and Psychiatry* 68:571–576.

Raaymakers, T. W., G. J. Rinkel, M. Limburg, and A. Algra. 1998. Mortality and morbidity of surgery for unruptured intracranial aneurysms: a meta-analysis. 29:1531–1538.

Rao, S. M. 1986. Neuropsychology of multiple sclerosis: a critical review. *Journal of Clinical and Experimental Neuropsychology*, 8:503–542.

Rao, S. M. 1993. Cognitive and neuroimaging changes in multiple sclerosis. In: U. Halbreich, ed., *Multiple Sclerosis: A Neuropsychiatric Disorder* (pp. 55–71). Washington, DC: American Psychiatric Press.

Rao, S. M., G. J. Leo, and P. St. Aubin-Faubert. 1989. On the nature of memory disturbance in multiple sclerosis. *Journal of Clinical and Experimental Neuropsychology*, 11:699–712.

Rao, S. M., P. St. Aubin-Faubert, and G. J. Leo. 1989. Information processing speed in patients with multiple sclerosis. *Journal of Clinical and Experimental Neuropsychology*, 11:471–477.

Rapp, S. R., M. A. Espeland, S. A. Shumaker, V. M. Henderson, R. L. Brunner, J. E. Manson, M.L.S. Gass, M. L. Stefanick, D. S. Lane, J. Hays, K. C. Johnson, L. H. Coker, M. Dailey, and D. Bowen. 2003. Effect of estrogen plus progestin on global cognitive function in postmenopausal women: the Women's Health Initiative Memory Study: a randomized controlled trial, *Journal of the American Medical Association* 289:2663–2672.

Reding, M., J. Haycox, and J. Blass. 1985. Depression in patients referred to a dementia clinic. *Archives of Neurology* 42:894–896.

Reitan, R. M. 1958. Validity of the Trail Making Test as an indication of organic brain damage. *Perceptual and Motor Skills* 8:271–276.

Reitan, R. M., and L. A. Davison. 1974. *Clinical Neuropsychology: Current Status and Applications.* New York: Hemisphere.

Rey, A. 1941. L'examen psychologique dans les cas d'encephalopathie traumatique. *Archives de Psychologie* 28:286–340.

Rey, A. 1964. *L'examen clinique en psychologie.* Paris: Presses Universitaires de France.

Richter, R. W., and B. Z. Richter. 2002. *Alzheimer's Disease.* London: Mosby.

Riddoch, M. J., and G. W. Humphreys. 1987. A case of integrative visual agnosia. *Brain* 110:1431–1462.

Rimel, R. W., B. Giordani, J. T. Barth, T. J. Boll, and J. A. Jane. 1981. Disability caused by minor head injury. *Neurosurgery* 9:221–228.

Rizzolatti, G., and V. Gallese. 1988. Mechanisms and theories of spatial neglect. In: F. Boller and J. Grafman eds., *Handbook of Neuropsychology, vol 1*. Amsterdam: Elsevier Science Publishers (Biomedical Division).

Roberts, G. W., D. Allsop, and C. Bruton. 1990. The occult aftermath of boxing. *Journal of Neurology, Neurosurgery, and Psychiatry* 53:373–378.

Robertson, I. 1990. Does computerised cognitive rehabilitation work? A review. *Aphasiology* 4:381–405.

Robertson, I., and E. Cashman. 1991. Auditory feedback for walking difficulties in a case of unilateral neglect: a pilot study. *Neuropsychological Rehabilitation* 1:175–183.

Robertson, I. H., and K. Hawkins. 1999. Limb activation and unilateral neglect. *Neurocase* 5: 153–160.*a name uickmark*

Robertson, I. H., K. Hogg, and T. M. McMillan. 1998. Rehabilitation of unilateral neglect: improving function by contralesional limb activation. *Neuropsychological Rehabilitation* 8:19–29.

Robertson, I. H., J. B. Mattingley, C. Rorden, and J. Driver. 1998. Phasic alerting of neglect patients overcomes their spatial deficit in visual awareness. *Nature* 395:169–172.

Robertson, I. H., T. M. McMillan, E. MacLeod, J. Edgeworth, and D. Brock. 2002. Rehabilitation by limb activation training reduces left-sided motor impairment in unilateral neglect patients: a single-blind randomised control trial. *Neuropsychological Rehabilitation* 12: 439–454.

Robertson, I. H., and J.M.J. Murre. 1999. Rehabilitation of brain damage: brain plasticity and principles of guided recovery. *Psychological Bulletin* 125:544–575.

Robertson, I., and N. North. 1992. Spatio-motor cueing in unilateral left neglect: the role of hemispace, hand and motor activation. *Neuropsychologia* 30:553–563.

Robertson, I. H., and N. T. North. 1994. One hand is better than two: motor extinction of left hand advantage in unilateral neglect. *Neuropsychologia* 32:1–11.

Robertson, I., N. North, and C. Geggie. 1992. Spatio-motor cueing in unilateral left neglect: three case studies of its therapeutic effect. *Journal of Neurology, Neurosurgery, and Psychiatry* 55:799–805.

Robertson, I. H., V. Ridgeway, E. Greenfield, and A. Parr. 1997. Motor recovery after stroke depends on intact sustained attention: a 2-year follow-up study. *Neuropsychology* 11: 290–295.

Robertson, I. H., R. Tegnér, K. Tham, A. Lo, and I. Nimmo-Smith. 1995. Sustained attention training for unilateral neglect: Theoretical and rehabilitation implications. *Journal of Clinical and Experimental Neuropsychology* 17:416–430.

Roeltgen, D. P. 2003. Agraphia. In: K. M. Heilman and E. Valenstein, eds., *Clinical Neuropsychology, 4th Edition* (pp 126–145). New York: Oxford University Press.

Ropper, A. H., and Zervas N. T. 1984. Outcome 1 year after SAH from cerebral aneurysm. Management morbidity, mortality, and functional status in 112 consecutive good-risk patients. *Journal of Neurosurgery* 60:909–915.

Rosenbaum, M., and N. Palmon. 1984. Helplessness and resourcefulness in coping with epilepsy. *Journal of Consulting and Clinical Psychology* 52:244–253.

Ross, E. D. 1981. The aprosodias: functional-anatomical organisation of the effective components of language in the right hemisphere. *Archives of Neurology* 38:561–589.

Rossetti, Y., G. Rode, L. Pisella, A. Farne, L. Li, D. Boisson, and M. Perenin. 1998. Prism adaptation to a rightward optical deviation rehabilitates left hemispatial neglect. *Nature* 395:166–169.

Rudel, R. G., and H.-L. Teuber. 1971. Spatial orientation in normal children and in children with early brain injury. *Neuropsychologia* 9:401–407.

Russell, W. R. 1971. *The Traumatic Amnesias*. New York: Oxford University Press.

Rutherford, W. H. 1989. Postconcussion symptoms: relationships to acute neurological indices, individual differences, and circumstances of injury. In: H. S. Levin, H. M. Eisenberg, and A. L. Benton, eds., *Mild Head Injury* (pp. 217–228). New York: Oxford University Press.

Sachdev, P. S. 1989. Mana, Tapu, Noa: Maori cultural constructs with medical and psychosocial relevance. *Psychological Medicine* 19:959–969.

Sadovnick, A. D., and P. A. Baird. 1988. The familial nature of multiple sclerosis: age-corrected empiric recurrence risks for children and siblings of patients. *Neurology*, 38:990–991.

Sacks, O. 1991. *Awakenings*. Rev. Ed. London: Picador.

Sagar, H. J., N. J. Cohen, S. Corkin, and J. H. Growdon. 1985. Dissociations among processes in remote memory. In: D. S. Olton, E. Gamzu, and S. Corkin, eds., *Memory Dysfunctions: An Integration of Animal and Human Research from Preclinical and Clinical Perspectives*, vol 4 (pp. 533–535). New York: Annals of the New York Academy of Sciences.

Sarazin, M., N. Horne, and B. Dubois. 2002. Natural history of Alzheimer's disease and other dementing illnesses. In: S. Gauthier and J. L. Cummings, eds., *Alzheimer's Disease and Related Disorders Annual 2002* (pp. 183–197). London: Martin Dunitz Ltd.

Sattler, J. M. 1992. *Assessment of Children, Revised and updated 3rd Edition*. San Diego, CA: Jerome M. Sattler.

Schacter, D. L. 1987. Implicit memory: history and current status. *Journal of Experimental Psychology (Learning, Memory, and Cognition)* 13:501–517.

Schneck, M. K., B. Reisberg, and S. H. Ferris. 1982. An overview of current concepts of Alzheimer's disease. *American Journal of Psychiatry* 139:165–173.

Schneider, J. W., and P. Conrad. 1980. In the closet with illness: epilepsy, stigma potential and information control. *Social Problems* 28:32–44.

Schwartz, M. L., and R. D. Dennerll. 1970. Neuropsychological assessment of children with and without questionable epileptogenic dysfunction. *Perceptual and Motor Skills* 30:111–121.

Scott, J. J. M. G. Williams, and A. T. Beck. 1989. *Cognitive therapy in clinical practice. An illustrative casebook*. London: Routledge.

Scoville, W. B. 1968. Amnesia after bilateral mesial temporal-lobe excision: Introduction to case H.M. *Neuropsychologia* 6:211–213.

Scoville, W., and B. Milner. 1957. Loss of recent memory after bilateral hippocampal lesions. Journal of Neurology, Neurosurgery, and Psychiatry 20:11–21.

Searleman, A. 1977. A review of right hemisphere linguistic abilities. Psychological Bulletin 84:503–528.

Sekino, H., N. Nakamura, K. Yuki, J. Satoh, K. Kikuchi, and S. Sanada. 1981. Brain lesions detected by CT scans in cases of minor head injuries. *Neurologia Medico-Chirurgica (Tokyo)* 21:677–683.

Sergent, J., E. Zuch, S. Terriah, and B. McDonald. 1992. Distributed neural network underlying musical sight-reading and keyboard performance. *Science* 257:106–109.

Seron, X., F. Coyette, and R. Bruyer. 1989. Ipsilateral influences on contralateral processing in neglect patients. *Cognitive Neuropsychology* 6:475–498.

Semmes, J., S. Weinstein, L. Ghent, and H.-L. Teuber. 1963. Correlates of impaired orientation in personal and extrapersonal space. *Brain* 86:747–772.

Shallice, T., and W. P. Burgess. 1991. Deficits in strategy application following frontal-lobe damage in man. *Brain* 114:727–741.

Shewan, C. M., and D. L. Bandur. 1986. *Treatment of Aphasia. A Language-Oriented Approach.* London: Taylor and Francis.

Shores, E. A., J. E. Marosszeky, J. Sandanam, and J. Batchelor. 1986. Preliminary validation of a clinical scale for measuring the duration of post-traumatic amnesia. *Medical Journal of Australia* 144:569–572.

Shoulson, I., and S. Fahn. 1979. Huntington's disease: clinical care and evaluation. *Neurology* 29:1–3.

Shumaker, S. A., C. Legault, S. R. Rapp, L. Thal, R. B. Wallace, J. K. Ockene, S. L. Hendrix, B. N. Jones, A. R. Assaf, R. D. Jackson, J. M. Kotchen, S. Wassertheil-Smoller, and J. Wactawski-Wende. 2003. Estrogen plus progestin and the incidence of dementia and mild cognitive impairment in postmenopausal women: the Women's Health Initiative Memory Study: a randomized controlled trial. *Journal of the American Medical Association* 289: 2651–2662.

Smith, A. 1966. Speech and other functions after left (dominant) hemispherectomy. *Journal of Neurology, Neurosurgery, and Psychiatry* 29:467–471.

Smith, A. 1978. Dominant and nondominant hemispherectomy. In: W. L. Smith, ed., *Drugs and Cerebral Function* (pp. 37–68). Springfield, IL: Ch. C. Thomas.

Smith, B. 1963. Cerebral pathology in subarachnoid haemorrhage. *Journal of Neurology, Neurosurgery, and Psychiatry* 26:535–539.

Smith, C. R., L. M. Samkoff, and L. C. Scheinberg. 1993. Clinical features, assessment, and differential diagnosis of multiple sclerosis. In: U. Halbreich, ed., *Multiple Sclerosis: A Neuropsychiatric Disorder* (pp. 1–31). Washington, DC: American Psychiatric Press.

Smith, D. H., K. A. Quaid, R. B. Dworkin, G. P. Gramelspacher, J. A. Granbois, and G. H. Vance. 1998. *Early Warning. Cases and ethical guidance for presymptomatic testing in genetic diseases.* Bloomington: Indiana University Press.

Smith, M. L. 1988. Recall of spatial location by the amnesic patient H.M. *Brain and Cognition* 7:178–183.

Smith, M. L., and B. Milner. 1981. The role of the right hippocampus in the recall of spatial location. *Neuropsychologia* 19:781–793.

Snow, P., and J. Ponsford. 1995. Assessing and managing impairment of consciousness following traumatic brain injury. In: J. Ponsford, S. Sloan, and P. Snow, eds., *Traumatic Brain Injury: Rehabilitation for Everyday Living* (pp. 33–64). Hove: Lawrence Erlbaum Associates.

Snowdon, D. A., S. J. Kemper, J. A. Mortimer, L. H. Greiner, D. R. Wekstein, and W. R. Markesbery. 1996. Linguistic ability in early life and cognitive function and Alzheimer's disease in late life. Findings from the Nun Study. *Journal of the American Medical Association* 275:528–532.

Sohlberg, M. M., and C. A. Mateer. 1989. *Introduction to Cognitive Rehabilitation: Theory and Practice* (pp. 159–170). New York: Guilford Press.

Sonesson, B., B. Ljunggren, H. Saveland, and L. Brandt. 1987. Cognition and adjustment after late and early operation for ruptured aneurysm. *Neurosurgery* 21:279–287.

Sperry, R. 1974. Lateral specialization in the surgically separated hemispheres. In: F. O. Schmitt and F. G. Worden, eds., *The Neurosciences: Third Study Program* (pp. 5–19). Cambridge, MA: MIT Press.

Sperry, R. W. 1982. Some effects of disconnecting the cerebral hemispheres. *Science* 217:1223–1226.

Sperry, R. W., E. Zaidel, and D. Zaidel. 1979. Self recognition and social awareness in the deconnected minor hemisphere. *Neuropsychologia* 17:153–166.

Sperry, R. W., M. S. Gazzaniga, and J. E. Bogen. 1969. Interhemispheric relationships: the neocortical commissures; syndromes of hemispheric disconnection. In: P. J. Vinken and G. W. Bruyn, eds., *Handbook of Clinical Neurology, vol 4* (pp 273–290). Amsterdam: North-Holland Publishing.

Spielberger, C. D. 1983. *Stait-Trait Anxiety Inventory Manual.* Palo Alto, California: Mind Garden.

Spreen, O., and A. L. Benton. 1977. *The Neurosensory Center Comprehension Examination for Aphasia (NCCEA) (Revised ed.).* University of Victoria: Neuropsychology Laboratory.

Spreen, O., and E. Strauss. 1991. *A Compendium of Neuropsychological Tests. Administration, Norms, and Commentary.* New York: Oxford University Press.

Spreen, O., and E. Strauss. 1998. *A Compendium of Neuropsychological Tests. Administration, Norms, and Commentary, 2nd Edition.* New York: Oxford University Press.

Spreen, O., A. T. Risser, and D. Edgell. 1995. *Developmental Neuropsychology.* New York: Oxford University Press

Squire, L. R. 1986. Mechanisms of memory. *Science* 232:1612–1619.

St. James-Roberts, I. 1981. A reinterpretation of hemispherectomy data without functional plasticity of the brain. *Brain and Language* 13:31–53.

Stabell, K. E. 1991. *Neuropsychological Investigation of Patients with Surgically Treated Aneurysm Rupture at Different Sites.* Unpublished doctoral dissertation, Oslo, Norway, University of Oslo.

Stenhouse, L. M., R. G. Knight, B. E. Longmore, and S. N. Bishara. 1991. Long-term cognitive deficits in patients after surgery on aneurysms of the anterior communicating artery. *Journal of Neurology, Neurosurgery, and Psychiatry* 54:909–914.

Stern, Y., B. Gurland, T. K. Tatemichi, M. X. Tang, D. Wilder, and R. Mayeux. 1994. Influence of education and occupation on the incidence of Alzheimer's disease. *Journal of the American Medical Association* 271:1004–1010.

Stolk, P. J. 1968. Adolf Hitler: his life and his illness. *Psychiatria, Neurologia, Neurochirurgia* 71:381–398.

Strub, R. L., and N. Geschwind. 1983. Localisation in Gerstmann syndrome. In: A. Kertesz, ed., *Localization in Neuropsychology* (pp. 295–321). New York: Academic Press.

Stuss, D. T. 1987. Contribution of frontal lobe injury to cognitive impairment after closed head injury: methods of assessment and recent findings. In: H. S. Levin, J. Grafman, and H. M. Eisenberg, eds., *Neurobehavioral Recovery from Head Injury* (pp. 166–177). New York: Oxford University Press.

Stuss, D. T., and R. T. Knight. 2002. *Principles of frontal lobe function.* Oxford: Oxford University Press.

Sullivan, E. V., H. J. Sagar, J.D.E. Gabrielli, S. Corkin, and J. H. Growdon. 1985. Sequencing deficits in Parkinson's disease. *Journal of Clinical and Experimental Neuropsychology* 7: 160.

Taha, A., K. P. Ball, and R. D. Illingworth. 1982. Smoking and subarachnoid hemorrhage. *Journal of the Royal Society of Medicine* 75:332–335.

Taylor, A., and R. S. Taylor. 1998. Neuropsychologic aspects of multiple sclerosis. *Physical Medicine and Rehabilitation Clinics of North America.* 9, 643–656.

Taylor, A. E., J. A. Saint-Cyr, and A. E. Lang. 1986. Frontal lobe dysfunction in Parkinson's disease. *Brain* 109:845–883.

Taylor, L. B. 1969. Localisation of cerebral lesions by psychological testing. *Clinical Neurosurgery* 16:269–287.

Teasdale, G., and B. Jennett. 1974. Assessment of coma and impaired consciousness. A practical scale. *Lancet* 2:81–83.

Teasdale, G., and B. Jennett. 1976. Assessment and prognosis of coma after head injury. *Acta Neurochirurgica (Wien)* 34:45–55.

TenHouten, W. D., K. D. Hoppe, J. E. Bogen, and D. O. Walter. 1986. Alexithymia: an experimental study of cerebral commissurotomy patients and normal control subjects. *American Journal of Psychiatry*, 143:312–316.

Teuber, H. L. 1955. Physiological psychology. *Annual Review of Psychology* 6:267–296.

Thompson, J. C., J. S. Snowden, D. Craufurd, and D. Neary. 2002. Behavior in Huntington's disease: dissociating cognition-based and mood-based changes. *Journal of Neuropsychiatry and Clinical Neuroscience*, 14:37–43.

Tomlinson, B. E., G. Blessed, and M. Roth. 1970. Observations on the brains of demented old people. *Journal of Neurological Science* 11:205–242.

Towgood, K., J. A. Ogden, and E. Mee. 2004. Neurological, neuropsychological and psychosocial outcome following treatment of unruptured intracranial aneurysms: a review and commentary. *Journal of the International Neuropsychological Society* 10:1–21.

Troy, C. M., and M. L. Shelanski. 2002. Aopotosis and its role in Alzheimer's disease. In: S. Gauthier and J. L. Cummings, eds., *Alzheimer's Disease and Related Disorders Annual 2002* (pp. 23–37). London: Martin Dunitz Ltd.

Tucker, D. M. 1981. Lateral brain function, emotion and conceptualization. *Psychological Bulletin* 89:19–46.

Tucker, D. M., R. T. Watson, and K. M. Heilman. 1977. Affective discrimination and evocation in patients with right parietal disease. *Neurology* 17:947–950.

Tulving, E. 1972. Episodic and semantic memory. In: E. Tulving and W. Donaldson, eds., *Organization of Memory* (pp. 381–403). New York: Academic Press.

Tulving, E. 1983. *Elements of Episodic Memory.* Oxford: Oxford University Press.

Utley, T.F.M., J. A. Ogden, A. Gibb, N. McGrath, and N.E. Anderson. 1997. The long-term neuropsychological outcome of herpes simplex encephalitis in a series of unselected survivors. *Neuropsychiatry, Neuropsychology, and Behavioral Neurology* 10:180–189.

Van Praag, H., G. Kempermann, and F. H. Gage. 1999. Running increases cell proliferation and neurogenesis in the adult mouse dentate gyrus. *Nature Neuroscience*, 2, 266–270.

Vaughan, I. 1986. *Ivan. Living with Parkinson's Disease.* London: Macmillan London Ltd.

Vilkki, J. 1985. Amnesic syndromes after surgery of anterior communicating artery aneurysms. *Cortex* 21:432–444.

Vilkki, J., P. Holst, J. Ohman, A. Servo, and O. Heiskanen. 1989. Cognitive deficits related to computed tomographic findings after surgery for a ruptured intracranial aneurysm. *Neurosurgery* 25:166–172.

Vilkki, J., P. Holst, J. Ohman, A. Servo, and O. Heiskanen. 1990. Social outcome related to cognitive performance and computed tomographic findings after surgery for a ruptured intracranial aneurysm. *Neurosurgery* 26:579–585.

Voller, B., T. Benke, K. Benedettos, P. Schnider, E. Auff, and F. Aicher. 1999. Neuropsychological, MRI and EEG findings after mild traumatic brain injury. *Brain Injury* 123:821–827.

Wada, J., and T. Rasmussen. 1960. Intracarotid injection of sodium Amytal for the lateralization of cerebral speech dominance: experimental and clinical observations. *Journal of Neurosurgery* 17:226–282.

Walker, M., and S. Salek. 2002. Quality of life assessment in dementia research. In: S. Gauthier and J. L. Cummings, eds., *Alzheimer's Disease and Related Disorders Annual 2002* (pp. 113–146). London: Martin Dunitz Ltd.

Walsh, K. W. 1985. *Understanding Brain Damage. A Primer of Neuropsychological Evaluation.* Edinburgh: Churchill Livingstone.

Walsh, K. W. 1994. *Neuropsychology. A Clinical Approach, 3rd Edition.* Edinburgh: Churchill Livingstone.

Warrington, E. K. 1984. *Recognition Memory Test.* Windsor, UK: NFER-Nelson.

Wassertheil-Smoller, S., S. Hendrix, M. Limacher, G. Heiss, C. Kooperberg, A. Baird, T. Kotchen, J. D. Curb, H. Black, J. E. Rossouw, A. Aragaki, M. Safford, E. Stein, S. Laowattana, and W. J. Mysiw (for the WHI Investigators). 2003. Effect of Estrogen plus progestin on stroke in postmenopausal women. The Women's Health Initiative: a randomized trial, *Journal of the American Medical Association* 289:2673–2684.

Watson, R. T., and K. M. Heilman. 1979. Thalamic neglect. *Neurology* 29:690–694.

Wechsler, D. A. 1945. A standardized memory scale for clinical use. *Journal of Psychology* 19: 87–95.

Wechsler, D. 1955. *Wechsler Adult Intelligence Scale.* New York: The Psychological Corporation.

Wechsler, D. 1974. *Wechsler Intelligence Scale for Children-Revised (WISC-R).* New York: Psychological Corporation.

Wechsler, D. 1981. *Wechsler Adult Intelligence Scale-Revised (WAIS-R).* San Antonio, TX: Psychological Corporation.

Wechsler, D. 1987. *Wechsler Memory Scale-Revised.* San Antonio, TX: The Psychological Corporation.

Wechsler, D. 1997a. *Wechsler Adult Intelligence Scale, 3rd Edition* (WAIS-III). San Antonio, TX: Psychological Corporation.

Wechsler, D. 1997b. *Wechsler Memory Scale, 3rd Edition* (WMS-III). San Antonio, TX: Psychological Corporation.

Wechsler, D. 2003. *Wechsler Intelligence Scale for Children, 4th Edition* (WISC-IV). San Antonio, TX: Psychological Corporation.

Weeks, D. J. 1988. *The Anomalous Sentences Repetition Test.* Manual. Windsor, UK: NFER-Nelson.

Weingartner, H., S. Burns, R. Diebel, and P. A. LeWitt. 1984. Cognitive impairments in Parkinson's disease: distinguishing between effort-demanding and automatic cognitive processes. *Psychiatry Research* 11:223–235.

Wells, K. C., S. M. Turner, A. D. Bellack, and M. Hersen. 1978. Effects of cue-controlled relaxation on psychomotor seizures. *Behaviour Research and Therapy* 16:51–53.

Wernicke, K. 1874. Der aphasische Symptomenkomplex. Breslau. Translated in *Boston Studies in Philosophy of Science* 4:34–97.

West, H., R. L. Maru, R. L. Eisenberg, K. Tuerk, and T. B. Stuker. 1977. Normal cerebral arteriography in patients with spontaneous SAH. *Neurology* 27:592–594.

Wexler, A. 1995. *Mapping Fate.* New York: Times Books.

Wexler, N. S., A. B. Young, and R. E. Tanzi. 1987. Homozygotes for Huntington's disease. *Nature* 326:194–197.

Wexler, N. S. 1979. Genetic Russian roulette: the experience of being at risk for Huntington's disease. In: S. Kessler, ed., *Genetic Counselling, Psychological Dimensions* (pp. 201–217). London: Academic Press.

White, M. 1986. Negative explanation, restraint, and double description: a template for family therapy. *Family Process* 25:169–184.

White, R. F., R. G. Feldman, and P. H. Travers. 1990. Neurobehavioral effects of toxicity due to metals, solvents, and insecticides. *Clinical Neuropharmacology* 13:392–412.

Wickelgren, W. A. 1968. Sparing of short-term memory in an amnesic patient: Implications for a strength theory of memory. *Neuropsychologia*, 6:235–244.

Willer, B and J. Corrigan. 1994. Whatever it takes: a model for community-based services. *Brain Injury*, 8, 647–659.

Williams, W. H., J. J. Evans, and S. Fleminger. 2003. Neurorehabilitation and cognitive-behaviour therapy of anxiety disorders after brain injury: an overview and a case illustration of obsessive-compulsive disorder. *Neuropsychological Rehabilitation* 13: 133–148.

Williamson, J., I. H. Stokoe, and S. Gray. 1964. Old people at home: their unreported needs. *Lancet* 1:1117–1120.

Wilson, B. 1997. Cognitive rehabilitation: how it is and how it might be. *Journal of the International Neuropsychological Society* 3:487–500.

Wilson, B. 1999. Case Studies in Neuropsychological Rehabilitation. New York: Oxford University Press.

Wilson, B., and D. Wearing. 1995. Prisoner of Consciousness: a state of just awakening following herpes simplex encephalitis. In: R. Campbell and M. A. Conway, eds., *Broken Memories. Case Studies in Memory Impairment* (pp. 14–30). Oxford: Blackwell Publishers.

Wilson, B., N. Alderman, P. Burgess, H. Emslie, and J. Evans. 1996. *Behavioural Assessment of the Dysexecutive Syndrome*. Bury St. Edmonds: Thames Valley Test Company.

Wilson, D. H., A. Reeves, and M. Gazzaniga. 1978. Division of the corpus callosum for uncontrolled epilepsy. *Neurology* 28:649–653.

Wilson, J.T.L. 1990. Significance of MRI in clarifying whether neuropsychological deficits after head injury are organically based. *Neuropsychology* 4:261–269.

Wilson, R. S., A. W. Kaszniak, H. L. Klawans, and D. C. Garron. 1980. High speed memory scanning in parkinsonism. *Cortex* 16:67–72.

Wilson, S., P. Bladin, and M. Saling. 2001. The "burden of normality". concepts of adjustment after surgery for seizures. *Journal of Neurology, Neurosurgery, and Psychiatry* 70:649–656.

Wimo, A., and B. Winblad. 2002. Pharmacoeconomics of dementia: impact of cholinesterase inhibitors. In: S. Gauthier and J. L. Cummings, eds., *Alzheimer's Disease and Related Disorders Annual 2002* (pp. 147–169). London: Martin Dunitz Ltd.

Wishart, H., and D. Sharpe. 1997. Neuropsychological aspects of multiple sclerosis: a quantitative review. Journal of Clinical and Experimental Neuropsychology, 19:810–824.

Wood, A. G., M. M. Saling, D. F. Abbott, and G. D. Jackson. 2001. A neurocognitive account of frontal involvement in orthographic lexical retrieval: an fMRI study. *NeuroImage* 14: 162–169.

Woolford, P. R. 1990. A cultural response to depression. *The New Zealand Family Physician* Winter:129–130.

World Health Organization and Commission of the European Communities. 1985. *Environmental Health Document 6: Neurobehavioral Methods in Occupational and Environmental Health: Symposium Report*. Copenhagen: WHO Regional Office for Europe and Commission of the European Communities.

World Health Organization/Nordic Council of Ministers 1985. *Organic Solvents and the Central Nervous System, EH5*. Copenhagen, Denmark: WHO.

Wrightson, P., and D. Gronwall. 1999. *Mild Head Injury: A Guide to Management* New York: Oxford University Press.

Young, D., P. A. Lawlor, P. Leone, M. Dragunow, and M. J. During. 1999. Environmental enrichment inhibits spontaneous apoptosis, prevents seizures and is neuroprotective. *Nature Medicine* 5:448–453.

Zaidel, D. W. 1988. Observations on right hemisphere language function. In: F. C. Rose, R. Whurr, and M. Wyke, eds., *Aphasia* (pp. 170–187). London: Whurr Publishers.

Zaidel, D., and R. W. Sperry, 1974. Memory impairment after commissurotomy in man. *Brain* 97:263–272.

Zaidel, E. 1983. A response to Gazzaniga. Language in the right hemisphere, convergent perspectives. *American Psychologist* May 1983:525–537.

Zaidel, E., D. W. Zaidel, and J. E. Bogen. 1990. Testing the commissurotomy patient. In: A. A. Boulton, G. B. Baker, and M. Hiscock, eds., *Neuromethods, vol 17: Neuropsychology* (pp. 147–201). Clifton, NJ: Humana Press.

Zaidel, E., M. Jacoboni, D. W. Zaidel, and J. E. Bogen. 2003. Neglect and related disorders. In: K. M. Heilman and E. Valenstein, eds., *Clinical Neuropsychology*, *4th Edition* (pp 347–403). New York: Oxford University Press.

Zola-Morgan, S., N. J., Cohen, and L. R. Squire. 1983. Recall of remote episodic memory in amnesia. *Neuropsychologia* 21:487–500.